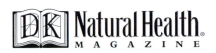

Natural Health
MAGAZINE

COMPLETE
GUIDE TO
SAFE
HERBS

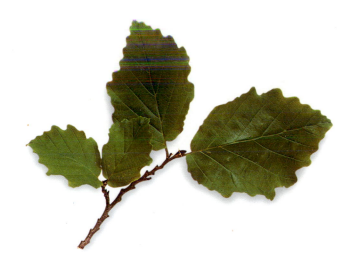

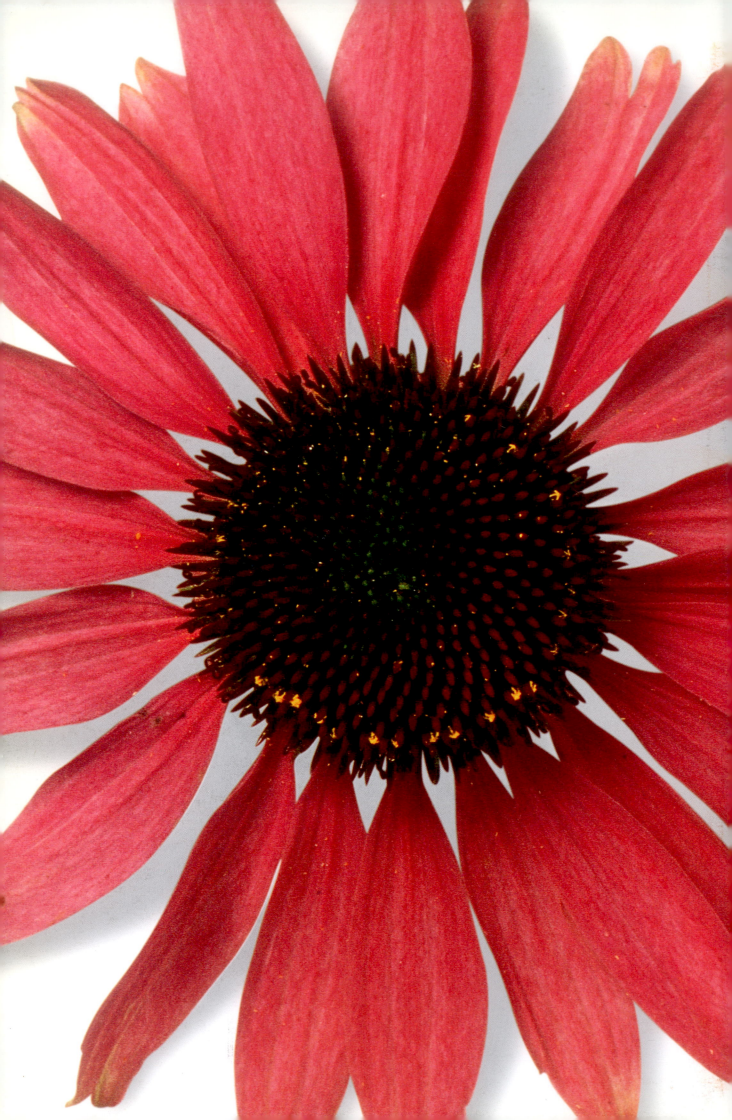

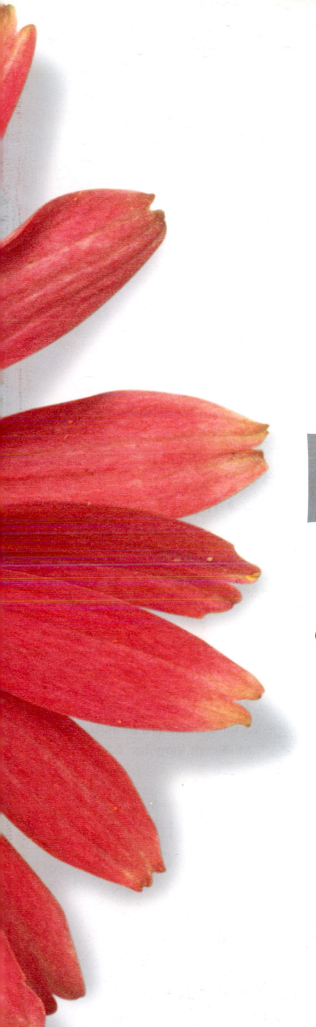

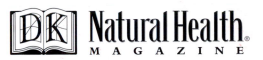
Natural Health® MAGAZINE

COMPLETE GUIDE TO

SAFE HERBS

CHRIS D. MELETIS, N.D.

AND THE EDITORS OF
Natural Health® MAGAZINE
WITH SHEILA BUFF

PRODUCED BY
THE PHILIP LIEF GROUP, INC.

LONDON, NEW YORK, MUNICH, MELBOURNE and DELHI

Author's dedication:
To my wonderful and supportive wife, Kathy:
You are my inspiration.
To God: Thanks for blessing this planet
with the bountiful natural
pharmacy that has sustained humanity
over the centuries.

Category Publisher LaVonne Carlson
Creative Director Tina Vaughan
Senior Editor Jill Hamilton **Art Editor** Claire Legemah
Editor Susannah Steel **Cover Design** Dirk Kaufman
Production Sara Gordon, Chris Avgherinos
DTP Design Russell Shaw
Picture Research Mark Dennis, Jo Walton

Natural Health® magazine is the leading publication in the field of
natural self-care. For subscription information call 800-526-8440 or visit
www.naturalhealthmag.com. Natural Health® is a registered trademark
of Weider Publications, Inc.

AUTHOR'S NOTE
The author strongly recommends that you consult a licensed healthcare
practitioner before following any complementary therapies if you have any
symptoms of illness, any diagnosed ailment, or are receiving conventional
treatment or medication for any condition. Do not cease conventional
treatment or medication without first consulting your physician. Always
inform your physician and your complementary practitioner of any
treatments, medication, or remedies that you
are taking or intend to take.

First American Edition, 2002
2 4 6 8 10 9 7 5 3 1
Published in the United States by DK Publishing, Inc.
DK Publishing, Inc., 375 Hudson Street, New York, NY 10014

Library of Congress cataloging-in-publication data

Meletis, Chris D., 1965- and the editors of *Natural Health*® magazine
Complete guide to safe herbs / [Chris Meletis].
    p. cm.
Includes index.
ISBN 0-7894-8073-5 (alk. paper)
    1. Herbs--Therapeutic use--Handbooks, manuals, etc. I. Title. II.
Natural Health® magazine

RM666.H33 M656 2001
615'.321--dc21

2001042263

Produced by The Philip Lief Group, Inc.
Reproduced by Colourscan in Singapore.
Printed and bound in Spain by Artes Graficas, Toledo SA

See our complete product line at
www.dk.com

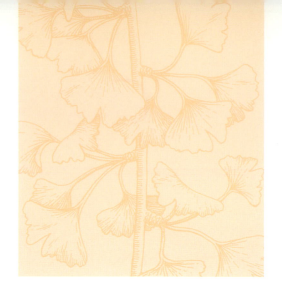

FOREWORD 6

INTRODUCTION 8

CONTENTS

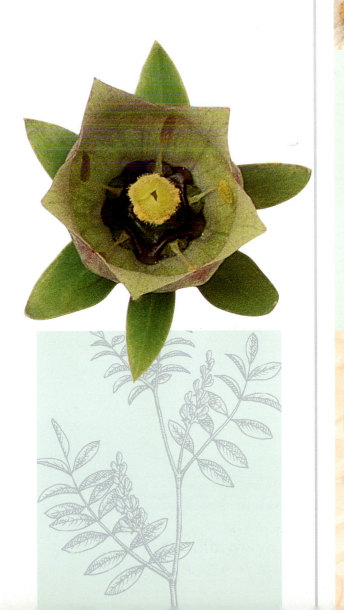

HERBAL USE IS ON THE RISE

I CAN'T RECALL a single issue of *Natural Health* magazine that hasn't discussed the issue of herbal safety. And it isn't surprising when you consider how popular herbs have become; sales of herbal products in the United States totaled nearly $15 billion in 2000 alone.

The National Nutritional Foods Association estimates that growth in the use of herbal products will continue at the astonishing rate of 20 percent a year. In fact, 50 percent of all adults living in America take dietary supplements of various kinds, including herbs, vitamins, and minerals.

However, according to recent industry surveys, more than half of the people buying herbs aren't really sure about how to use them. The Food and Drug Administration is charged with ensuring that the medications you take are safe, but herbs fall into a separate category that isn't monitored by any government agency. That means you are pretty much on your own when it comes to herbal safety. That's why this book is so important – it provides you with the information you need for consuming herbs safely to self-treat a variety of health problems.

❖ TAKING CHARGE OF ❖ YOUR HEALTH, NATURALLY

One reason herbs are so widely used is that they are considered to be generally safer and gentler than drugs. They typically present less risk of unpleasant, or even dangerous, side effects. When it comes to treating many minor ailments, such as an upset stomach, a cough, or a sore throat, herbs often work just as well as, or better than, prescription or over-the-counter medications. When used under

READ THE LABEL

WE always advise our readers to look carefully at the information on any herbal product. The container should be clearly labeled with both the scientific and common names of all herbs the product contains. Any standardized ingredients and their percentages should be included, along with recommended dosages.

We also recommend that consumers check herbal products to see if companies adhere to "Good Manufacturing Practices," or GMPs. A GMP seal means that the company is certified by the National Nutritional Foods Association, a trade organization that works with herbal suppliers to ensure high standards in such areas as staff training, cleanliness, equipment maintenance, and record keeping.

the supervision of an experienced physician, herbs can also be very effective in treating more serious ailments, such as high blood pressure and prostate problems, often with fewer side effects than conventional medications.

❖ WHY THIS BOOK NOW? ❖

Many of us have a lot of unanswered questions about herbs. Newspapers and the nightly news often report about someone who used a natural product to improve their health – only to compromise it. And a trip to your neighborhood health food store, food market, or pharmacy, with their rows and rows of herbal products, can be an overwhelming experience. Which of these products can you consume with confidence? Will a particular herb interact with a medication prescribed by your physician? Can you take standard doses of both echinacea and elderberry when you feel a cold coming on? How do the foods in your daily diet affect the herbs you consume?

This book addresses your concerns about herbal safety and provides all the information you need to receive the maximum benefit from herbal remedies. I think you'll find *Natural Health's Complete Guide to Safe Herbs* a vital tool for your family's health, and a trusted friend you'll refer to time and time again.

– *Rachel Streit*
Editor in Chief,
Natural Health® magazine

HERBAL SAFETY: WHAT'S THE FUSS ABOUT?

As A NATUROPATHIC PHYSICIAN, I always tell my patients to make herbal safety a priority. Although most herbs are very safe when used properly, they must be used with caution. Many herbs that are safe when used alone may be dangerous when combined with drugs or other supplements.

A good example is the popular herb St. John's wort *(Hypericum perforatum)*. A number of studies have shown St. John's wort to be an effective natural treatment for mild depression. But when it is combined with certain drugs, including some medications used to treat AIDS and other illnesses, St. John's wort actually prevents the drugs from working properly.

Some herbs are dangerous and should be used only under your physician's supervision or not at all. For example, in small amounts and under medical supervision, the stimulant herb ephedra *(Ephedra sinica)*, also known as ma huang, can be an effective appetite suppressant. In larger amounts, this herb can cause high blood pressure, anxiety, irritability, rapid heartbeat, and heart rhythm problems. Overdoses of ephedra have even resulted in the deaths of several people who used it as an herbal version of the illegal drug Ecstasy.

Whenever you use herbs to treat a health problem, no matter how minor, it is important to understand exactly what the herb is and how to use it correctly. You also need to know if the herb will interact positively or negatively with any other foods, herbs, supplements, or medications you take.

Before trying any herb, consult this book to find the information you need to use it safely. If you are not sure whether the herb is safe for you, or if you're uncertain about the dosage, don't use it.

The dosages in this book are for the occasional treatment of minor health problems. Always start with the smallest dose, increasing it gradually if needed. To use herbs to treat more serious conditions, such as asthma, diabetes, or heart disease, consult your physician. Never stop taking any medication that your physician has prescribed for a health problem. If you think you'd like to try using herbs instead of drugs, you should always discuss them with your physician first.

❖ A WORD ABOUT OUR SOURCES ❖

In recent years, as interest in natural remedies has grown, a wider variety of herbs has been scientifically studied. These studies often back up the traditional uses of the herbs, and explain their action in the body. The information in this book is based on the latest scientific research available, but many herbs have not yet been carefully studied. Supplementing the science in this book is the clinical information I've amassed over the years as a naturopathic physician and in my own research and writings on the safety and effectiveness of herbs.

Other valuable sources of scientific information about herbs are the reports conducted by the German Commission E. In 1978, the German Federal Health Agency appointed a number of scientists to a commission charged with examining the safety and effectiveness of more than 300 herbs widely used in the German health care system. These reports, published as *The Complete German Commission E Monographs*, are widely used around the world to assess the value of medicinal herbs and to determine the most effective dosages. Wherever possible, information from this source has been incorporated into the herbal discussions in this book. For more information about this and other herbal references, see the Additional Reading list on page 248.

❧ STANDARDIZED PRODUCTS ❧

Because herbs are organic, their chemical makeup can vary considerably. Where the herb is grown, when it is harvested, and how it is stored and processed are just some of the factors that can significantly affect the strength of the final product. A small amount of an herb grown under optimal conditions might be highly effective, while a larger amount of a poorer-quality product might be required to obtain the same herbal effect. To solve this problem of variability, some companies are now processing herbs to ensure that each batch they produce contains the same percentage of each of the herb's constituents. This process is called standardization (or guaranteed potency), and each dose of a product prepared in this way is chemically identical.

But standardization poses some problems. A typical herb can contain a variety of constituents, and the active ones are not always known. The constituent that is chosen for standardization may not be the one that

GROWING AND HARVESTING YOUR OWN HERBS

SOME herbs are easy to grow yourself. Many common kitchen herbs, such as parsley *(Petroselinum crispum)*, oregano *(Origanum vulgare)*, basil *(Ocimum basilicum)*, and thyme *(Thymus vulgaris)* can be grown from seed or seedlings. These herbs do well year-round in pots on a sunny windowsill. Fragrant and attractive herbs that will grow outdoors include angelica *(Angelica archangelica)*, chamomile *(Matricaria recutita)*, calendula *(Calendula officinalis)*, lavender *(Lavandula* spp.), lemon balm *(Melissa officinalis)*, peppermint *(Mentha piperita)*, sage *(Salvia officinalis)*, and others. Books on herb gardening will include details about which herbs are appropriate for your growing region and how to harvest them.

Some familiar herbs can be gathered in the wild, a practice known as wildcrafting. Anyone with a lawn can find dandelion roots and leaves *(Taraxacum* spp.), while herbs such as burdock *(Arctium lappa)*, mugwort *(Artemisia vulgaris)*, mullein *(Verbascum thapsus)*, and shepherd's purse *(Capsella bursa-pastoris)* are found along roads and in fields.

Grow a selection of common kitchen herbs to use fresh or dried.

is most effective – and it's also possible that several compounds in an herb must work together to provide maximum benefit. In general, however, manufacturers standardize their products based upon scientific evidence found in *The Commission E Monographs* and other reliable sources *(p. 248)*.

Not every product has been studied enough to allow standardization, so the quality of products varies considerably. In addition, there is little government regulation of the supplement industry. To be sure you buy a safe product, purchase your herbs at a reputable natural products store or pharmacy, and choose products from reliable manufacturers.

Herbs in tablet, caplet, or capsule form sometimes contain additional ingredients such as lactose, which are added to help in the processing. Capsule shells are made of gelatin. If you wish to avoid certain additives, such as wheat, corn, dairy, or animal products, check the label. Many manufacturers provide herbs that are free of animal products and other additives. When buying herbs in bulk, buy only from reputable suppliers, and double-check the Latin name of the herb to be sure you've correctly identified it. To maintain the herbs' freshness, buy only enough to meet your needs for a few weeks at a time and store them in a cool, dry, dark place, out of the reach of children. To avert any potential problems, consult a pharmacist in addition to your physician: these professionals are usually very knowledgeable about herbs, particularly the way they interact with drugs. Above all, this book will help point you in the right direction for using herbs safely and effectively – so use it in good health!

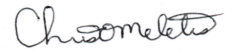

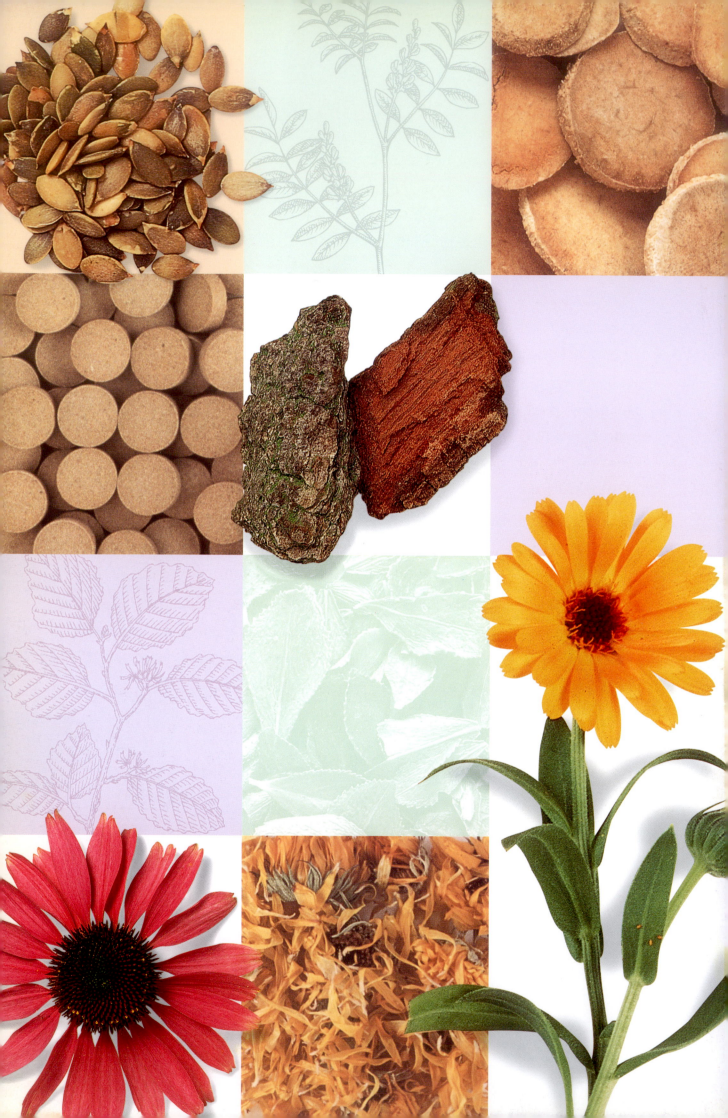

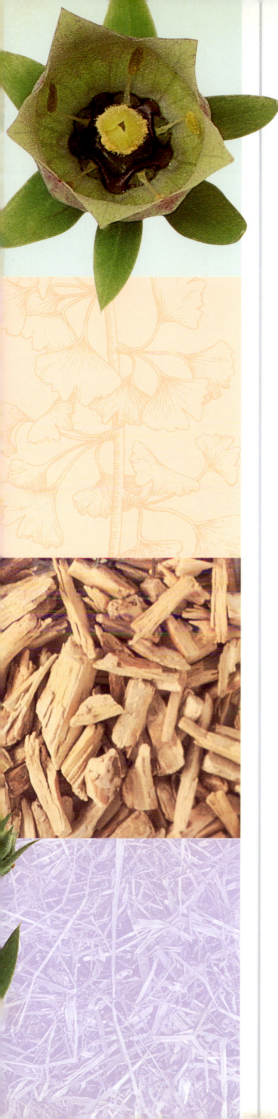

CHAPTER 1

SAFE AND EFFECTIVE HERBS

INTEREST IN HERBAL MEDICINE
has risen dramatically in recent years
for a variety of reasons: in comparison
with many prescription drugs, herbs are
often safer and cause fewer side effects;
they are frequently less expensive;
and, perhaps most importantly,
herbs enable you to treat yourself
for occasional, minor health problems.
In this chapter you'll find the uses,
dosages, and cautions for 176 safe herbs,
with explanations of how they work.

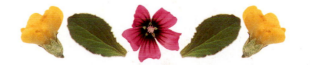

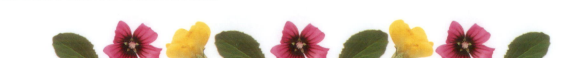

UNDERSTANDING HERBAL MEDICINE

HERBS – the leaves, flowers, seeds, bark, roots, and other parts of plants – contain a wide range of complex chemical compounds that have a variety of benefits on our health. In fact, many of these compounds are used in a concentrated form to create powerful drugs.

The best known of these drugs is probably the heart medication digoxin *(p. 147)*, which is derived from the leaves of the foxglove plant *(Digitalis purpurea)*. In comparison to drugs, herbs are usually gentler on your body, are less likely to cause any side effects, and are slower to act (the benefits can sometimes take weeks or months to be felt).

✤ CHOOSING THE RIGHT ✤ HERBAL REMEDY

With so many different herbal products now available to buy, it can sometimes be difficult to choose an herb that's right for you and to treat your particular condition. Based upon up-to-date clinical data and empirical observation, the selection of herbs discussed in this first chapter are generally considered to be safe and effective.

Foxglove

FRESH PEPPERMINT
Peppermint leaf is known to be an effective, natural remedy for treating minor digestive problems in adults.

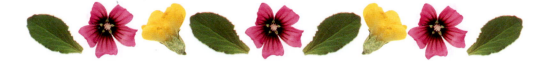

WORDS OF CAUTION

ALTHOUGH most herbs are generally very safe to use and carry few side effects, some people will be sensitive to certain herbs. Stop using an herb immediately if you experience an upset stomach, headache, skin rash, or any other unpleasant symptoms within two hours of taking it.

If you would like to try an herbal remedy to treat a chronic health problem, or to use herbs instead of a medication, always discuss it with your physician first to make sure the herb is right for you.

However, some herbs should be avoided by people with certain medical conditions. For example, dozens of herbs can be taken to relieve mild digestive problems, but some of them may aggravate ulcers or gallstones. Check the "Comments and cautions" section in every entry to be sure you can safely take the herb. Once you have selected an herb, begin with the smallest recommended dose; increase it gradually if needed, but don't exceed the maximum dosage.

✤ DOSAGE GUIDELINES ✤

The dosages listed in this book are guidelines for the safe treatment of minor, occasional problems. You will note that a particular herbal form is often recommended for a certain disorder – for example, herbal teas or decoctions are usually recommended for digestive upsets. Liquid extracts and tinctures, however, are generally beneficial for a wide variety of ailments, and can even be applied to the skin in some cases. Because these products can vary in strength, you should always remember to consult the package for other dosage information.

IDENTIFYING HERBS

EVERY herb is known by two names: its scientific, or Latin name, and the name by which it is commonly known. The Latin name eliminates any potential confusion by pinpointing the exact plant species. In cases where there are several members of an herb family, the second word in the Latin name consists of the letters spp., meaning "more than one species." Although common names are often easier to remember, double-check the Latin name of any herbs you might want to use – many plants are known by more than one common name, and that name may apply to several herbs.

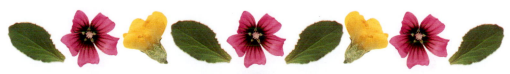

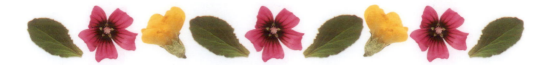

 TEAS, DECOCTIONS, AND TINCTURES

HERBAL TEAS AND DECOCTIONS

OFTEN the simplest way to take an herbal remedy is in the form of a tea or decoction. The aerial parts – the leaves or flowers – of most herbs can be easily brewed into teas, but the roots, bark, and seeds usually require a more vigorous extraction process of the plant's active ingredients, so these are usually heated in boiling water and made into decoctions.

Herbal teas and decoctions are easy to prepare. The amount of herb you use will vary (see the dosage instructions in each herbal entry) but in general, the guidelines are simple:

For an herbal tea: Bring 1 cup of water to a boil in a small pot. Add the loose herb. Steep for 3–5 minutes. Strain before drinking.

For a decoction: Combine the herb and 1 cup of water in a small pot. Bring to a boil. Reduce the heat and simmer for 10–15 minutes. Strain the mixture before drinking.

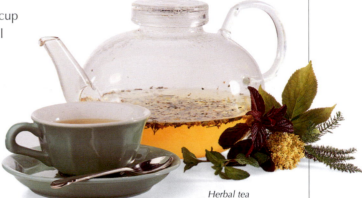

Herbal tea

Herbal teas and decoctions can sometimes taste bitter. Sweeten the liquid with a little sugar, honey, or maple syrup if desired, but do not add milk as it can reduce the effectiveness of some herbs' active ingredients.

TINCTURES

NATUROPATHIC practitioners often recommend tinctures because they permit variable dosages. The tinctures are usually made by soaking herbs in alcohol. The alcohol base preserves the herb's potency for a long time, often for two years or more. Since sunlight can destroy the effectiveness of herbs, tinctures are packaged in dark bottles that should always be stored in a cool, dark place. As they contain alcohol and highly concentrated ingredients, they should always be kept out of the reach of children.

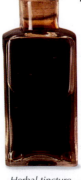

Always follow the directions on the package to determine the right dosage. The different substances within a tincture may separate, so always shake the bottle vigorously before measuring out the dose. If you are avoiding alcohol for any reason, or if you wish to give a tincture to a child, add the appropriate dose of tincture to one-half cup of very warm water; let it stand for 10 minutes. By the time the water is cool enough to drink, *Herbal tincture* most of the alcohol will have evaporated.

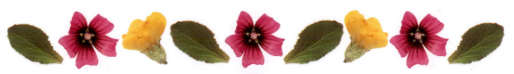

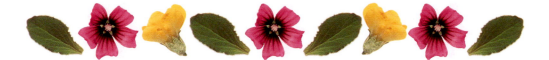

For the long-term use of herbal remedies, or to treat more serious conditions, consult an experienced naturopathic or holistic physician. When developing your treatment plan, your physician will consider many factors, including your age, your weight, your gender, and the medications and supplements you may already be taking.

✦ USING HERBS SAFELY ✦

Always buy herbs from reliable manufacturers, and store them in a cool, dry, dark place out of the reach of children. Many people keep their herbs in the bathroom cabinet, which may seem logical and within easy reach. However, because bathrooms can get warm and moist, this isn't such a good idea. To maintain the herb's freshness, buy only enough of an herb to last for a few weeks at a time.

HOW TO USE THIS CHAPTER

THE herbal entries in this chapter are all listed in alphabetical order according to their Latin, or scientific, name, with their common names underneath. Before using any herb, read each entry thoroughly to check you have selected the most appropriate herb, and to be sure that it is safe to take for your particular condition.

Latin name

Common name

Each entry carries a short explanation of how an herb works in the body

The dosages listed are all considered safe for treating occasional problems. Consult your physician for more personalized dosage instructions

Rubus fruticosus, R. villosus
BLACKBERRY LEAF

WHY IT'S USED Blackberry leaf is used to treat mild diarrhea, sore throats, mouth sores, minor cuts and scrapes, and hemorrhoids.

HOW IT WORKS Astringent substances, called tannins, in blackberry leaves have a variety of therapeutic benefits.

COMMENTS AND CAUTIONS Drinking large amounts of blackberry leaf tea can cause nausea.

DOSAGE •**Tea:** Steep 1 tablespoon of dried leaves in 1 cup of boiling water for 15 minutes. Drink up to 1 cup daily to treat diarrhea. •**Tincture:** 1 teaspoon 2 to 3 times daily or as directed on the package. Use the cooled tea or tincture as a gargle for sore throats and mouth sores. For cuts, scrapes, and hemorrhoids, soak a clean cloth in the tea or tincture and apply externally.

Brief description of the main benefits of taking an herb

Always check the "Comments and cautions" section to ensure that an herb is safe for you to take

Herbs can be purchased in different forms: as tablets or capsules (with or without an enteric coating, which allows the herb to pass unabsorbed through the stomach until it reaches the intestine), liquid extract, syrups, or dried herbs. The dried herbs can be made into teas, decoctions, and tinctures (see also pp. 10–11 for information on standardized products)

The berries can be prepared as a gargle for swallowing

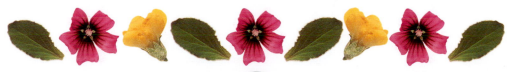

SAFE HERBS CATALOG

Achillea millefolium
YARROW

WHY IT'S USED Yarrow is used to prevent colds and flu and stop the bleeding resulting from cuts and scrapes.

HOW IT WORKS Researchers do not fully understand how yarrow works.

COMMENTS AND CAUTIONS Yarrow is used to treat upper respiratory infections, menstrual problems, and indigestion in Europe, but there is modest scientific evidence to show that it works to remedy these conditions. It may cause miscarriage in pregnant women and allergic reactions in some children.

DOSAGE •**Tea:** Steep 1–2 teaspoons of dried herb in 1 cup of boiling water for 10 minutes; drink up to 3 cups daily to prevent colds and flu. To treat minor cuts and scrapes, soak a clean cloth in cooled tea and apply to the skin for 15 minutes up to 3 times daily. •**Tincture:** See package directions.

Yarrow flower heads contain a volatile oil

WOUND HEALER
Yarrow, a native European herb, is known to have been valued for its ability to stop bleeding since classical times, when it was used to staunch war wounds.

Aesculus hippocastanum
HORSE CHESTNUT

WHY IT'S USED Horse chestnut, which is also available in the form of horse chestnut seed extract (HCSE), is used to treat varicose veins, leg swelling caused by poor circulation, hemorrhoids, and bruising.

HOW IT WORKS This herb contains aescin, a substance that strengthens the walls of veins and reduces swelling.

COMMENTS AND CAUTIONS Horse chestnut occasionally causes itching or nausea. If you have a liver or kidney disease, discuss this herb with your physician first before you try it. Horse chestnut can be poisonous.

DOSAGE •**Capsules:** 50–75 mg of aescin 2 times daily. •**Cream or gel:** Rub a small amount into the skin to treat sports injuries, varicose veins, and hemorrhoids.

VENOUS DISORDERS
While the bark and leaves of the horse chestnut tree can be useful medicinally, it is the seeds that are used as the main herbal remedy for poor circulation and veins.

Agrimonia eupatoria
AGRIMONY

WHY IT'S USED Agrimony is used to relieve minor mouth irritation and sore throat, mild diarrhea, and skin irritation such as sunburn.

HOW IT WORKS Agrimony contains tannins, astringent substances with therapeutic benefits.

COMMENTS AND CAUTIONS Do not use in a poultice – sun sensitivity or skin rashes may occur. Large or frequent doses can cause stomach upset or constipation, especially in children.

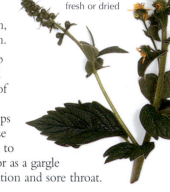

The aerial parts are used, either fresh or dried

DOSAGE •**Tea:** Steep 3 teaspoons of dried agrimony in 1 cup of boiling water for 10 minutes. Drink 2 cups daily for diarrhea; use cooled tea as a wash to treat skin irritation, or as a gargle to treat mouth irritation and sore throat.

Agropyron repens, Elymus repens
COUCH GRASS

WHY IT'S USED Couch grass is used to treat urinary tract infections (UTIs) and other urinary problems, including enlarged prostate, also called benign prostatic hypertrophy (BPH). Couch grass is also used to treat colds and coughs.

HOW IT WORKS Little is known about the active ingredients in couch grass. Research shows that the oils in the plant have an antimicrobial effect.

COMMENTS AND CAUTIONS To diagnose or treat BPH, consult your physician. Since couch grass is a diuretic, it could cause dehydration in children.

DOSAGE •**Capsules:** 1,000–2,000 mg 2 times daily. •**Tea:** Steep 1 teaspoon of couch grass in 1 cup of boiling water for 10 minutes. Drink up to 3 cups daily. •**Liquid extract:** 1 teaspoon 3 times daily or as directed on the package. •**Tincture:** ½–1 teaspoon 3 times daily or as directed on the package.

The roots, rhizomes, and short stems are all used medicinally

Couch grass is a cleansing diuretic

Allium cepa
ONION

WHY IT'S USED Onion is used to help prevent atherosclerosis (hardening of the arteries) by lowering cholesterol levels and thinning the blood.

HOW IT WORKS Onions are high in organic sulfur compounds, which have been shown to prevent blood clots and reduce cholesterol.

COMMENTS AND CAUTIONS Recent studies suggest that onions can also help reduce the risk of esophageal and stomach cancer.

DOSAGE •Fresh onions: at least ½ cup 4 or more times weekly. **•Tea:** Steep 3 teaspoons of chopped fresh onions in 1 cup of boiling water. **•Juice:** 1 teaspoon of fresh onion juice 3 to 4 times daily; combine with honey or syrup if desired. **•Tincture:** 1 teaspoon 3 to 4 times daily or as directed on the package.

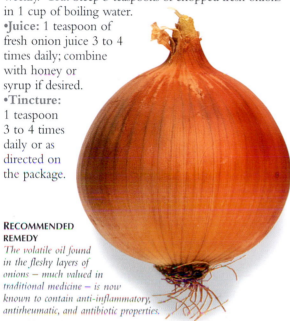

RECOMMENDED REMEDY
The volatile oil found in the fleshy layers of onions — much valued in traditional medicine — is now known to contain anti-inflammatory, antirheumatic, and antibiotic properties.

Allium sativum
GARLIC

WHY IT'S USED Garlic is used to treat a wide variety of health problems such as cardiovascular disease (including high cholesterol, high blood pressure, and atherosclerosis), intermittent claudication (a circulatory problem in the legs), microbial infection, and inflammation.

HOW IT WORKS Researchers believe that alliin, allinase, and allicin are the active ingredients in garlic; these substances have a wide variety of therapeutic actions.

COMMENTS AND CAUTIONS Do not combine with blood-thinning drugs (*e.g., warfarin, p. 195*). Large doses can cause uterine bleeding or miscarriage in pregnant women.

DOSAGE •Capsules: 300 mg 3 times daily of an extract standardized to contain 1.3 percent alliin or 1 percent total allicin potential. **•Fresh garlic:** 1 clove daily.

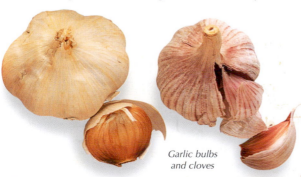

Garlic bulbs and cloves

Aloe vera
ALOE VERA GEL

WHY IT'S USED The clear gel contained in the fleshy leaves of the aloe plant helps relieve pain from minor burns including sunburn, and may also help cuts and scrapes heal faster. Studies have shown that an ointment containing aloe gel can help relieve the symptoms of mild psoriasis and seborrhea.

HOW IT WORKS A number of different complex sugars in aloe vera may stimulate the body's skin repair process.

COMMENTS AND CAUTIONS Use fresh gel externally for minor skin burns and cuts. To treat psoriasis and seborrhea, consult your physician. Internal use can cause uterine bleeding and miscarriage in pregnant women.

DOSAGE Dab a few drops of gel onto the affected area and let dry. Repeat up to 4 times daily. Stop using if irritation occurs or if your symptoms get worse.

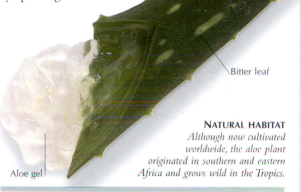

Bitter leaf

NATURAL HABITAT
Although now cultivated worldwide, the aloe plant originated in southern and eastern Africa and grows wild in the Tropics.

Aloe gel

Aloe barbadensis, A. vera
ALOE VERA JUICE

WHY IT'S USED Aloe vera juice is used to enhance immunity and to treat bacterial infections, viral infections including HIV, psoriasis, mild cases of Type 2 diabetes, Crohn's disease, ulcerative colitis, canker sores, and constipation. Some evidence suggests that it may help control asthma symptoms and some types of cancer.

HOW IT WORKS Aloe vera juice contains acemannan, a substance with an antiviral effect that appears to work synergistically with AZT *(p. 130)*, a drug used in the treatment of HIV/AIDS. Anti-inflammatory substances in aloe vera may alleviate the symptoms of asthma.

COMMENTS AND CAUTIONS External use is safe; internal use can cause severe diarrhea in children. Do not confuse aloe vera juice with aloe vera latex, a bitter yellow liquid made from the rind of the plant, which is a dangerous laxative.

DOSAGE •Liquid: 6 teaspoons (30 ml) 1 to 3 times daily. **•Capsules:** 50–200 mg daily for up to 10 days, or as directed by a physician.

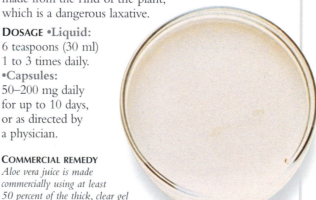

COMMERCIAL REMEDY
Aloe vera juice is made commercially using at least 50 percent of the thick, clear gel naturally produced by the aloe plant.

Althaea officinalis
MARSHMALLOW LEAF

WHY IT'S USED Marshmallow leaf is used to treat upper respiratory infections, asthma, and minor digestive problems. It is sometimes used to relieve discomfort from ulcers and Crohn's disease.

HOW IT WORKS Marshmallow leaf contains large amounts of complex sugars that soothe mucous membranes such as those in the throat and digestive tract.

COMMENTS AND CAUTIONS Because marshmallow leaves have a naturally high sugar content, they should not be used by people who have diabetes.

DOSAGE •**Capsules:** 1,000–2,000 mg 2 to 3 times daily. •**Tea:** Steep 1 teaspoon of dried leaves in 1 cup of boiling water for 10 minutes. Sip up to 2 cups daily. •**Liquid extract or tincture:** See package directions.

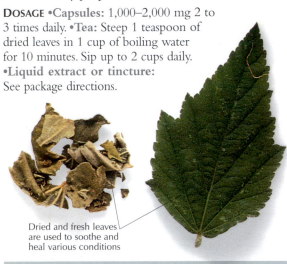
Dried and fresh leaves are used to soothe and heal various conditions

Althaea officinalis
MARSHMALLOW ROOT

WHY IT'S USED Marshmallow root is used in the treatment of sore throats and dry coughs. The root is also used to relieve discomfort from ulcers, gastritis, and other intestinal problems.

HOW IT WORKS Marshmallow root contains large quantities of complex sugars, which soothe mucous membranes such as those in the throat and digestive tract.

COMMENTS AND CAUTIONS Marshmallow root can slow the absorption of other medications. Take it two hours before or after drugs or other herbs.

DOSAGE •**Capsules:** 2,000–3,000 mg per day. •**Decoction:** Steep 2 teaspoons of ground marshmallow root in 1 cup of cold water for 30 minutes, stirring often. Warm before drinking; sip up to 2 cups throughout the day. •**Liquid extract or tincture:** See package directions.

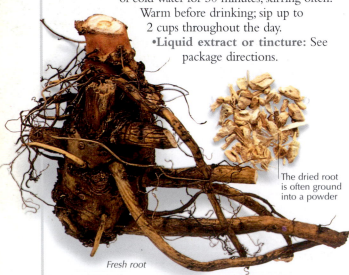
The dried root is often ground into a powder

Fresh root

Ananas comosus
BROMELAIN

WHY IT'S USED Bromelain is used to aid protein digestion and treat minor digestive problems, sports injuries, asthma, and sinusitis. Bromelain has also been shown to reduce pain from shingles and to speed postsurgical healing.

HOW IT WORKS Bromelain is a proteolytic enzyme, a natural substance that helps digest the proteins in food and reduces inflammation.

COMMENTS AND CAUTIONS Do not combine bromelain with antibiotics or with blood-thinning medications such as warfarin (*p. 195*). Do not take it if you are sensitive to pineapple, or have gastritis, ulcers, or esophagitis, since it may increase your blood pressure and heart rate. It can also cause severe irritation to the gastrointestinal tract and excess bleeding in children. If you have high blood pressure or heart disease, consult your physician. If you have a sensitive stomach, select a product with an enteric coating (*see p. 17*).

DOSAGE •**Capsules:** Bromelain's strength is typically measured in units called MCU (milk-clotting units) or GDU (gelatin-dissolving units). Take 500 MCU or 300 GDU 3 to 4 times daily.

The fruit contains the enzyme bromelain

The fruit, juice, and leaves all have different medicinal uses

Anethum graveolens
DILL SEED

WHY IT'S USED Dill seed is used to treat minor digestive problems. It can also be used to help relieve bad breath.

HOW IT WORKS Oils in dill seeds relax muscles in the digestive tract. Chlorophyll in the seeds freshens breath.

COMMENTS AND CAUTIONS Since dill seed relaxes the muscles linking the esophagus with the stomach, it may cause heartburn or acid reflux. It may also cause sun-sensitivity in fair-skinned children.

DOSAGE •**Tea:** Steep 2 teaspoons of dill seeds in 1 cup of boiling water. Drink up to 3 cups daily. •**Tincture:** ½–1 teaspoon up to 3 times daily or see package directions.

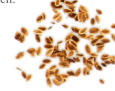
NORSE ORIGINS
The name dill derives from the Norse word dylla, *"to soothe."*

Angelica archangelica
ANGELICA ROOT

WHY IT'S USED Angelica is used to treat loss of appetite, mild stomach cramps, feelings of fullness, bloating, or gas.

HOW IT WORKS Angelica root contains terpenes and furocoumarins, oily substances that stimulate the secretion of gastric juices and help relax muscles.

COMMENTS AND CAUTIONS Angelica is also known as European angelica to distinguish it from Chinese angelica, known as dong quai *(Angelica sinensis, below)*. Angelica can make skin sensitive to light, especially children's skin; avoid prolonged exposure to sunlight when taking it. It may also cause hormonal imbalance in children. Do not use this herb if you are pregnant.

DOSAGE •**Tea:** Steep 1 tablespoon of finely chopped root in 1 cup of boiling water for 10 minutes. Drink 30 minutes before a meal. •**Tincture:** ½–1 teaspoon 3 times daily or as directed on the package.

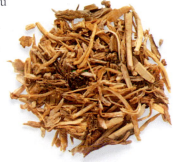

HARVESTING ANGELICA
Angelica root is often harvested in the fall of the first year of growth.

Angelica sinensis
DONG QUAI

WHY IT'S USED In Chinese medicine, dong quai is used to treat a variety of women's problems such as fibrocystic breast disease, menstrual cramps, premenstrual syndrome (PMS), irregular menstruation, and menopausal symptoms.

HOW IT WORKS Scientists have not yet fully determined how dong quai works.

COMMENTS AND CAUTIONS Dong quai is also known as Chinese angelica; it is closely related to European angelica. Although studies have not conclusively proven its effectiveness for hot flashes, many women find it helpful. Dong quai can cause uterine contractions and uterine relaxation in pregnant women. It may also cause hormonal imbalance and sun-sensitivity.

DOSAGE •**Capsules:** 1 or 2 250-mg capsules 3 times daily. •**Tincture:** ½–1 teaspoon 3 times daily or as directed on the package.

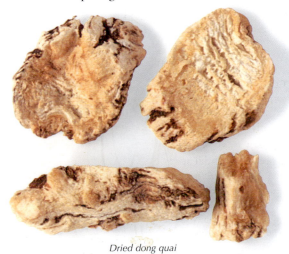

Dried dong quai

Arctium lappa, A. minus
BURDOCK ROOT

WHY IT'S USED Burdock root is used to treat urinary tract and skin infections, acne, psoriasis, and fungal infections such as ringworm. It is also sometimes used to treat rheumatoid arthritis.

HOW IT WORKS Substances in burdock root have been found to have antibacterial and antifungal effects.

COMMENTS AND CAUTIONS This herb is a stimulant that can cause miscarriage in pregnant women. Moderate dietary consumption of the fresh root is safe for children.

DOSAGE •**Tea:** Steep 1 teaspoon of dried burdock root in 3 cups of water for 30 minutes. Drink up to 3 cups daily. •**Capsules:** 1 500-mg capsule 2 to 3 times daily. •**Tincture:** ¼ teaspoon twice daily, or as directed on the package.

EDIBLE ROOT
Fresh burdock root is edible and can be prepared in small amounts as a vegetable.

Arctostaphylos uva-ursi
UVA URSI

WHY IT'S USED The leaves of the low-lying evergreen uva ursi bush are used to treat urinary tract infections (UTIs) and bladder problems.

HOW IT WORKS Uva ursi contains substances that are thought to have an antiseptic effect in the bladder.

COMMENTS AND CAUTIONS Uva ursi, also known as bearberry, works best in alkaline urine; do not take cranberry juice or vitamin C at the same time, since they raise urine acidity. Do not use for more than five days. May cause uterine contractions in pregnant or nursing women. Prolonged use may cause dehydration and urinary tract infections in children.

DOSAGE •**Capsules:** 2–4 200-mg capsules, standardized to contain at least 20 percent arbutin, 4 times daily. •**Tea:** Steep 2 teaspoons of dried leaves in 1 cup of boiling water for 15 minutes. Drink ½ cup 4 times daily. •**Liquid extract or tincture:** See package directions.

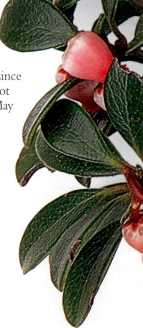

NATURAL ANTISEPTIC
Uva ursi is considered to be one of the best natural urinary antiseptics.

Armoracia rusticana
HORSERADISH

WHY IT'S USED Horseradish is used to treat upper respiratory tract infections, sinus congestion, sore throat, and urinary tract infections (UTIs) in conjunction with medication.

HOW IT WORKS
The pungent oils in horseradish have antibiotic properties.

COMMENTS AND CAUTIONS
Horseradish can cause vomiting, sweating, or upset stomach in high doses or in sensitive individuals, and gastrointestinal irritation in children; keep root away from the eyes, nose, and mucous membranes. Pregnant women with a high risk of miscarriage or bleeding disorders should avoid it. Do not use if you have hypothyroidism, ulcers, or kidney disease. Stop use after seven days.

DOSAGE •Fresh root: Eat ½ teaspoon of fresh, grated root 2 to 3 times daily. **•Tea:** Steep 1 teaspoon of grated root in 1 cup of boiling water for 5 minutes. Drink no more than 3 cups daily. **•Tincture:** ¼ teaspoon 2 to 3 times daily or as directed on the package.

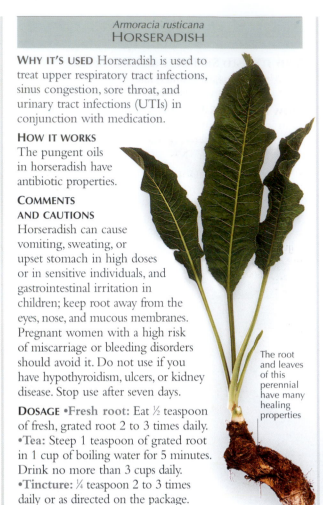

The root and leaves of this perennial have many healing properties

Artemisia vulgaris
MUGWORT

WHY IT'S USED Mugwort is most often used for minor digestive ailments. It is sometimes recommended for alleviating insomnia.

HOW IT WORKS Mugwort contains oils that are believed to help stimulate the flow of digestive juices.

COMMENTS AND CAUTIONS
Do not use mugwort if you are pregnant. This herb may cause diarrhea in children. It may also have a sedative effect; take appropriate precautions. Do not take it in combination with alcohol or other sedative herbs, supplements, or any medications.

DOSAGE •Tea: Steep 3 teaspoons of dried herb in 1 cup of boiling water for 5 minutes. For indigestion, drink 1 cup before meals, or for insomnia, drink 1 cup 1 hour before bedtime. **•Tincture or liquid extract:** See package directions.

Mugwort has a bitter taste and pungent aroma

The plant grows in temperate northern regions

Arnica chamissonis, A. montana
ARNICA

WHY IT'S USED Arnica is used to treat and heal minor injuries such as bruises, bumps, swelling, and sore muscles.

HOW IT WORKS Arnica contains helenalin, a substance that has an anti-inflammatory effect.

COMMENTS AND CAUTIONS Arnica should never be used internally. Do not use it on broken skin. Frequent use of arnica can lead to skin sensitization and irritation. In theory, arnica could interact with the blood-thinning drug warfarin (*p. 195*); if you take this drug, do not use arnica. If you are pregnant, consult a physician first before using this herb.

DOSAGE Rub a small amount of arnica tincture or ointment into the painful area 4 times daily. Choose an ointment that contains no more than 20–25 percent arnica tincture or 15 percent arnica oil.

FIRST-AID HERB
Arnica is commonly used as a first-aid topical remedy to help speed recovery after an injury.

The whole aromatic plant, including the root, is used topically

Asparagus officinalis
ASPARAGUS ROOT

WHY IT'S USED Asparagus root is used as a diuretic and in the treatment of urinary tract infections (UTIs). It is sometimes used to help prevent kidney stones.

HOW IT WORKS The complex sugar inulin, one of the many active ingredients in asparagus root, has a diuretic effect.

COMMENTS AND CAUTIONS Do not use asparagus root if you have a kidney disease or heart disease. Asparagus root can irritate the urinary tract. Do not confuse asparagus root with the edible part of the plant.

DOSAGE •Capsules: 250–350 mg twice daily.

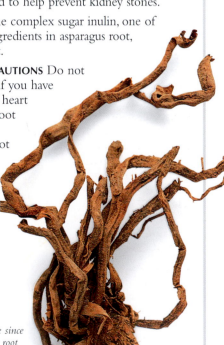

STRONG DIURETIC
Used in herbal medicine since ancient times, asparagus root is the part of the plant that is most effective as a diuretic.

...

Asparagus racemosus
SHATAVARI

WHY IT'S USED In Ayurveda (traditional Indian medicine), shatavari is used to strengthen the female reproductive system and to treat menopausal symptoms such as hot flashes. Shatavari is also used as a diuretic, to reduce inflammation, and to treat genital herpes.

HOW IT WORKS *Inulin, one of many active ingredients in shatavari, has a diuretic effect. It is not yet understood how shatavari relieves other problems.*

COMMENTS AND CAUTIONS Shatavari is a member of the asparagus family. Be sure to consume potassium-rich foods such as orange juice or bananas while taking shatavari because diuretics such as this can deplete your levels of potassium. Do not use it if you are pregnant.

DOSAGE •Powder: ½ teaspoon mixed with 4 ounces of milk or water 2 times daily. **•Capsules:** 250 mg 2 times daily.

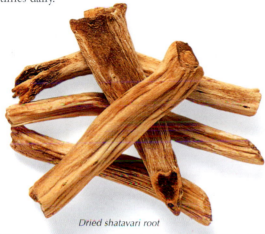

Dried shatavari root

Astragalus membranaceus
ASTRAGALUS

WHY IT'S USED In traditional Chinese medicine, astragalus (also called huang qi) is used to strengthen the immune system. It has antiviral effects, stimulates the immune system, protects the liver, and thins the blood.

HOW IT WORKS *Researchers do not yet fully understand how astragalus works.*

COMMENTS AND CAUTIONS Astragalus is best used to help prevent infection, not to treat it. Do not use astragalus if you are also receiving immunosuppressive therapy, including drugs to treat cancer or autoimmune illnesses such as lupus. Do not combine with blood-thinning drugs such as warfarin (*p. 195*). Astragalus is high in the mineral selenium; large doses of this herb may cause selenium poisoning.

DOSAGE •Capsules: 250–500 mg 1 to 3 times daily for up to 30 days or as directed by your physician. **•Fluid extract:** 1–3 teaspoons daily for up to 30 days or as directed by your physician.

Sliced, dried astralagus root

Atriplex halimus
SALT BUSH

WHY IT'S USED Salt bush, a woody shrub from the Mediterranean region, is used to treat mild cases of Type 2 diabetes.

HOW IT WORKS Salt bush leaves are high in the mineral chromium, which is often used to control blood sugar levels.

COMMENTS AND CAUTIONS If you have diabetes and you want to try salt bush, discuss it first with your physician; increased blood sugar monitoring and adjustment of your medication may be needed.

DOSAGE Take as directed by your physician.

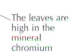

The leaves are high in the mineral chromium

DIABETES AID
The leaves from the salt bush plant are sometimes recommended by physicians to control Type 2 diabetes.

Avena sativa
OAT BRAN

WHY IT'S USED Oat bran, which is a good source of dietary fiber, is used to lower cholesterol and to treat constipation, irritable bowel syndrome (IBS), and other intestinal problems.

HOW IT WORKS Oat bran is high in soluble fiber, which provides bulk to the stool, promotes regularity, and contains beta glucan – a substance that absorbs cholesterol in the intestine and helps eliminate it.

COMMENTS AND CAUTIONS Oat bran can interfere with your absorption of other herbs and medications; take oat bran 2 hours before or after them. For constipation, take oat bran in the early evening; results should occur the next morning.

DOSAGE 3–6 tablespoons of oat bran daily prepared as a breakfast cereal, added to food, or stirred into 16 ounces of juice or water.

Oat bran

Avena sativa
OAT STRAW

WHY IT'S USED Oat straw is added to bathwater to treat skin problems including eczema, poison ivy, seborrhea, chicken pox, and sunburn.

HOW IT WORKS Oat straw is high in silicic acid and zinc, both of which help soothe irritated, itchy skin.

COMMENTS AND CAUTIONS Oat straw is also known as green oats and green tops.

DOSAGE •**Decoction:** Steep 1 cup of chopped oat straw in 3 quarts of boiling water for 20 minutes. Then add to the bathwater.

Oat straw

Avena sativa
WILD OATS

WHY IT'S USED Wild oats are used to relieve anxiety and nicotine withdrawal.

HOW IT WORKS Oats contain alkaloids, substances that appear to act as mild sedatives.

COMMENTS AND CAUTIONS This herb may have a sedative effect; take appropriate precautions. Do not take it in combination with alcohol or other sedative herbs, supplements, or medications. For information about dietary oats, see oat bran (*Avena sativa, above*).

DOSAGE •**Capsules:** 500 mg up to 3 times daily. •**Tincture:** ½ teaspoon 3 times daily or as directed on the package.

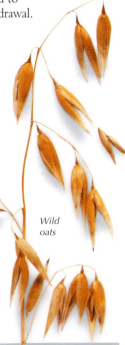
Wild oats

Azadirachta indica
NEEM

WHY IT'S USED Neem is used to treat fevers, inflammation, and infections.

HOW IT WORKS Researchers do not understand how neem works.

COMMENTS AND CAUTIONS In addition to its medicinal uses, neem is considered a safe natural insecticide. It is also used as an ingredient in toothpastes.

DOSAGE Commercial preparations vary in strength; follow package directions.

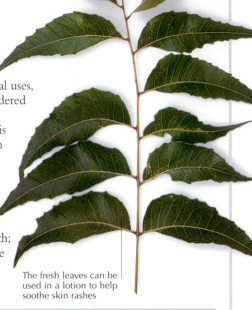
The fresh leaves can be used in a lotion to help soothe skin rashes

Barosma betulina, B. crenulata, B. serratifolia
BUCHU

WHY IT'S USED Buchu is used to treat kidney and bladder problems and to relieve bloating from premenstrual syndrome (PMS).

HOW IT WORKS Buchu contains substances that are antiseptic, diuretic, and anti-inflammatory.

COMMENTS AND CAUTIONS Buchu is an ingredient in some over-the-counter diuretic formulas. Be sure to consume potassium-rich foods such as orange juice and bananas while taking the herb, unless your physician advises otherwise, because diuretics such as buchu can deplete your levels of potassium. May cause dehydration in children and miscarriage in pregnant women.

DOSAGE •**Tea:** Steep 1 teaspoon of dried buchu leaves in 1 cup of boiling water for 15 minutes. Drink up to 3 cups daily. •**Capsules:** 500–750 mg twice daily. •**Tincture:** 1 teaspoon up to 3 times daily or see package directions.

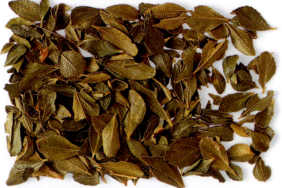
Dried buchu leaves

Berberis acquifolium, Mahonia acquifolium
OREGON GRAPE

WHY IT'S USED
Oregon grape is used primarily to treat the symptoms of psoriasis, including itching and burning.

HOW IT WORKS Oregon grape contains berberine, a substance that has been shown to fight infections and appears to slow down accelerated skin cell growth common in psoriasis.

COMMENTS AND CAUTIONS Oregon grape is closely related to barberry *(Berberis vulgaris, below)*. Do not combine Oregon grape with other berberine-containing herbs such as goldenseal *(Hydrastis canadensis, p. 39)*. Oregon grape may cause uterine bleeding and miscarriage in pregnant women.

DOSAGE •Cream or ointment: Apply a thin layer of a product standardized to contain 10 percent Mahonia extract to the affected area 3 times daily.
•Capsules or tablets: 250 mg 2 to 3 times daily.
•Tea: Steep 1–2 teaspoons of dried herb in 2 cups of boiling water for 10 minutes. Drink up to 3 cups daily. **•Tincture:** ½ teaspoon up to 3 times daily or as directed on the package.

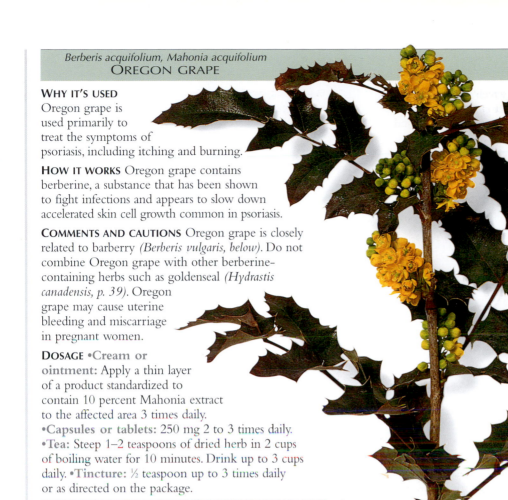

MOUNTAIN GRAPE
Oregon grape can grow at high altitudes – up to 7,000 ft (2,000 m). Its natural habitat is the Rocky Mountains, as well as the woodland area stretching from Colorado to the Pacific coast.

Berberis vulgaris
BARBERRY

WHY IT'S USED Barberry is used to treat sore throats, minor mouth irritations, and minor digestive problems.

HOW IT WORKS Berberine, a substance found in barberry, has an antibiotic effect, relaxes muscles, and increases the flow of bile, which facilitates digestion.

COMMENTS AND CAUTIONS
Overdoses can cause lethargy, nosebleeds, and kidney irritation. Do not use barberry if you have heart disease, liver disease, jaundice, or if you are nursing or pregnant; it may cause uterine bleeding and miscarriage. Do not combine with other berberine-containing herbs such as bloodroot *(Sanguinaria canadensis, p. 53)*, goldenseal *(Hydrastis canadensis, p. 39)*, or Oregon grape *(Berberis spp., above)*.

DOSAGE •Tea: Steep ½ teaspoon of powdered barberry root bark in 8 ounces of boiling water for 15 minutes. Sweeten lightly if desired and drink up to 1 cup daily. Use cooled tea as a gargle or mouthwash. **•Capsules:** 250 mg 1 to 2 times daily. **•Tincture:** 1 to 2 teaspoons daily or as directed on the package.

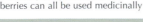
The stem, bark, root bark, and berries can all be used medicinally

Beta vulgaris rubra
BEET LEAF

WHY IT'S USED Beet leaves are used to treat minor digestive problems such as loss of appetite, mild nausea, bloating, and gas.

HOW IT WORKS Beet leaves contain the B vitamins choline and inositol and a related substance called betaine, which are believed to stimulate the production of bile. Bile facilitates digestion.

COMMENTS AND CAUTIONS
Do not use beet leaf if you have gallstones, gallbladder disease, or biliary duct disease. Large doses may increase the chances of uterine bleeding and miscarriage in pregnant women.

DOSAGE •Capsules: 3,000–5,000 mg each day.

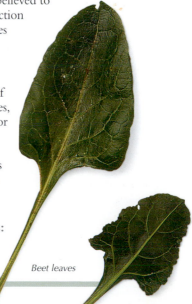
Beet leaves

Borago officinalis
BORAGE OIL

WHY IT'S USED Borage oil is used to treat a range of different problems, including premenstrual syndrome (PMS), diabetic neuropathy (a painful nerve condition), eczema and other skin problems, and rheumatoid arthritis.

HOW IT WORKS Pressed from the seeds of the borage plant, borage oil is a good source of gamma linolenic acid (GLA) – an essential fatty acid that plays an important role in inflammatory conditions.

COMMENTS AND CAUTIONS Borage seeds contain pyrrolizidine alkaloids (PAs), substances that can cause liver damage. Select a product that is labeled PA-free. Those who have liver disease should not use borage oil because of the possible presence of PA; borage oil should not be used by children or pregnant and nursing women.

DOSAGE 500 mg, twice per day, of a product labeled PA-free.

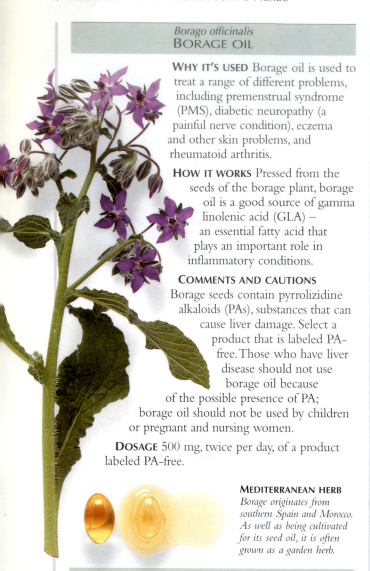

MEDITERRANEAN HERB
Borage originates from southern Spain and Morocco. As well as being cultivated for its seed oil, it is often grown as a garden herb.

Boswellia serrata
BOSWELLIA

WHY IT'S USED Boswellia, a gummy resin from the boswellia tree of northern India, is used to treat arthritis, tendinitis, bursitis, and other joint problems.

HOW IT WORKS Boswellia contains substances known as boswellic acids that have an anti-inflammatory effect.

COMMENTS AND CAUTIONS The beneficial effects of boswellia usually take up to eight weeks to show results. Boswellia is safe, however, some people using it may experience a mild stomach upset, diarrhea, or skin irritation, especially in children.

DOSAGE •**Capsule:** 1 400-mg capsule standardized to 37.5 percent boswellic acids 3 times daily.

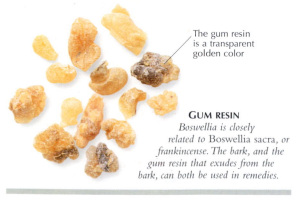

The gum resin is a transparent golden color

GUM RESIN
Boswellia is closely related to Boswellia sacra, or frankincense. The bark, and the gum resin that exudes from the bark, can both be used in remedies.

Bupleurum spp.
BUPLEURUM

WHY IT'S USED In traditional Chinese medicine, bupleurum (also known as thoroughwax or chai hu) is used to treat a wide variety of ailments, including liver disease such as hepatitis, and AIDS.

HOW IT WORKS Soapy substances known as saponins are thought to stimulate the body's immune system.

COMMENTS AND CAUTIONS Although bupleurum is safe, it is found in some dangerous herbal combination formulas for treating liver disease, including Asian products known as sho-saiko-to, and xino-chai-hu-tang. Such formulas have been associated with a serious form of lung disease and should not be used. Stop using bupleurum if it causes stomach upset or diarrhea. Do not use bupleurum if you are pregnant or nursing; it may also cause stomach upset and diarrhea in children.

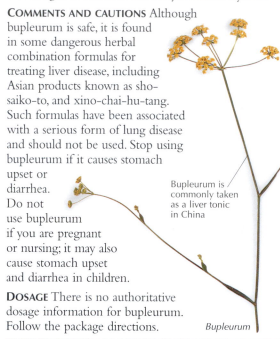

Bupleurum is commonly taken as a liver tonic in China

DOSAGE There is no authoritative dosage information for bupleurum. Follow the package directions.

Bupleurum

Calendula officinalis
CALENDULA

WHY IT'S USED Calendula ointment, tincture, or spray is used externally to treat skin problems, especially cuts, sores, rashes, and slow-healing wounds.

HOW IT WORKS A variety of complex substances in calendula help stimulate wound healing and have anti-inflammatory effects.

COMMENTS AND CAUTIONS Calendula is also known as pot marigold. Do not use calendula on deep wounds or severe injuries. Stop using it if irritation or redness occurs. See your physician if it does not help within a few days.

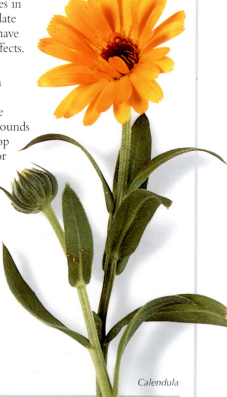

DOSAGE Apply a small amount of calendula ointment or spray, standardized to contain at least 5 percent calendula, to the affected area 3 times daily. Calendula tincture can be used as a wash or poultice.

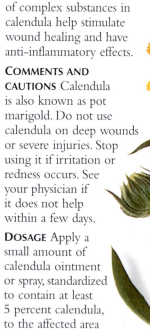

Calendula

Camellia sinensis
GREEN TEA

WHY IT'S USED Green tea has been found to help protect against cancer and heart disease.

HOW IT WORKS Green tea contains powerful antioxidants that are thought to offer even more protection against free radicals than vitamins C and E.

COMMENTS AND CAUTIONS A cup of green tea contains 30 mg caffeine; decaffeinated products are also available. Moderate amounts are safe for pregnant and nursing women; the caffeine may overstimulate children.

DOSAGE •Tea: Steep 1 teaspoon of green tea leaves in 1 cup of boiling water for 5 minutes. Drink up to 6 cups daily. **•Capsules:** 100–150 mg, twice daily, of a product standardized to contain 97 percent green tea polyphenols.

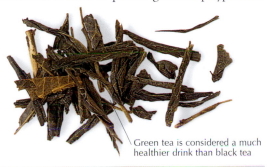

Green tea is considered a much healthier drink than black tea

Capsella bursa-pastoris
SHEPHERD'S PURSE

WHY IT'S USED Shepherd's purse is used to reduce heavy menstrual bleeding and bleeding between periods, prevent nosebleeds, and treat minor skin wounds.

HOW IT WORKS Researchers don't yet fully understand how shepherd's purse reduces bleeding.

COMMENTS AND CAUTIONS Do not use this herb if you have kidney stones. It may also cause uterine bleeding or miscarriage in pregnant women, and irritate sensitive skin.

DOSAGE •Tea: Steep 1 teaspoon of dried herb in 1 cup of boiling water for 15 minutes. Drink up to 2 cups daily between meals. Soak a clean cloth in the cooled tea and apply to wounds for 15 minutes up to 4 times daily. **•Liquid extract:** ½ teaspoon 3 times daily or as directed on the package.

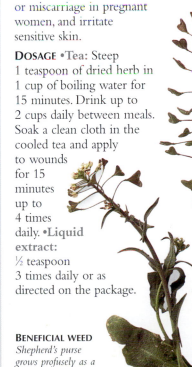

BENEFICIAL WEED
Shepherd's purse grows profusely as a weed in many temperate regions, and can be harvested throughout the year.

Capsicum annuum
CAPSAICIN CREAM

WHY IT'S USED Capsaicin cream is used to relieve the pain and itching of shingles (herpes zoster), trigeminal neuralgia (a painful facial disorder), surgical wounds, diabetic neuropathy (a painful nerve condition), arthritis, and psoriasis.

HOW IT WORKS Capsaicin, the compound that gives cayenne pepper its heat, helps deplete the body's level of Substance P, a chemical that transmits the sensation of pain to the central nervous system.

COMMENTS AND CAUTIONS Wear gloves when applying cream, or wash hands thoroughly after use. Avoid mucous membranes, eyes, and broken skin. Discontinue use if redness or irritation occurs; it may cause skin burns in children. For best results, use regularly and consistently; effects can take several days.

DOSAGE Apply small amounts of cream containing 0.025–0.075 percent capsaicin to the affected area. A burning sensation that lasts for several minutes is normal. When the sensation diminishes, apply a larger amount as needed.

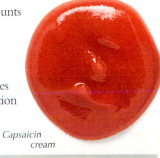

Capsaicin cream

Capsicum frutescens
CAYENNE PEPPER

WHY IT'S USED Cayenne pepper is used to treat many minor digestive problems (such as loss of appetite and gas), and may prevent stomach irritation from nonsteroidal anti-inflammatory drugs. Cayenne may also help improve circulation and is sometimes used to treat heart disease.

HOW IT WORKS Capsaicin, the compound that gives cayenne pepper its heat, may have a protective effect on the lining of the stomach.

COMMENTS AND CAUTIONS If you have ulcers, gastritis, esophagitis, or a sensitive stomach, use cayenne with caution. Do not use cayenne if you take the drug theophylline for asthma; the cayenne may increase your absorption of the drug to dangerous levels. Stop using cayenne pepper if stomach irritation or nausea occurs.

DOSAGE •Capsules: Strengths vary among products; follow package directions. **•Tincture:** ⅛ teaspoon 1 to 3 times daily or as directed on the package.

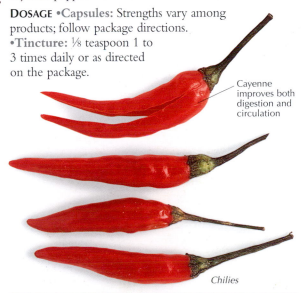

Cayenne improves both digestion and circulation

Chilies

Carica papaya
PAPAYA

WHY IT'S USED Papaya leaf is used to treat minor digestive problems such as nausea and mild diarrhea. Papain, an enzyme concentrated from papaya, is also used to treat minor digestive problems such as nausea, bloating, and gas, especially from eating high-protein foods. Papain has also been used to treat inflammation following surgery.

HOW IT WORKS Papaya leaf is high in papain, an enzyme that aids digestion by breaking down proteins.

COMMENTS AND CAUTIONS Do not use papaya or papain if you take a blood-thinning drug such as warfarin (*p. 195*), or have gastritis, acid reflux, or ulcers; it could further damage irritated tissue. It may cause uterine bleeding or miscarriage in pregnant women.

DOSAGE Commercial products are available containing papaya powder or papain, often in combination with other proteolytic enzymes such as bromelain *(Ananas comosus, p. 20)*. Follow the package directions on each of these products.

Papaya leaves can be used to tenderize meat

Centella asiatica
GOTU KOLA

WHY IT'S USED Gotu kola is used primarily to treat varicose veins, poor leg circulation, and hemorrhoids. It is also used to speed up the healing of wounds and burns, to prevent scarring, and to relieve the symptoms of scleroderma, a disease of the connective tissues.

HOW IT WORKS Soapy substances in gotu kola called triterpene saponins are believed to strengthen the body's connective tissue.

COMMENTS AND CAUTIONS It may take up to six weeks to realize the benefits of gotu kola.

DOSAGE •**Capsules:** 30–60 mg, twice daily, of an extract standardized to contain 40 percent asiaticoside, 29–30 percent asiatic acid, 29–30 percent madecassic acid, and 1–2 percent madecassoside. •**Tea:** Steep 1 teaspoon of dried leaves in ½ cup of boiling water for 10 minutes. Drink up to 1 cup daily. •**Liquid extract:** ½–1 teaspoon daily or as directed on the package. •**Tincture:** 1–1½ teaspoons twice daily.

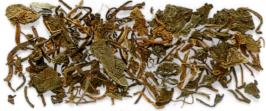

Dried aerial parts

Ceratonia siliqua
CAROB

WHY IT'S USED Carob is used to treat acute diarrhea.

HOW IT WORKS Carob contains sugars that absorb liquid, and astringent substances called tannins that reduce intestinal inflammation and have a mild antimicrobial action.

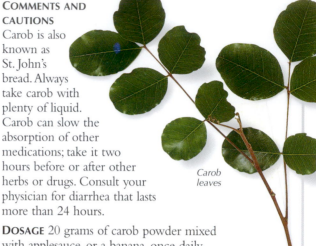

COMMENTS AND CAUTIONS Carob is also known as St. John's bread. Always take carob with plenty of liquid. Carob can slow the absorption of other medications; take it two hours before or after other herbs or drugs. Consult your physician for diarrhea that lasts more than 24 hours.

Carob leaves

DOSAGE 20 grams of carob powder mixed with applesauce, or a banana, once daily. Follow each dose with at least 8 ounces of liquid.

Chamaemelum nobile (Roman), *Matricaria recutita* (German)
CHAMOMILE

WHY IT'S USED Chamomile is used to relieve a wide variety of ailments, including mild digestive problems, stress, insomnia, gingivitis (gum disease), asthma and other lung problems, and many skin conditions.

HOW IT WORKS Chamomile flowers contain complex substances including apigenin, which may help relax muscles.

COMMENTS AND CAUTIONS Do not use chamomile if you take blood-thinning drugs such as warfarin (*p. 195*), or if you are allergic to ragweed or to plants in the daisy family such as cornflower *(Centaurea cyanus)* or mugwort *(Artemisia vulgaris, p. 22)*. Large doses can increase the risk of complications in pregnancy.

DOSAGE •**Capsules and tablets:** Follow package directions to treat stress and insomnia. •**Tea:** Steep 2 teaspoons of chamomile flowers in 1 cup of boiling water for 10 minutes; drink up to 3 cups daily for digestive problems. Use cooled tea as a mouthwash 3 times daily for gingivitis. •**Cream:** For skin conditions, apply a small amount of chamomile cream to the affected area up to 4 times daily.

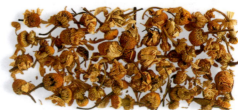

Dried chamomile flowers

Cichorium intybus
CHICORY

WHY IT'S USED Chicory is used to treat minor digestive problems such as loss of appetite, mild nausea, bloating, and gas, and relieve the symptoms of gallbladder disease.

HOW IT WORKS Bitter compounds in chicory act as an appetite stimulant and increase the flow of saliva and gastric juices in the body.

COMMENTS AND CAUTIONS Long-term use of chicory could make your skin sensitive to light. Avoid prolonged exposure to sunlight or tanning lamps while using this herb. Large amounts of chicory may cause uterine bleeding or miscarriage in pregnant women.

DOSAGE •**Capsules:** 1,000–3,000 mg daily before meals. •**Tea:** Steep 1 teaspoon of dried chicory in 1 cup of boiling water for 10 minutes. Drink before meals.

Chicory root can be roasted and used as a coffee substitute

Chamomile flower heads have a slightly bitter, aromatic taste

This herb is safe for use both internally and externally

FLOWERS IN BLOOM
Chamomile flower heads are picked in full bloom on the day they open, when the active compounds they contain are most potent. The flower heads can be used either fresh or dried in infusions and other herbal preparations.

Cimicifuga racemosa rhizoma
BLACK COHOSH ROOT

WHY IT'S USED Black cohosh root is used to treat the symptoms of menopause, especially hot flashes, headache, irritability, vaginal dryness, and sleep disturbances.

HOW IT WORKS The active ingredient in black cohosh root is still unknown.

COMMENTS AND CAUTIONS Black cohosh has few if any side effects. Do not confuse it with blue cohosh, a potentially dangerous herb unrelated to black cohosh. Black cohosh may cause miscarriage in pregnant women. Do not take it continuously for more than six months without a physician's supervision.

DOSAGE •**Capsules:** 150–500 mg twice daily. •**Tincture:** ½–1 teaspoon 3 times daily or as directed on the package.

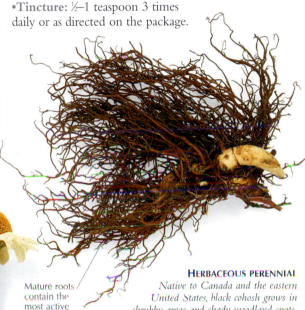

Mature roots contain the most active properties

HERBACEOUS PERENNIAL
Native to Canada and the eastern United States, black cohosh grows in shrubby areas and shady woodland spots. The root is a Native American remedy.

Cinnamomum aromaticum
CHINESE CINNAMON BARK

WHY IT'S USED Chinese cinnamon bark is used to treat minor digestive problems and to relieve bad breath.

HOW IT WORKS Oils in Chinese cinnamon are believed to increase the flow of gastric juices.

COMMENTS AND CAUTIONS Chinese cinnamon can cause gastrointestinal irritation, and may damage tooth enamel. Do not use Chinese cinnamon if you are pregnant.

DOSAGE •**Capsules:** 600 mg, 3 times daily, with meals. •**Tea:** Steep ½ teaspoon of ground bark in 1 cup of water for 10 minutes. Drink ½ cup before meals. Use cooled tea as a mouthwash to relieve bad breath. •**Liquid extract and tincture:** Follow package directions. Take 3 times daily before meals.

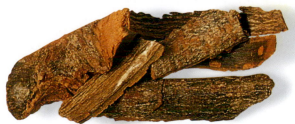

Dried Chinese cinnamon bark

Cinnamomum camphora
CAMPHOR

WHY IT'S USED Camphor ointments are used on the skin to relieve sore muscles. Inhaling camphor vapor helps relieve chest congestion and reduce coughing.

HOW IT WORKS Camphora, a substance extracted from the oil in the wood of the camphor tree, increases blood flow to the skin and creates a sensation of warmth.

COMMENTS AND CAUTIONS Camphor is potentially toxic. In 1980, the FDA banned camphorated oil containing 20 percent camphor after cases of poisoning were reported. Commercial products (e.g., Ben-Gay and Vicks VapoRub) containing up to 11 percent camphor are considered safe. Camphor may cause uterine bleeding and miscarriage in pregnant women, birth defects, and choking in infants.

DOSAGE Apply small amounts of a cream containing less than 11 percent camphor as directed on the package.

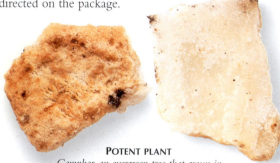

POTENT PLANT
Camphor, an evergreen tree that grows in tropical and subtropical regions, has long been valued by the Chinese for its volatile oil. The white crystalline substance derived from the stems, roots, and other parts of the tree (above), is known to have antiseptic, stimulant, and antispasmodic properties.

Cinnamomum verum
CINNAMON

WHY IT'S USED Cinnamon bark is used to help treat minor digestive problems (such as loss of appetite, mild nausea, stomach cramps, bloating, and gas) and also to relieve bad breath. Recent research suggests cinnamon may help people with mild cases of Type 2 diabetes regulate their blood sugar.

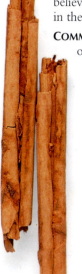

HOW IT WORKS The oils in cinnamon bark are believed to increase the flow of gastric juices in the stomach.

COMMENTS AND CAUTIONS Cinnamon is often added as a flavoring agent to herbal mixtures and other preparations. Large amounts of cinnamon may cause uterine bleeding and miscarriage in pregnant women and gastrointestinal irritation in children.

DOSAGE •Capsules: 0.5–1 gram 3 times daily with meals. **•Tea:** Steep ½ teaspoon of ground bark in 1 cup of water for 10 minutes. Drink ½ cup before meals. Use cooled tea as a mouthwash to relieve bad breath. **•Liquid extract and tincture:** Follow the package directions. Take 3 times daily before meals.

Cinnamon sticks and powder

Citrus aurantium
BITTER ORANGE PEEL

WHY IT'S USED Bitter orange peel is used to treat heartburn and other minor digestive problems.

HOW IT WORKS Oily substances found in bitter orange peel increase bile flow, which facilitates digestion.

COMMENTS AND CAUTIONS Bitter orange peel can make skin sensitive to light, especially children's skin. Avoid prolonged exposure to sunlight or tanning lamps when taking it. This herb can cause birth defects, uterine bleeding, and miscarriage in pregnant women.

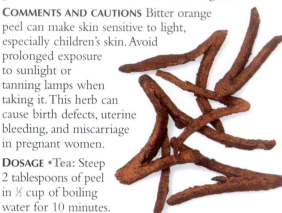

DOSAGE •Tea: Steep 2 tablespoons of peel in ½ cup of boiling water for 10 minutes. Take 1 to 3 times daily.

Bitter orange peel

Cnicus benedictus
BLESSED THISTLE

WHY IT'S USED Blessed thistle, also known as holy thistle, is used to treat minor digestive problems such as loss of appetite, bloating, or gas.

HOW IT WORKS Blessed thistle contains bitter substances that stimulate the flow of saliva and digestive juices.

The spiny, leathery leaves and flowering tops are both used in preparations

COMMENTS AND CAUTIONS Do not use this herb if you are allergic to plants in the daisy family such as mugwort *(Artemisia vulgaris, p. 22)*, cornflower *(Centaurea cyanus)*, or milk thistle *(Silybum marianum, p. 54)*. It can also cause gastrointestinal irritation in children.

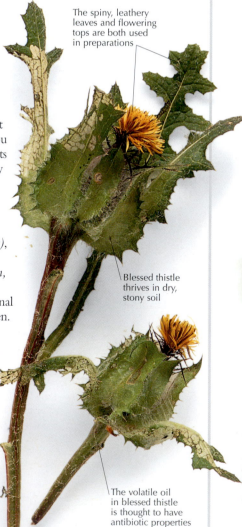

Blessed thistle thrives in dry, stony soil

DOSAGE •Tea: Steep 2 teaspoons of dried herb in ½ cup boiling water for 10 minutes. Drink up to 3 times daily. **•Tincture:** ½ teaspoon 2 to 3 times daily or as directed on the package.

The volatile oil in blessed thistle is thought to have antibiotic properties

Codonopsis spp.
CODONOPSIS

WHY IT'S USED Codonopsis is used to treat HIV infection, and as a supportive treatment for cancer patients receiving radiation treatment. In traditional Chinese medicine, codonopsis is sometimes used as an inexpensive substitute for ginseng.

HOW IT WORKS Substances in codonopsis seem to stimulate weight gain, improve endurance, increase red blood cell counts, and stimulate the immune system.

COMMENTS AND CAUTIONS If you have an autoimmune disease such as HIV or lupus, or if you have cancer, discuss codonopsis with your physician before you try it.

DOSAGE •Decoction: Simmer ½ cup of codonopsis in 4 cups of water until the liquid is reduced to 2 cups. Take 1 cup twice daily on an empty stomach, or as directed by your physician.

MILD SUBSTITUTE *Though milder than ginseng, codonopsis is thought to carry the same qualities, of helping the body adapt to stress, fatigue, and cold.*

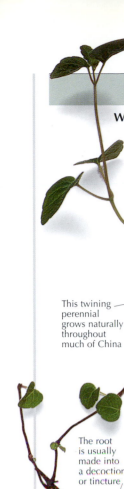

This twining perennial grows naturally throughout much of China

The root is usually made into a decoction or tincture

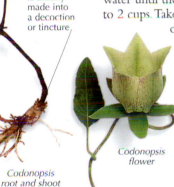

Codonopsis flower

Codonopsis root and shoot

Cola acuminata, C. nitida
KOLA NUT

WHY IT'S USED Kola nut is a mild stimulant.

HOW IT WORKS Kola nut contains caffeine and other compounds that have a stimulating effect on the body.

COMMENTS AND CAUTIONS Kola nut is approved by the FDA as a food additive and as a flavoring in cola drinks. Do not take it if you have ulcers or should avoid caffeine, which raises blood pressure and heart rate, and can cause miscarriage, birth defects, premature delivery, low birth weight, and overstimulation in sensitive individuals.

DOSAGE •Capsules: 500 mg 2 to 3 times daily. **•Tea:** Steep 1 teaspoon of kola nut in 1 cup of boiling water for 10 minutes; drink 1 to 2 cups daily.

Kola nuts

Between 10 and 15 kola nuts, or seeds, are contained within the large, woody seed pods of the kola tree

Coleus forskohlii
COLEUS

WHY IT'S USED Coleus is used primarily to treat asthma, eczema, psoriasis, high blood pressure, and angina.

HOW IT WORKS The active ingredient in coleus is forskolin, a substance that relaxes muscles and acts as a natural antihistamine.

COMMENTS AND CAUTIONS If you take blood-thinning drugs such as warfarin (*p. 195*) or drugs for high blood pressure, consult your physician. Coleus can cause uterine bleeding or miscarriage in pregnant women, and may interfere with children's proper muscle functioning.

DOSAGE Use as directed by your physician.

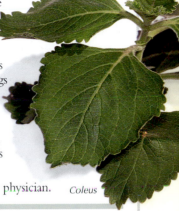

Coleus

Commiphora molmol
MYRRH

WHY IT'S USED Myrrh is used primarily to treat sore throat and tonsillitis, and to prevent and treat gum disease.

HOW IT WORKS Myrrh contains a number of complex substances, including furanosesquiterpenes, which are believed to give myrrh its characteristic antiseptic action.

COMMENTS AND CAUTIONS Myrrh may cause uterine bleeding or miscarriage in pregnant women, and gastrointestinal irritation in children. It has been used in perfume and incense and as a medicine for centuries.

DOSAGE •Capsules or tablets: 500–1,000 mg 2 to 3 times daily. **•Gargle or mouthwash:** 5–10 drops of myrrh tincture in 8 ounces of warm water; use up to 3 times daily.

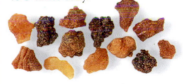

Myrrh resin and capsules

Commiphora mukul
GUGGUL

WHY IT'S USED Guggul is used to treat arthritis, high cholesterol, indigestion, and arteriosclerosis.

HOW IT WORKS Researchers don't yet understand how guggul works.

COMMENTS AND CAUTIONS Research shows that guggul can lower cholesterol by as much as 11 percent; benefits may take up to four weeks to be felt. Guggul may cause diarrhea. If you want to treat high cholesterol with guggul, consult your physician.

DOSAGE 1 750-mg capsule, 3 times daily, of a capsule standardized to contain 2.5 percent guggulsterones.

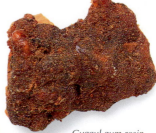

Guggul gum resin

Coriolus versicolor
TURKEY TAIL

WHY IT'S USED Turkey tail, a type of mushroom, is used to stimulate the immune system, especially in people suffering from hepatitis, AIDS, and chronic fatigue syndrome, and patients undergoing cancer treatment.

HOW IT WORKS Turkey tail contains polysaccharides (complex sugars) that stimulate the body's immunity and have antitumor effects.

COMMENTS AND CAUTIONS Turkey tail is also called coriolus mushroom. It has been extensively studied in Japan.

DOSAGE Consult your physician about your individual dosage.

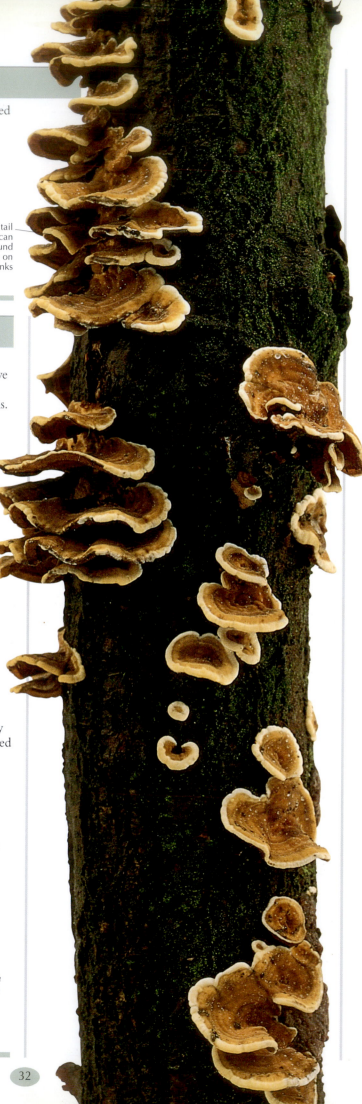

Turkey tail fungi can be found growing on tree trunks

Crataegus oxyacantha
HAWTHORN

WHY IT'S USED Hawthorn is used to help maintain cardiovascular health, treat the early stages of congestive heart failure, lower high blood pressure, relieve mild angina symptoms, and reduce benign heart palpitations.

HOW IT WORKS Hawthorn contains complex mixtures of chemicals that work in combination to improve the heart's pumping ability.

COMMENTS AND CAUTIONS If you have heart disease and want to try hawthorn, consult your physician, even if you don't take medication. Unlike drugs such as digoxin (p. 147), hawthorn does not increase the risk of heart rhythm problems. It may take four to 12 weeks for the benefits to be felt. Hawthorn may cause a dangerous drop in blood pressure and altered heart function.

DOSAGE •Capsules: 100–300 mg, 2 to 3 times daily, of an extract of leaves and flowers standardized to contain 2–3 percent flavonoids or 18–20 percent procyandins.
•Tincture: 1 teaspoon 3 times daily or as directed on the package.

Hawthorn helps maintain a healthy heart

Flowers can also be used in an infusion to improve poor circulation

HEART TONIC
The thorny hawthorn bush, which grows in the temperate regions of the Northern Hemisphere, is considered an extremely valuable medicinal herb, and has been used since the Middle Ages as a remedy for many conditions.

Curcuma longa
TURMERIC ROOT

WHY IT'S USED Turmeric is used in Ayurveda (traditional Indian medicine) to treat minor digestive problems such as loss of appetite, bloating, and gas, and help relieve the symptoms of rheumatoid arthritis.

HOW IT WORKS Turmeric contains curcumin, a substance with an anti-inflammatory effect that helps relieve the pain and swelling of arthritis, and oils that stimulate the flow of digestive juices.

COMMENTS AND CAUTIONS Turmeric has a stimulating effect on the gallbladder; do not use it if you have ulcers, gallstones, or gallbladder disease. Large doses can cause miscarriage and uterine bleeding in pregnant women.

DOSAGE Capsules: 400–600 mg curcumin 3 times daily. •**Tea:** Steep 1 teaspoon of ground root in 1 cup of boiling water for 10 minutes. Drink ½ cup 2 times daily. •**Liquid extract:** ½ teaspoon 2 times daily or as directed on the package. •**Tincture:** ¼ teaspoon 2 times daily or as directed on the package.

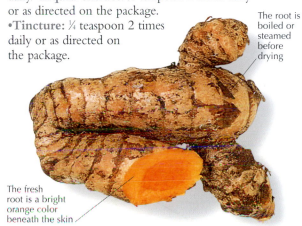

The root is boiled or steamed before drying

The fresh root is a bright orange color beneath the skin

Curcurbita pepo
PUMPKIN SEED

WHY IT'S USED Pumpkin seed extract is used to treat the symptoms of an enlarged prostate gland, called benign prostatic hypertrophy (BPH), including frequent urination and urinary urgency. It is also used as a traditional remedy for tapeworm.

HOW IT WORKS The active ingredients that help BPH are unknown. An amino acid, called curcubitacin, is believed to be effective against tapeworm. The seeds may cause gastrointestinal irritation in children.

COMMENTS AND CAUTIONS To diagnose or treat tapeworm or BPH, consult your physician. Pumpkin seeds only relieve the symptoms of BPH; they do not reduce prostate enlargement. Because diuretics, including pumpkin seeds, can deplete levels of potassium, consume potassium-rich foods such as orange juice or bananas.

DOSAGE •**Capsule:** 80 mg pumpkin seed extract 3 to 4 times daily. •**Seeds:** 1–2 heaped tablespoons of ground hulled seeds, stirred into 8 ounces of cold water or juice. Take morning and evening.

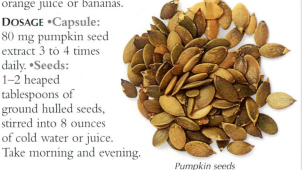

Pumpkin seeds

Cynara scolymus
ARTICHOKE LEAF

WHY IT'S USED Artichoke leaf is used for minor digestive problems. Recent studies have shown that artichoke leaf extract can help lower cholesterol. Artichoke may also protect your liver from toxic chemicals.

HOW IT WORKS Substances in artichoke leaf increase bile flow, help remove toxins from the liver, and may interfere with cholesterol production.

COMMENTS AND CAUTIONS Do not use artichoke leaf if you have gallstones, gallbladder disease, or biliary duct disease because it may have a stimulating effect on the gallbladder.

DOSAGE •**Capsules:** For indigestion, 1 250-mg capsule, standardized to 2.5–5.0 percent caffeoylquinic acids, 3 times daily. **For high cholesterol:** 1 320-mg capsule, standardized to 2.5–5.0 percent caffeoylquinic acids, 4 to 5 times daily. •**Tincture:** 1 teaspoon 3 times daily or as directed on the package.

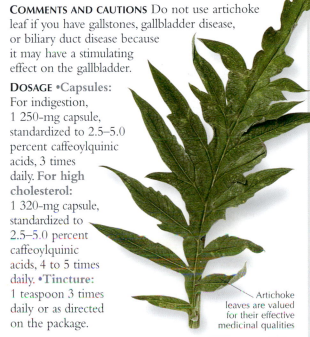

Artichoke leaves are valued for their effective medicinal qualities

Echinacea angustifolia, E. purpurea
ECHINACEA

WHY IT'S USED Echinacea helps prevent and treat colds, bronchitis, gingivitis, cold sores, yeast and ear infections.

HOW IT WORKS Echinacea contains a number of complex immune-stimulating substances.

COMMENTS AND CAUTIONS Echinacea is also known as purple coneflower. A numbing of the tongue is normal when using liquid forms. Do not use it if you have an autoimmune disease or if you are allergic to plants in the daisy family such as mugwort *(Artemisia vulgaris, p. 22)*. Echinacea may trigger autoimmune disorders in pregnant women.

DOSAGE •**Capsules:** 1 200–300-mg capsule 3 times daily.

•**Juice:** ½–¾ teaspoon 3 times daily of echinacea juice standardized to contain 2.4 percent fructo-furanosides. •**Liquid extract or tincture:** See package directions.

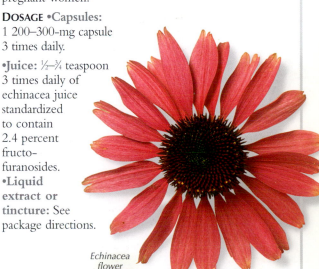

Echinacea flower

Elettaria cardamomum
CARDAMOM

Cardamom pod and seeds

WHY IT'S USED Cardamom seeds are used to treat minor digestive problems such as loss of appetite, heartburn, mild nausea, bloating, and gas. The seeds are also used to help treat colds, coughs, flu, and bronchitis.

HOW IT WORKS Complex oils in the seeds aid digestion by stimulating the gallbladder, and fight viral infections.

COMMENTS AND CAUTIONS Do not use cardamom if you have gallstones, gallbladder disease or biliary duct disease. Cardamom seeds can also interfere with children's digestion.

DOSAGE •**Tea:** Steep 1 teaspoon of crushed cardamom seeds in 1 cup of boiling water for 10 minutes. Drink up to 3 cups daily. •**Tincture:** ½–1 teaspoon up to 3 times daily or as directed on the package.

Eleutherococcus senticosus
ELEUTHERO

WHY IT'S USED Eleuthero is used as a stress reliever and a mild stimulant to help improve concentration, physical stamina, and memory, to speed recovery from illness or surgery, and to support the immune and adrenal systems.

HOW IT WORKS Eleuthero contains at least 29 natural chemical compounds. Researchers still don't fully understand how they work.

COMMENTS AND CAUTIONS Eleuthero is also known as Siberian ginseng and is used in Chinese medicine when ginseng would be too stimulating. Do not use eleuthero if you have high blood pressure or heart problems; it may also cause overstimulation and altered hormonal balance in children. Buy only from a reputable source.

DOSAGE •**Capsules or tablets:** 1,000 mg up to 2 to 3 times daily. •**Tea:** Steep ½ teaspoon of powdered or dried root in 1 cup of boiling water for 10 minutes. Drink no more than 1 cup a day in divided doses. •**Liquid extract:** ½ teaspoon daily or as directed on the package. •**Tincture:** 1–1½ teaspoons twice daily or as directed on the package.

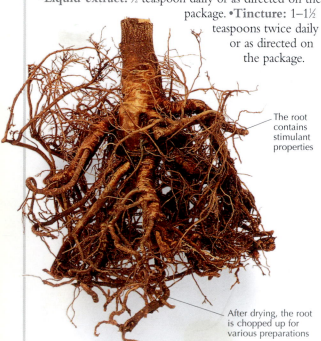

The root contains stimulant properties

After drying, the root is chopped up for various preparations

Equisetum arvense
HORSETAIL

WHY IT'S USED Horsetail is used to treat arthritis and urinary tract infections (UTIs), and to help strengthen nails and bones.

HOW IT WORKS Horsetail is a diuretic and contains silicon, which is important in nail and bone health.

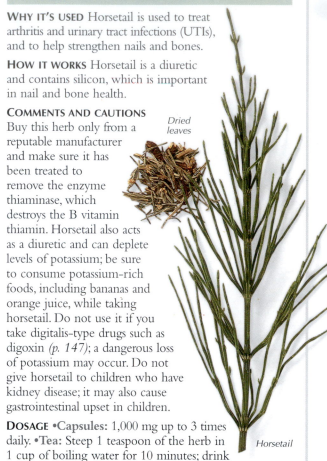
Dried leaves

Horsetail

COMMENTS AND CAUTIONS Buy this herb only from a reputable manufacturer and make sure it has been treated to remove the enzyme thiaminase, which destroys the B vitamin thiamin. Horsetail also acts as a diuretic and can deplete levels of potassium; be sure to consume potassium-rich foods, including bananas and orange juice, while taking horsetail. Do not use it if you take digitalis-type drugs such as digoxin *(p. 147)*; a dangerous loss of potassium may occur. Do not give horsetail to children who have kidney disease; it may also cause gastrointestinal upset in children.

DOSAGE •**Capsules:** 1,000 mg up to 3 times daily. •**Tea:** Steep 1 teaspoon of the herb in 1 cup of boiling water for 10 minutes; drink ½ cup up to 3 times daily. •**Liquid extract or tincture:** ½ teaspoon up to 3 times daily, or see package directions.

Eriodictyon californicum
YERBA SANTA

WHY IT'S USED Yerba santa leaf is used to treat respiratory problems such as asthma, bronchitis, and coughs related to colds and flu.

HOW IT WORKS Yerba santa contains eriodictyol, a mild expectorant that helps relieve congestion.

COMMENTS AND CAUTIONS The leaves of yerba santa, an evergreen tree native to southwestern America, have a pleasant, sweet taste, which is approved by the FDA as a flavoring agent.

DOSAGE •**Tincture:** Follow package directions.

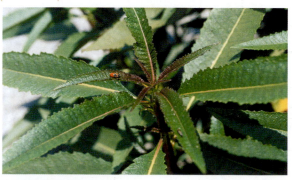

COUGH RELIEVER
The lance-shaped leaves of the yerba santa plant contain a mild expectorant that relieves coughs caused by many different conditions.

Eschscholzia californica
CALIFORNIA POPPY

WHY IT'S USED California poppy has a mild antianxiety effect. It is used as a sedative in Native American medicine.

HOW IT WORKS Complex sugars and other ingredients in California poppy are sleep-inducing.

COMMENTS AND CAUTIONS California poppy is not addictive. It has a sedative effect; take appropriate precautions. Do not combine with other sedative herbs, supplements, medications, or alcohol. This herb may increase the risk of miscarriage in pregnant women, and cause excessive drowsiness in children. Consult a physician if your insomnia lasts for more than two weeks.

DOSAGE •Tea: Steep 1 teaspoon of dried California poppy flower in 1 cup of boiling water for 5 minutes. Drink no more than 1 cup daily 1 hour before bedtime. **•Liquid extract:** ¼ teaspoon 1 hour before bedtime or see package directions.

SOOTHING BENEFITS
California poppy is a close relative of the opium poppy (Papaver somniferum), *a narcotic. However, California poppy has a beneficial, rather than disorientating, effect on the body.*

Eucalyptus globulus
EUCALYPTUS

WHY IT'S USED Eucalyptus oil is used to treat chest congestion, sore muscles, and joint pain from arthritis.

HOW IT WORKS The herb stimulates bronchial tubes and brings relief from coughs and colds. If used topically, it increases blood flow to give a warm, soothing sensation.

COMMENTS AND CAUTIONS Never use it internally – even small amounts can cause poisoning – and do not use it if you are pregnant or nursing. For best results, choose a product that contains at least 70 percent eucalyptol oil. Discontinue use if you develop skin irritation or a rash occurs.

DOSAGE •For chest congestion: Add a few drops of oil to hot water or a vaporizer and inhale the steam. Rub a small amount of tincture, or an ointment containing 5–20 percent essential oil, onto the chest up to 3 times daily. **•For muscle and joint pain:** Rub a few drops of tincture or eucalyptus oil mixed with 1 teaspoon of olive oil, or an ointment containing 5–20 percent essential oil onto the chest area up to 3 times daily.

Eucalyptus leaves

Filipendula ulmaria
MEADOWSWEET

WHY IT'S USED Meadowsweet is used to reduce inflammation and to relieve cold and flu symptoms, including fever and pain.

HOW IT WORKS Meadowsweet contains salicylates, aspirin-like substances that reduce fever and inflammation.

COMMENTS AND CAUTIONS Do not use meadowsweet if you are allergic to salicylates or aspirin. Do not give meadowsweet to children; salicylates have been related to a serious brain and liver condition called Reye syndrome.

DOSAGE
•Capsules: 1,000 mg once or twice daily.
•Tea: Steep 2 teaspoons of dried meadowsweet in 1 cup of boiling water for 10 minutes. Sweeten and drink as hot as possible up to 4 times daily.

Meadowsweet

•Liquid extract: ½ teaspoon up to 3 times daily or as directed on the package. **•Tincture:** ½ teaspoon up to 3 times daily or as directed on the package.

Foeniculum vulgare
FENNEL SEED

WHY IT'S USED Fennel seed is used to treat minor digestive problems and is also helpful for treating irritable bowel syndrome.

HOW IT WORKS The oils in fennel seed, particularly terpenoid anethole, help relax the intestinal tract.

COMMENTS AND CAUTIONS If indigestion persists for more than two weeks, consult a physician. Fennel may cause uterine contractions in pregnant women, and large amounts can cause an hormonal imbalance in children.

DOSAGE •Tea: Steep ½ teaspoon of crushed fennel seeds in 1 cup of boiling water for 10 minutes. Drink up to 3 cups daily between meals. **•Liquid extract:** ½ teaspoon up to 3 times daily between meals or as directed on the package. **•Tincture:** ½ teaspoon up to 3 times daily between meals or as directed on the package.

Fennel seeds

Foeniculum vulgare
FENNEL OIL

WHY IT'S USED Fennel oil is used to treat minor digestive problems such as loss of appetite, heartburn, mild nausea, stomach cramps, bloating, and gas.

HOW IT WORKS Fennel oil has a relaxing effect on the intestinal tract.

COMMENTS AND CAUTIONS Do not use during pregnancy. For persistent indigestion, see your physician.

DOSAGE •Fennel oil: Add 1–3 drops of oil to 1 cup of hot water or ½ teaspoon of honey; take up to 3 times daily between meals.

Fennel oil

Fucus vesiculosus, Laminaria, Macrocytis, Nereocystis spp.
KELP

WHY IT'S USED Kelp, a form of seaweed, is used to treat fibrocystic breast disease, and is sometimes also recommended as a weight loss aid.

HOW IT WORKS Kelp is high in iodine, a trace mineral that is needed for normal thyroid gland function.

COMMENTS AND CAUTIONS Kelp is also known as kombu. It is a good source of folic acid (folate) and a number of other vitamins and minerals. If you are being treated for a thyroid condition, use kelp only under your physician's supervision. Large doses of kelp may trigger hyperthyroid disease. Kelp is also high in sodium; do not use it if your salt intake is restricted.

DOSAGE The iodine content of kelp products varies considerably among products. Read the label and take only enough kelp to provide 100 mcg of iodine daily.

Kelp

Gentiana lutea
GENTIAN ROOT

WHY IT'S USED Gentian is used to treat minor digestive problems.

HOW IT WORKS Bitter substances in gentian stimulate the flow of digestive juices.

COMMENTS AND CAUTIONS Do not use gentian if you have frequent heartburn, acid reflux, gallstones, gallbladder disease, ulcers, or biliary duct disease. Gentian root can cause gastrointestinal irritation, especially in children.

DOSAGE •Capsule or tablet: 1 500-mg tablet before meals. **•Decoction:** Boil 1 teaspoon of powdered gentian root in 3 cups of water for 30 minutes. Sweeten if needed; take 1 tablespoon 1 hour before meals. **•Tincture:** ½–1 teaspoon 1 hour before meals or as directed on the package.

Yellow gentian

Ginkgo biloba
GINKGO

WHY IT'S USED Ginkgo is used widely to help improve memory and mental functioning, to improve circulation (especially to the brain, legs, and reproductive organs), to treat dizziness and tinnitus (ringing in the ear), and sometimes to treat asthma and other ailments.

HOW IT WORKS Ginkgo contains powerful antioxidants that limit the damage of free radicals, and compounds that help to keep blood vessels open.

COMMENTS AND CAUTIONS Because ginkgo may have a blood-thinning effect, do not take it if you are also taking a blood-thinning drug such as warfarin (*p. 195*).

DOSAGE 60–120 mg, twice daily, of a product standardized to contain 24 percent ginkgo flavonol glycosides and 6 percent terpene lactones.

Ginkgo leaf

Ganoderma lucidum
REISHI

WHY IT'S USED Reishi, a tree fungus native to China and Japan, has been used for centuries as an adaptogen – a substance that helps the body cope with stress and fight off infection. Research into other health claims, including cancer treatment, continues.

HOW IT WORKS Reishi has been extensively studied, but researchers still do not fully understand how it works.

COMMENTS AND CAUTIONS Benefits may take up to two weeks to be felt.

DOSAGE •Raw reishi 500–2,000 mg 3 times daily with meals. **•Capsules:** 1 150-mg capsule standardized to contain 4 percent tripertenes and 10 percent polysaccharides 4 times daily. **•Reishi extract:** Follow package directions.

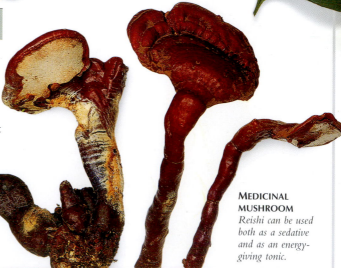

MEDICINAL MUSHROOM
Reishi can be used both as a sedative and as an energy-giving tonic.

Glycine max
SOY ISOFLAVONES

WHY IT'S USED Soy isoflavones, substances found in soy products such as tofu (soybean curd) and soy milk, are classified as phytoestrogens – plant substances that act as a mild form of estrogen. They help relieve menopausal symptoms and reduce high cholesterol in women.

HOW IT WORKS Researchers have identified daidzein and genistein as two of the active ingredients in soy that have a mild estrogenic benefit.

COMMENTS AND CAUTIONS Research suggests that soy foods offer greater benefit than supplements, especially for lowering cholesterol. If you have thyroid disease, a history of breast or reproductive cancer, or are pregnant, discuss soy isoflavones first with your physician. Daidzein and genistein are also found in red clover *(Trifolium pratense, p. 56)*. Soy may cause hormonal imbalance and diarrhea in children.

DOSAGE 100–200 mg of soy isoflavones daily from supplements and soy food.

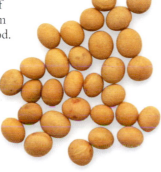

SOY BEANS
These highly nutritious beans are also known to benefit the circulatory system. They are now grown throughout the world as a staple crop.

Glycine max
SOY LECITHIN

WHY IT'S USED Soy lecithin helps reduce cholesterol and treat liver disease. It is also currently being studied as a treatment for Alzheimer's disease and bipolar disorder.

HOW IT WORKS Soy lecithin contains phospholipids – fatty acids that are important in the generation of cell membranes and in brain function. Soy lecithin appears to improve cholesterol metabolism.

COMMENTS AND CAUTIONS More research is needed to investigate the benefits of soy lecithin. Soy lecithin may cause hormonal imbalance and diarrhea.

DOSAGE 1,200 mg of lecithin 2 to 3 times daily with food.

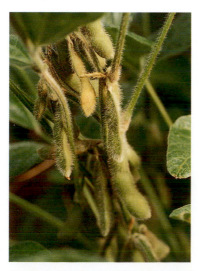

ASIAN STAPLE
Soy is a dietary mainstay in many Asian countries and has been used medicinally for thousands of years.

Glycyrrhiza glabra
LICORICE ROOT

WHY IT'S USED Licorice root is used to treat ulcers, upper respiratory infections, minor digestive problems, and AIDS.

HOW IT WORKS Glycyrrhizin, the main active ingredient in licorice, is antiviral and anti-inflammatory.

COMMENTS AND CAUTIONS Research shows deglycyrrhizinated licorice (DGL) works best for ulcers. To treat upper respiratory infections and digestive problems, use regular licorice. Discuss licorice with your physician before using it to treat AIDS or a serious viral infection. Do not use it if you have high blood pressure, kidney disease, or take a drug such as digoxin *(p. 147)*. Licorice may cause high blood pressure in children and pregnant and nursing women, and also uterine bleeding.

DOSAGE •**For ulcers:** 2–4 100-mg chewable DGL tablets 20 minutes before meals. •**For upper respiratory and digestive problems:** Steep 1 teaspoon of powdered licorice root in 1 cup of boiling water for 5 minutes; drink ½ cup after meals, or take liquid extract after meals according to the package directions.

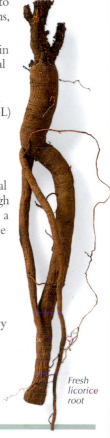

Fresh licorice root

Gritola trondosa
MAITAKE

WHY IT'S USED Maitake is a medicinal mushroom from Japan that is used to fight off infection and improve your resistance to stress.

HOW IT WORKS Maitake contains a complex sugar called beta-D-glucan that appears to stimulate the body's immune system.

COMMENTS AND CAUTIONS Other health claims for maitake, including its use in treating cancer and HIV, are not well documented.

DOSAGE •**Capsules or tablets:** 3,000–7,000 mg daily in divided doses. •**Liquid extract:** Follow the directions on the package.

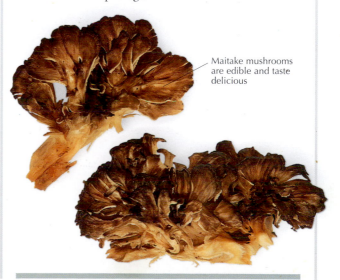

Maitake mushrooms are edible and taste delicious

Grindelia spp.
GUMWEED

WHY IT'S USED Gumweed is used to treat coughs related to colds and bronchitis.

HOW IT WORKS Compounds in gumweed appear to relax the respiratory tract.

COMMENTS AND CAUTIONS People allergic to ragweed may also be allergic to gumweed. Gumweed is toxic if taken in excessive doses. Do not give this herb to children as it may cause diarrhea.

DOSAGE •**Capsules:** 2,000–3,000 mg daily. •**Liquid extract:** 1–2 teaspoons daily or as directed on the package. •**Tincture:** ½ teaspoon daily or as directed on the package.

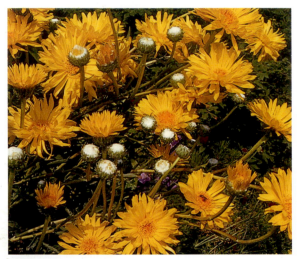

DAISIES IN THE DESERT
Gumweed, a perennial herb with triangular leaves and yellow-orange flowers that closely resemble daisies, grows in arid and saline soil and is native to the southern United States and Mexico. It was traditionally used by North American Indians to treat bronchial problems such as colds, coughs, and tuberculosis, and to help speed the healing of skin irritation and burns.

Gymnema sylvestre
GYMNEMA

WHY IT'S USED Gymnema, an Asian evergreen climbing plant, is used in Ayurveda (traditional Indian medicine) to treat mild cases of Type 2 diabetes.

HOW IT WORKS Recent scientific research has shown that gymnema may help lower blood sugar by increasing insulin production and lowering insulin resistance.

COMMENTS AND CAUTIONS If you have diabetes, take gymnema only under your physician's supervision. Likewise, always consult your physician before giving gymnema to children with diabetes. Gymnema is also known by its Hindi name, gurmar.

DOSAGE 400–600 mg daily of gymnema extract standardized to 24 percent gymnemic acid. In Ayurvedic medicine the dose is 2,000–4,000 mg of powdered gymnema daily.

Gymnema is believed to decrease cravings for sweets

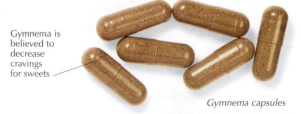

Gymnema capsules

Hamamelis virginiana
WITCH HAZEL

WHY IT'S USED Witch hazel is used to treat minor injuries (such as cuts, scrapes, bruises, burns, sunburn, and insect bites), hemorrhoids, sore throat, and mouth irritation.

HOW IT WORKS Witch hazel is high in astringent substances called tannins, which have a variety of therapeutic benefits.

COMMENTS AND CAUTIONS To relieve hemorrhoids, use one of the commercially prepared treatments containing witch hazel. This herb may cause skin irritation in some children.

The bark is much higher in tannins than the leaves

DOSAGE •**For minor injuries:** Apply distilled witch hazel directly to the skin as a compress up to 4 times daily. Apply ointment directly to the skin up to 4 times daily. •**For sore throat and mouth irritation:** Combine 1 ounce of witch hazel distillate with 4 ounces of warm water. Gargle or rinse up to 4 times daily; do not swallow.

SKIN SOOTHER
Distilled witch hazel, made from leaves and young twigs, is used to treat inflamed and tender skin.

Harpagophytum procumbens
DEVIL'S CLAW

WHY IT'S USED Devil's claw is a South African herb used to treat arthritis, gout, back pain, and minor digestive problems such as loss of appetite and mild nausea.

HOW IT WORKS Complex substances in devil's claw may have an anti-inflammatory and analgesic effect. Its bitter taste stimulates the flow of saliva and gastric juices.

COMMENTS AND CAUTIONS Do not use devil's claw if you have acid reflux or ulcers. Enteric-coated tablets and capsules are best (see p. 17), but plain ones also work well. Devil's claw may cause stomach upset and vomiting, especially in children.

DOSAGE •**Capsules or tablets** (for arthritis, back pain, and gout): 300–400 mg, 3 times daily, of devil's claw standardized to 2–3 percent iridoid glycosides or 1–2 percent harpagoside. •**Tea:** Steep 1 teaspoon of the herb in 1½ cups of boiling water and let stand overnight. Drink up to 3 cups daily for indigestion.

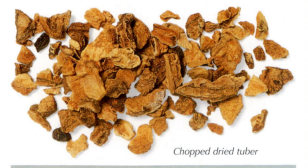

Chopped dried tuber

Humulus lupulus
HOPS

WHY IT'S USED Hops are used to treat anxiety, insomnia, and minor digestive problems.

HOW IT WORKS Researchers believe that the mild sedating effect of hops derives from a substance known as methybutenol. The bitter taste of hops stimulates the flow of saliva and digestive juices.

COMMENTS AND CAUTIONS It is the bitterness of the hops that gives beer its flavor. This herb has a sedative effect; take appropriate precautions. Do not take it in combination with alcohol or other sedative herbs, supplements, or medications. For indigestion, take hops before meals and for insomnia, one hour before bedtime. Fresh hops may cause excessive drowsiness.

DOSAGE •Capsules: 500 mg 1 to 3 times daily. **•Tea:** Steep 1–2 teaspoons of dried hops in 1 cup of boiling water for 5 minutes. Sweeten lightly if needed; drink up to 3 cups daily. **•Tincture:** ½–1 teaspoon 1 to 3 times daily or as directed on the package.

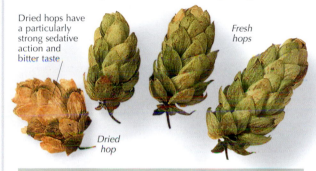

Dried hops have a particularly strong sedative action and bitter taste

Fresh hops

Dried hop

Hydrastis canadensis
GOLDENSEAL

WHY IT'S USED Goldenseal is used to treat slow-healing wounds, fungal infections, sore throat, bladder infections, bronchitis, Crohn's disease, gastritis, and diarrhea.

HOW IT WORKS The key ingredients in goldenseal are berberine and hydrastine, which have an antibiotic effect.

COMMENTS AND CAUTIONS Do not use goldenseal for more than two weeks. Pregnant women should not use goldenseal since it can cause uterine contractions.

DOSAGE •Ointment, cream, or powder: Apply a small amount of a product containing at least 10 percent alkaloids to wounds or fungal infections. **•Capsules:** 250–500 mg, 3 times daily, of a product standardized to contain 10 percent alkaloids, for bronchitis or digestive problems. **•Tea:** Steep ½ teaspoon of goldenseal root in 1 cup of boiling water for 10 minutes; drink up to two cups daily for bronchitis or digestive problems. Use cooled tea as a gargle to treat a sore throat.

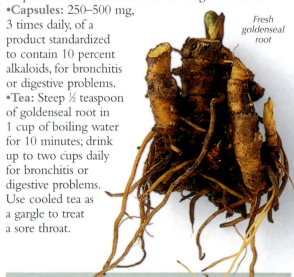

Fresh goldenseal root

Hypericum perforatum
ST. JOHN'S WORT

WHY IT'S USED St. John's wort is used to treat mild to moderate depression, seasonal affective disorder (SAD), anxiety, and insomnia.

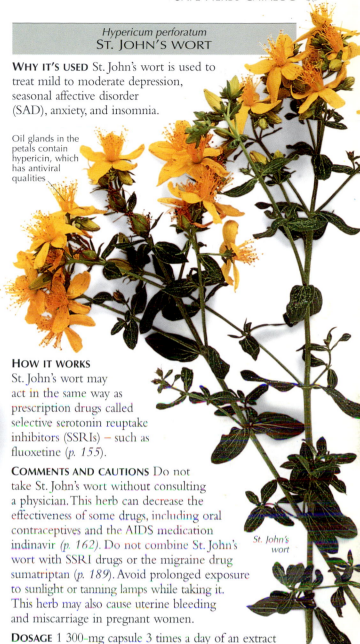

Oil glands in the petals contain hypericin, which has antiviral qualities

HOW IT WORKS St. John's wort may act in the same way as prescription drugs called selective serotonin reuptake inhibitors (SSRIs) – such as fluoxetine (p. 155).

COMMENTS AND CAUTIONS Do not take St. John's wort without consulting a physician. This herb can decrease the effectiveness of some drugs, including oral contraceptives and the AIDS medication indinavir (p. 162). Do not combine St. John's wort with SSRI drugs or the migraine drug sumatriptan (p. 189). Avoid prolonged exposure to sunlight or tanning lamps while taking it. This herb may also cause uterine bleeding and miscarriage in pregnant women.

St. John's wort

DOSAGE 1 300-mg capsule 3 times a day of an extract standardized to contain 0.3 percent hypericin and 4 percent hyperforin, or as recommended by a physician.

Ilex paraguariensis
MATÉ

WHY IT'S USED Maté, native to South America, is a mild stimulant used to relieve headaches caused by fatigue.

HOW IT WORKS Maté is high in caffeine, a stimulant.

COMMENTS AND CAUTIONS Maté is a popular beverage in South America. Pregnant and nursing women and children especially should avoid maté because of its caffeine content.

DOSAGE •Tea: Steep 1 teaspoon of dried leaves in cup of boiling water for 5 minutes. Drink up to 2 cups daily. **•Liquid extract:** ½ teaspoon 1 to 2 times daily or as directed on the package. **•Tincture:** 2 teaspoons 1 to 2 times daily or as directed on the package.

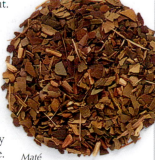

Maté

Juglans regia
WALNUT LEAF

WHY IT'S USED Walnut leaf is used to treat minor burns and sunburn.

HOW IT WORKS Walnut leaf is high in astringent substances called tannins, which soothe the skin and decrease irritation.

COMMENTS AND CAUTIONS When using walnut leaf, begin with small doses and increase gradually as needed. It may cause skin irritation in children.

DOSAGE •**Decoction:** Combine ½ cup of dried walnut leaf with ½ cup of cold water. Bring to a boil and simmer for 15 minutes; allow to cool. Add to bathwater or apply to the affected area for 15 minutes with a clean cloth.

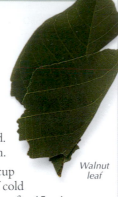

Walnut leaf

Larix spp.
LARCH

WHY IT'S USED Larch bark is used to treat colds, flu, coughs, ear infections, and sore throat.

HOW IT WORKS Larch contains large amounts of arabinogalactan, a complex sugar that stimulates the immune system.

COMMENTS AND CAUTIONS Do not use larch if you have liver or kidney disease; arabinogalactan can accumulate in the liver and damage the kidneys. Larch works best for colds and flu if you begin taking it as soon as the symptoms appear. Do not inhale larch powder; it can cause inflammation of the airway.

DOSAGE Mix 1–3 teaspoons of larch powder in 8 ounces of juice or water. Take 2 to 3 times daily.

European larch

Lavendula angustifolia
LAVENDER

WHY IT'S USED Lavender is used to help treat mild anxiety and insomnia, soothe sore muscles, bruises, mild burns, and eczema, and treat minor digestive problems.

HOW IT WORKS Lavender contains a complex oil that has a mild sedative effect and stimulates the flow of digestive juices.

COMMENTS AND CAUTIONS Lavender oil may irritate broken skin, and can cause skin irritation in children. Do not use undiluted oil internally; it can cause severe gastrointestinal distress and may cause uterine bleeding in pregnant women.

DOSAGE •**Tea:** Steep 2 teaspoons of dried lavender flowers in 1 cup of boiling water for 5 minutes, or add 1 drop of oil to 1 cup of hot water. Drink up to 3 cups daily to treat anxiety or digestive problems; drink 1 cup 1 hour before bedtime for insomnia. •**Oil:** Rub 1 drop of lavender oil onto sore muscles, bruises, burns, and eczema up to 3 times daily. Add several drops of oil to warm bathwater to reduce anxiety and soothe sore muscles.

Lentinus edodes
SHIITAKE MUSHROOM

WHY IT'S USED Shiitake is a Japanese medicinal mushroom that is used to treat hepatitis and to stimulate the immune systems of AIDS patients and those undergoing chemotherapy for cancer.

HOW IT WORKS Shiitake contains a complex sugar called lentinan that appears to stimulate immune activity in your body.

COMMENTS AND CAUTIONS Shiitake mushrooms are edible and taste delicious. They are widely used in Japanese and Chinese cuisine and are now cultivated in the US. For medicinal purposes, lentinan extract is more effective than mushrooms.

DOSAGE •**Capsules or tablets:** 1,000–3,000 mg 3 times daily of an extract standardized to contain 3.2 percent KS-2 polysaccharides, or as directed by your physician. •**Tincture:** ½ teaspoon 2 times daily or as directed on the package.

COOKING CURE *Cooked shiitake mushrooms can be used to help stimulate the immune system and combat colds and flu and other infections.*

The flowers contain a volatile oil that has antiseptic and antibacterial qualities

Lavender is grown for use as a perfume and for medicinal purposes

Dried lavender is valued for its soothing effects

40

Leonurus cardiaca
MOTHERWORT

WHY IT'S USED Motherwort is used to treat heart problems caused by anxiety and stress, especially irregular or rapid heartbeat, and to relieve menstrual discomfort and cramps. It is sometimes used in conjunction with medication to treat hyperthyroidism (overactive thyroid gland).

HOW IT WORKS Motherwort contains a number of alkaloids that appear to benefit the heart and uterus.

COMMENTS AND CAUTIONS Do not use motherwort to treat heart conditions without the supervision of your physician. It should not be used by children or those with a history of breast cancer, and may cause uterine bleeding and contractions in pregnant women.

Motherwort

DOSAGE •Capsules: 1,500 mg twice daily, or as directed by your physician. **•Tea:** Steep 2 teaspoons of dried herb in 1 cup of boiling water for 5 minutes. Drink up to 2 cups daily. **•Liquid extract or tincture:** Follow the directions on the package.

Ligusticum porteri
OSHA

WHY IT'S USED Osha is used to treat coughs and sore throats related to colds and flu, minor digestive problems such as loss of appetite, stomach cramps, and gas, and viral infections such as colds, herpes, and AIDS.

HOW IT WORKS Osha root contains a variety of substances that are antibiotic and antiviral, and that help relieve coughs, relax the intestinal tract, and stimulate the flow of digestive juices.

COMMENTS AND CAUTIONS Osha is also known as bear root, Colorado cough root, and mountain lovage. Osha leaves look similar to poison hemlock, an extremely toxic plant. Buy osha from a reliable source. Osha may cause uterine bleeding and miscarriage in pregnant women.

DOSAGE •Tincture: Follow package directions.

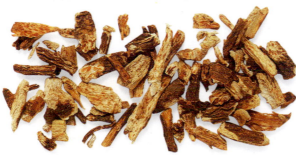

Dried osha root

Ligustrum lucidum
LIGUSTRUM

WHY IT'S USED Ligustrum berries are used to improve immunity and treat infections.

HOW IT WORKS Ligustrum berries contain ligustrin, also known as oleanolic acid, which appears to stimulate the immune system.

COMMENTS AND CAUTIONS Ligustrum is also known as glossy privet. Do not confuse it with other members of the *Ligustrum* family.

DOSAGE •Capsules: 2,500 mg of encapsulated berries once or twice daily. **•Tea:** Steep 1 teaspoon of crushed berries in 1 cup of boiling water for 10 minutes. Drink up to 3 cups daily. **•Tincture:** ½ teaspoon 3 times daily or as directed on the package.

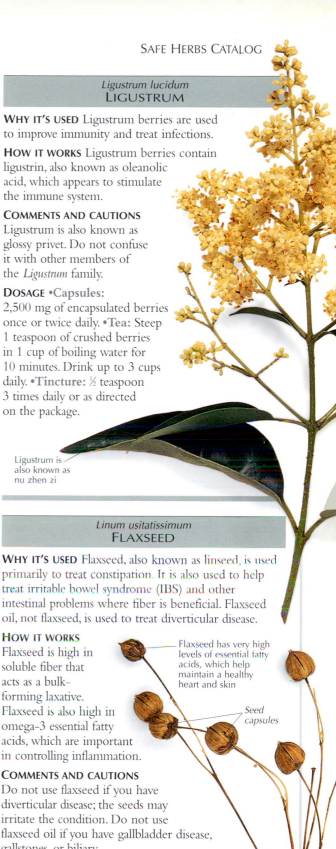

Ligustrum is also known as nu zhen zi

Linum usitatissimum
FLAXSEED

WHY IT'S USED Flaxseed, also known as linseed, is used primarily to treat constipation. It is also used to help treat irritable bowel syndrome (IBS) and other intestinal problems where fiber is beneficial. Flaxseed oil, not flaxseed, is used to treat diverticular disease.

HOW IT WORKS Flaxseed is high in soluble fiber that acts as a bulk-forming laxative. Flaxseed is also high in omega-3 essential fatty acids, which are important in controlling inflammation.

Flaxseed has very high levels of essential fatty acids, which help maintain a healthy heart and skin

Seed capsules

COMMENTS AND CAUTIONS Do not use flaxseed if you have diverticular disease; the seeds may irritate the condition. Do not use flaxseed oil if you have gallbladder disease, gallstones, or biliary duct disease. Do not confuse flaxseed oil with linseed oil, a toxic wood preservative. Do not use during pregnancy unless your physician advises it.

Seeds must be split or ground up before being swallowed

DOSAGE •Seed: Run 1 tablespoon of flaxseed through a coffee grinder; add to ½ cup of water and drink. Repeat up to 3 times daily. **•Oil:** ½–1 tablespoon per day.

Marrubium vulgare
HOREHOUND

WHY IT'S USED Horehound is used to treat minor digestive problems such as loss of appetite, bloating, and gas.

HOW IT WORKS Horehound contains a bitter substance called marrubiin, which stimulates the flow of digestive juices.

COMMENTS AND CAUTIONS Do not use horehound if you have ulcers or gastritis – bitter compounds in the plant could worsen your symptoms. This herb may cause miscarriage in pregnant women.

DOSAGE •**Tea:** Steep ½ teaspoon of dried leaves in 1 cup of boiling water for 10 minutes. Sweeten if needed; drink up to 3 cups daily. •**Tincture:** ¼ teaspoon up to 3 times daily or as directed on the package.

MEDICINAL ACTION
Horehound is a soothing tonic for the body's mucous membranes – particularly beneficial for people who have bronchitis or whooping cough.

Medicago sativa
ALFALFA

WHY IT'S USED Research suggests that alfalfa may lower cholesterol and improve the symptoms of mild cases of Type 2 diabetes. It may be beneficial in treating menopausal symptoms, but more research is needed in this area.

HOW IT WORKS Soapy substances in alfalfa, called saponins, may reduce cholesterol and symptoms of mild Type 2 diabetes. Alfalfa also contains genistein and daidzein, which may act like a mild form of estrogen.

COMMENTS AND CAUTIONS Alfalfa contains L-canavine, which may aggravate or cause symptoms similar to the disease systemic lupus erythematosus (SLE). If you have SLE, do not use alfalfa. Many cases of food poisoning have been traced to fresh alfalfa sprouts. Those with diabetes or an autoimmune disease should not be given alfalfa.

DOSAGE 500–1,000 mg alfalfa tablets daily or up to 1 cup of fresh alfalfa sprouts daily.

The aerial parts, and also the sprouting seeds, are used medicinally and as a food

TEMPERATE GROWER
Also known as lucerne, alfalfa is native to Asia, Europe, and north Africa.

Melaleuca alternifolia
TEA TREE OIL

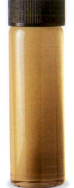
Tea tree oil

WHY IT'S USED Tea tree oil is used to treat skin conditions, including cuts and scrapes, insect stings, fungal infections such as athlete's foot, and acne blemishes.

HOW IT WORKS The leaves of the tea tree contain a complex oil that is an excellent antiseptic.

COMMENTS AND CAUTIONS This oil is used as an antiseptic ingredient in a wide variety of commercial products. Tea tree oil should not be used internally, or applied to the skin in undiluted form. When using cream or ointment, test by applying a small amount to healthy skin to determine your sensitivity. Discontinue if any irritation occurs.

DOSAGE Apply a few drops of tea tree oil or a small amount of cream or ointment containing 5–10 percent tea tree oil directly to the affected area and rub it in. Repeat up to 4 times daily.

Melissa officinalis
LEMON BALM

WHY IT'S USED Lemon balm is used to prevent and reduce the severity of herpes outbreaks, to treat insomnia, and relieve anxiety and minor digestive problems.

HOW IT WORKS Lemon balm inhibits the herpes virus. The plant's oils have a slight sedative effect and relax the intestinal tract.

COMMENTS AND CAUTIONS Lemon balm is also known as melissa. Do not use it if you have glaucoma; the herb can increase pressure within the eye. Internal use may lead to altered hormone balance and uterine bleeding in pregnant women.

DOSAGE •**Cream or ointment:** At the first sign of a herpes outbreak, apply a thick layer of a product standardized to 70:1, 4 times daily. For prevention, apply twice daily. •**Tea:** Steep 1 teaspoon of dried herb in 1 cup of boiling water for 5 minutes. Drink 1 cup 3 times daily before meals for anxiety or digestive problems; drink 1 cup 1 hour before bedtime for insomnia. •**Liquid extract:** As directed on the package.

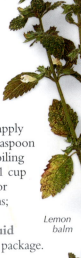
Lemon balm

Mentha arvensis
MINT OIL

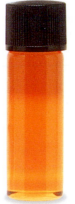

Mint essential oil

WHY IT'S USED Mint oil is used to treat minor digestive problems, irritable bowel syndrome (IBS), colds and flu, sore muscles, and aching joints.

HOW IT WORKS Mint oil, which contains menthol, relaxes the intestinal tract, dries mucous membranes, and has a cooling effect in your body.

COMMENTS AND CAUTIONS To treat IBS with mint oil, consult your physician. Do not use internally if you have reflux disease, gallstones, or gallbladder or liver disease. Do not use on broken skin or mucous membranes. Mint oil may cause choking and skin irritation in children.

DOSAGE •Oil: Add 3–4 drops of mint oil to hot water or a vaporizer; inhale the steam up to 4 times daily to treat colds and flu. Add 1–2 drops of oil to ½ cup of hot water; drink up to 2 cups daily for digestive problems. Rub 2–4 drops onto the area up to 3 times daily for painful muscles or joints. **•Ointment or cream:** Rub a small amount of a product containing 5–20 percent mint oil onto painful muscles and joints up to 4 times daily.

Mentha piperita
PEPPERMINT LEAF

WHY IT'S USED Peppermint is used to treat digestive problems such as loss of appetite, nausea, stomach cramps, bloating, gas, and irritable bowel syndrome (IBS).

HOW IT WORKS Peppermint leaves contain an oil that is high in menthol, which has a relaxing effect on the body's digestive tract.

COMMENTS AND CAUTIONS Do not use peppermint if you have frequent heartburn, acid reflux, ulcers, gallstones, or gallbladder disease, liver disease, or biliary duct disease. To treat IBS with peppermint oil, consult your physician. Do not give peppermint oil to children. Enteric-coated capsules (which remain intact until they pass through the stomach) containing peppermint oil may cause a sensation of rectal burning.

DOSAGE •Enteric-coated capsules: 1 0.2-ml capsule 2 to 3 times daily. **•Tea:** Steep 1 teaspoon of dried leaves in 1 cup of boiling water for 10 minutes. Drink up to 3 cups daily. **•Liquid extract or tincture:** ½ teaspoon 2 to 3 times daily or as directed on the package.

Fresh aerial parts are dried and distilled to extract the volatile oil

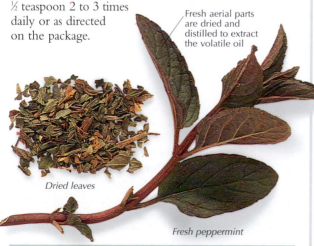

Dried leaves

Fresh peppermint

Momordica charantia
BITTER MELON

WHY IT'S USED In traditional Indian medicine and modern Western medicine, bitter melon is used to treat mild cases of Type 2 diabetes. Bitter melon is also used to provide immune system support for HIV patients.

HOW IT WORKS Bitter melon appears to stimulate the pancreas to release insulin. How bitter melon helps the immune system is not fully understood.

COMMENTS AND CAUTIONS Because it is used to treat chronic health conditions that require regular monitoring, bitter melon should be used under your physician's supervision.

DOSAGE Consult your physician for individual dosage recommendations.

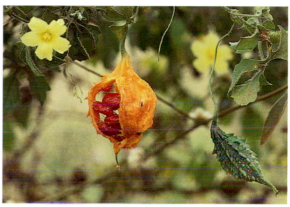

TROPICAL PICKINGS
The orange-yellow fruit, red seeds, and deeply lobed leaves of the bitter melon climbing plant can all be used in medicinal preparations.

Nepeta cataria
CATNIP

WHY IT'S USED Catnip is a mild sedative used to relieve anxiety and insomnia, minor digestive problems, and mild menstrual discomfort. It can be used to treat coughs under a physician's supervision.

HOW IT WORKS Nepetalactone, an active ingredient in catnip, has a sedative effect.

COMMENTS AND CAUTIONS This herb has a sedative effect; take appropriate precautions. Do not combine it with alcohol, supplements, medications, or other sedative herbs. Catnip may cause miscarriage in pregnant women.

DOSAGE •Tea: Steep 1–2 teaspoons of dried catnip in 1 cup of boiling water for 5 minutes. Drink up to 3 cups daily. **•Tincture:** 1 teaspoon up to 3 times daily or see package directions.

Aromatic herb has gray-green leaves and white and purple flowers

Rubus fruticosus, R. villosus
BLACKBERRY LEAF

WHY IT'S USED Blackberry leaf is used to treat mild diarrhea, sore throat, mouth sores, minor cuts and scrapes, and hemorrhoids.

HOW IT WORKS Astringent substances, called tannins, in blackberry leaves have a variety of therapeutic benefits.

COMMENTS AND CAUTIONS Drinking large amounts of blackberry leaf tea can cause nausea.

DOSAGE •Tea: Steep 1 tablespoon of dried leaves in 1 cup of boiling water for 15 minutes. Drink up to 1 cup daily to treat diarrhea. **•Tincture:** 1 teaspoon 2 to 3 times daily or as directed on the package. Use the cooled tea or tincture as a gargle for sore throat and mouth sores. For cuts, scrapes, and hemorrhoids, soak a clean cloth in the tea or tincture and apply externally.

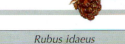

The berries can be prepared as a gargle for a sore throat

Rubus idaeus
RASPBERRY LEAF

WHY IT'S USED Raspberry leaf is used to treat diarrhea, sore throat, and mouth irritation.

HOW IT WORKS The leaves contain astringent substances called tannins that soothe mucous membranes, have a mild antimicrobial action, and reduce intestinal inflammation.

COMMENTS AND CAUTIONS If you are pregnant, drink raspberry leaf tea under the advice of a physician. Do not confuse raspberry leaf tea with raspberry-flavored black tea. This herb may cause diarrhea in children.

DOSAGE •Tea: Steep 1–2 teaspoons of dried raspberry leaves in 1 cup of boiling water for 10 minutes. Drink up to 3 cups daily for diarrhea. Use cooled tea as a gargle for sore throat and mouth irritation.
•Tincture: 1 teaspoon 3 times daily or as directed on the package.

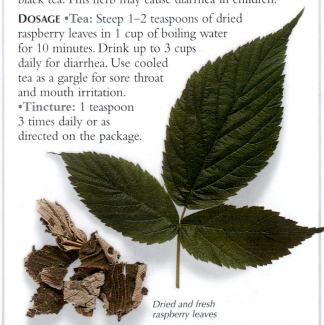

Dried and fresh raspberry leaves

Rumex crispus
YELLOW DOCK ROOT

WHY IT'S USED Yellow dock root is used to relieve constipation. It is sometimes used to treat chest congestion and hemorrhoids, but there is little scientific evidence to support these uses.

HOW IT WORKS Yellow dock is high in anthroquinones, which have a laxative effect.

COMMENTS AND CAUTIONS Yellow dock is a common ingredient in herbal laxative mixtures. Yellow dock contains oxalates; do not use it if you have a history of kidney stones. It may also cause diarrhea, especially in children.

DOSAGE •Capsules: 500–1,000 mg dried root 3 times daily. **•Tea:** Steep 1 teaspoon of ground root in 1 cup of boiling water for 10 minutes. Drink up to 3 cups daily. **•Liquid extract:** 1 teaspoon 3 times daily or as directed on the package. **•Tincture:** ¼ teaspoon 3 times daily or as directed on the package.

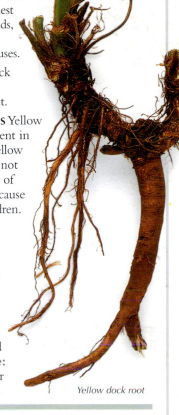

Yellow dock root

Ruscus aculeatus
BUTCHER'S BROOM

WHY IT'S USED Butcher's broom is used to treat hemorrhoids and varicose veins, and to nourish and strengthen the circulatory system.

HOW IT WORKS Soapy substances called saponins in butcher's broom have an anti-inflammatory action and constrict small veins.

COMMENTS AND CAUTIONS Butcher's broom is a diuretic and may cause dehydration.

DOSAGE •Capsules: Enough standardized capsules to provide 25–50 mg ruscogenins, taken twice a day. **•Suppositories or ointments:** For hemorrhoids, use suppositories and ointments standardized to 10 percent saponin glycosides (ruscogenins) as directed on the package.

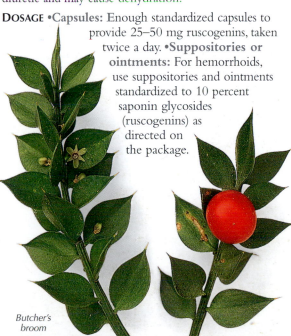

Butcher's broom

Salix spp.
WILLOW BARK

WHY IT'S USED Willow bark is used to treat headaches, symptoms of arthritis, and fever from colds and flu.

HOW IT WORKS Salicin, an anti-inflammatory substance in willow bark, reduces fever and relieves pain.

COMMENTS AND CAUTIONS Do not use if you are allergic to salicylates or aspirin. Prolonged or excessive use can lead to ulcers, bleeding, and bruising. Take as a tea for best results; the body absorbs less salicin from capsules. Children and teenagers should not use willow bark because of the risk of Reye syndrome.

DOSAGE •Tea: Steep ½ teaspoon of powdered bark in 1 cup of boiling water for 5 minutes; sweeten and drink up to 3 cups daily. **•Capsules:** 1–2 500-mg capsules standardized to at least 7 percent salicin, up to 3 times daily. **•Tincture or liquid extract:** ¼ teaspoon up to 3 times daily or as directed on the package.

Deeply fissured willow bark has anti-inflammatory properties

Salvia officinalis
SAGE

Leaves have antiseptic and astringent properties

WHY IT'S USED Sage is used to treat minor digestive disorders and relieve mouth irritation and sore throat.

HOW IT WORKS Sage contains thujone, which stimulates the flow of digestive juices and has a relaxing effect on the intestinal tract. It is also high in substances called tannins, which soothe the mucous membranes.

COMMENTS AND CAUTIONS Sage is safe in dietary amounts for pregnant women, but large doses could cause uterine contractions. Do not give sage to children with fevers.

Purple sage

Sage's scientific name, *salvia*, means "to cure" in Latin

DOSAGE •Capsules: 1,000–3,000 mg dried sage leaf 3 times daily before meals for digestive problems. **•Tea:** Steep 2 teaspoons of dried sage leaf in 1 cup of boiling water for 10 minutes. Drink up to 3 cups daily before meals for indigestion. Use cooled tea as a mouthwash or gargle. **•Tincture or liquid extract:** ½ teaspoon 3 times daily before meals for digestive problems; mix with 8 ounces of warm water for a mouth rinse or gargle to relieve sore throat or mouth irritation.

Sambucus nigra
ELDERBERRY

WHY IT'S USED Elderberries are used to prevent and shorten the duration of colds, flu, and respiratory illnesses. Elderberry is also used to treat mild tonsillitis and inflammation.

HOW IT WORKS Elderberries are very high in vitamin C, which may explain why they help ward off colds.

COMMENTS AND CAUTIONS Elderberries are used to flavor liqueurs such as Sambucca. Dried elder tree bark is a very powerful laxative and should not be used.

DOSAGE •Tea: Steep 3 teaspoons of dried elderberries in 1 cup of boiling water for 10 minutes. Drink 1 to 2 cups of very hot tea up to 3 times daily, preferably in the afternoon and evening.
•Liquid extract: 2 teaspoons twice daily or as directed on the package.
•Tincture: ½ teaspoon 2 to 3 times daily or as directed on the package.

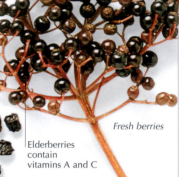

Fresh berries

Elderberries contain vitamins A and C

Dried berries

Sambucus nigra
ELDERBERRY FLOWER

WHY IT'S USED Elderberry flowers, also known as elder flowers, are used to prevent and treat colds, flu, fever, and bronchitis. They are also used to treat coughs and fever related to colds, bronchitis, and flu. In addition, elderberry flowers may be helpful for treating viral infections, including herpes and HIV.

HOW IT WORKS How elderberry flower works is not yet fully understood.

COMMENTS AND CAUTIONS Elderberry flowers promote the sweating that can reduce the symptoms of a fever.

DOSAGE •Tea: Steep 1 teaspoon of dried elderberry flowers in 1 cup of boiling water for 10 minutes. Drink 1 to 2 cups of very hot infusion up to 3 times daily, preferably in the afternoon and evening.
•Tincture: ¼–½ teaspoon 2 to 3 times daily or as directed on the package.

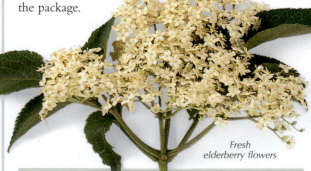

Fresh elderberry flowers

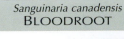
Sanguinaria canadensis
BLOODROOT

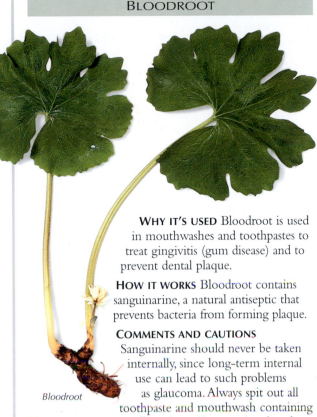

WHY IT'S USED Bloodroot is used in mouthwashes and toothpastes to treat gingivitis (gum disease) and to prevent dental plaque.

HOW IT WORKS Bloodroot contains sanguinarine, a natural antiseptic that prevents bacteria from forming plaque.

COMMENTS AND CAUTIONS Sanguinarine should never be taken internally, since long-term internal use can lead to such problems as glaucoma. Always spit out all toothpaste and mouthwash containing bloodroot; do not swallow them. Do not give dental products containing bloodroot to children; they may accidentally swallow them. Do not use bloodroot if you are pregnant or nursing.

DOSAGE Bloodroot can be found in a number of commercial toothpastes and mouthwashes. Use as directed on the label.

Bloodroot

Schisandra chinensis
SCHISANDRA

WHY IT'S USED Schisandra is used to treat liver problems, especially hepatitis. It is sometimes used to increase stamina and concentration, although there is little scientific research that supports this purpose.

HOW IT WORKS Researchers don't know how it works.

COMMENTS AND CAUTIONS Schisandra, a woody vine found in eastern Asia, is also known by its Chinese name, wu wei zi. Schisandra may cause skin rash and stomach upset, especially in children.

DOSAGE •Capsules and tablets: 700–3,000 mg twice daily. **•Tincture:** ½–1 teaspoon up to 3 times daily or as directed on the package.

Schisandra is one of China's most important tonic herbs

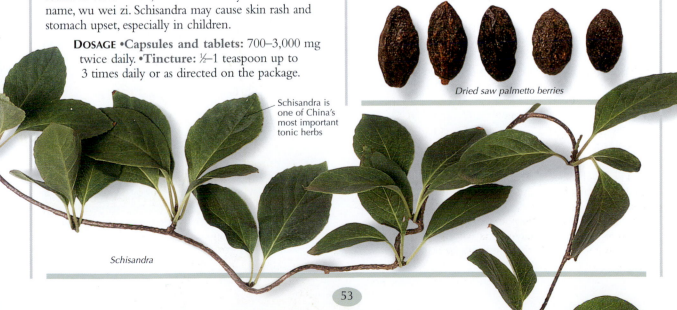

Schisandra

Senna alexandrina
SENNA

WHY IT'S USED Senna is used to treat constipation.

HOW IT WORKS Senna pods and leaves contain anthroquinones, which have a strong laxative effect.

COMMENTS AND CAUTIONS Senna is a powerful laxative that should be used for no more than seven days in a row except under a physician's supervision. It can cause severe abdominal cramps. Do not use senna if you have intestinal problems such as ulcers, irritable bowel syndrome (IBS), Crohn's disease, or ulcerative colitis. Do not use senna if you are pregnant or nursing. Do not give senna to children.

DOSAGE •Tea: Steep 1 teaspoon of dried senna leaves or 4 dried senna pods in 1 cup of boiling water for 10 minutes. Sweeten slightly; drink up to 1 cup daily first thing in the morning (for evening results) or at bedtime (for morning results).

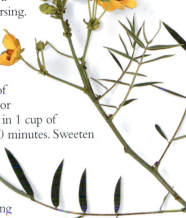

Senna

Serenoa repens
SAW PALMETTO

WHY IT'S USED Saw palmetto is used to treat urinary problems, such as frequent urination, nighttime urination, and difficulty urinating, caused by an enlarged prostate gland (also called benign prostatic hypertrophy, BPH).

HOW IT WORKS Substances contained in saw palmetto berries inhibit enzymes that contribute to BPH.

COMMENTS AND CAUTIONS The berries are the fruit of a palm tree found in the southeastern US. To diagnose or treat BPH, consult your physician. Saw palmetto relieves symptoms, but does not reduce prostate size. Saw palmetto may cause hormonal imbalance in children.

DOSAGE 160 mg 2 times daily of a product standardized to contain 85–95 percent fatty acids and sterols.

Dried saw palmetto berries

Silybum marianum
MILK THISTLE

WHY IT'S USED Milk thistle is used to treat liver problems such as hepatitis, jaundice, cirrhosis, and damage from exposure to toxins. Milk thistle may also be helpful for treating psoriasis and gallstones under a physician's supervision.

HOW IT WORKS Silymarin, a complex mixture of substances in milk thistle fruit, appears to improve bile flow, protect liver cells, and stimulate their regeneration.

COMMENTS AND CAUTIONS Studies of milk thistle show that it is very effective for treating liver disease. It may cause uterine bleeding in pregnant women.

DOSAGE 1 250-mg capsule, standardized to contain 70–80 percent silymarin, 2 times daily, or 10–15 grams of ground seeds, as directed by your physician.

Milk thistle

MILK THISTLE SEEDS
Since the seeds contain silymarin, they are the main part used, but the flower heads are used in remedies and can be eaten.

Smilax sarsaparilla
SARSAPARILLA

WHY IT'S USED Long used as a "blood purifier," sarsaparilla is used to treat psoriasis, eczema, arthritis, and irritable bowel syndrome (IBS).

HOW IT WORKS Sarsaparilla seems to improve digestion by reducing intestinal toxins. It also contains phytosterols, substances that help control inflammation in the body.

COMMENTS AND CAUTIONS Do not use sarsaparilla if you have gastritis, ulcers, or kidney disease. Do not combine it with digoxin *(p. 147),* or with pink bismuth *(p. 131);* a dangerous interaction may occur. Sarsaparilla may cause miscarriage in pregnant women, and irritate the skin, kidneys, and gastrointestinal tract.

DOSAGE •**Capsule:** 250–500 mg 2 to 3 times daily. •**Tincture:** ½ teaspoon 3 times daily or as directed on the package.

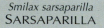

Sarsaparilla root was the original flavoring for root beer

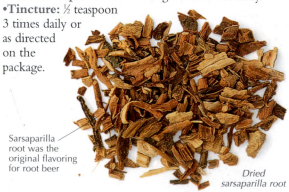

Dried sarsaparilla root

Solidago spp.
GOLDENROD

WHY IT'S USED Goldenrod is used as a diuretic and to treat mild bladder infections and kidney stones.

HOW IT WORKS Goldenrod appears to soothe and relax the urinary tract. Its active ingredients are still unknown.

COMMENTS AND CAUTIONS When taking goldenrod, drink plenty of water to flush bacteria from your urinary tract. Diuretics such as goldenrod can deplete your potassium; be sure to consume potassium-rich foods such as orange juice or bananas when using this herb. It may also cause dehydration, especially in children.

DOSAGE •**Capsules:** 2,000–3,000 mg 2 to 3 times daily. •**Tea:** Steep 1 teaspoon of dried herb in 1 cup of boiling water for 10 to 15 minutes; drink up to 2 cups daily between meals.

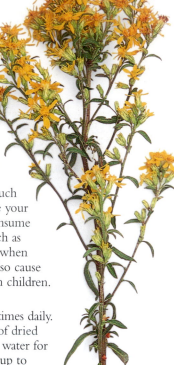

Goldenrod

Spilanthes oleracea
SPILANTHES

WHY IT'S USED Spilanthes is used to treat minor digestive problems such as loss of appetite, mild nausea, bloating, and gas.

HOW IT WORKS Unknown substances in spilanthes stimulate the flow of saliva and digestive juices.

COMMENTS AND CAUTIONS Spilanthes is a weedy plant native to South America.

DOSAGE •**Tincture:** ¼–½ teaspoon 3 times daily or as directed on the package.

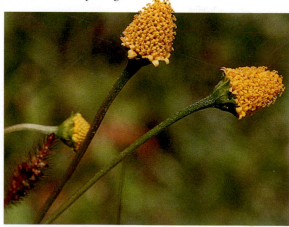

SOUTH AMERICAN NATIVE
This weedlike plant has a strong folk medicine following, but additional research is needed to understand how it works.

Stevia rebaudiana
STEVIA

WHY IT'S USED Stevia is used as a calorie-free sweetener. It is sometimes recommended to treat high blood pressure and high blood glucose levels, but more research is needed in this area.

HOW IT WORKS The active ingredient in stevia is stevioside, a substance that is 100 to 200 times sweeter than sugar but contains no calories.

COMMENTS AND CAUTIONS Stevia is native to Paraguay. Its faintly bitter taste is not noticeable when it is added to food or drink. Stevia may cause reduced blood pressure; use only under a physician's supervision.

Stevia

DOSAGE Use small amounts to sweeten foods or beverages. Take no more than 1,000 mg daily.

Syzygium aromaticum
CLOVE

WHY IT'S USED Clove is used to relieve minor digestive problems and to treat bad breath, gingivitis (gum disease), and mouth pain.

HOW IT WORKS The oil in cloves is antibacterial and may have a relaxing effect on the muscles of the intestinal tract. It is a soothing oral analgesic.

COMMENTS AND CAUTIONS Do not use clove medicinally during pregnancy. Clove may cause skin and mouth irritation in children.

DOSAGE Steep 1 teaspoon of crushed cloves in 1 cup of boiling water for 15 minutes. Drink up to 3 cups daily. Use cooled tea as a mouthwash.

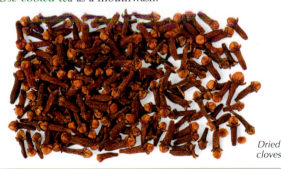

Dried cloves

Syzygium aromaticum
CLOVE OIL

WHY IT'S USED Clove oil is used as an oral antiseptic and to relieve toothache pain.

HOW IT WORKS Clove oil has a numbing effect when applied directly to the painful area.

COMMENTS AND CAUTIONS Clove oil can cause irritation, especially in children; use only occasionally. Do not use medicinally during pregnancy. Clove oil is the active ingredient in nonprescription toothache remedies.

DOSAGE Using a cotton swab, apply a small amount of clove oil to the painful tooth and surrounding area. Repeat as needed for up to 24 hours.

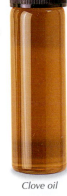

Clove oil

Tabebuia avellanedae, T. impetiginosa
LAPACHO

WHY IT'S USED Lapacho is used to treat mild yeast infections, colds and flu, diarrhea, and bladder infections.

HOW IT WORKS Lapacho bark contains a number of bitter compounds, including one called lapachol that has antibiotic properties.

COMMENTS AND CAUTIONS Lapacho is also known as taheebo and pau d'arco. To ensure a high-quality product, buy from a reputable manufacturer and look for the active ingredient lapachol. There are about 100 *Tabebuia* species, but only the bark of *T. avellanedae*, also known as *T. impetiginosa*, should be used.

DOSAGE
•**Capsules:** 300 mg 3 times daily. •**Tea:** Steep 1 teaspoon of lapacho in 1 cup of boiling water for 10 minutes. Drink up to 2 cups daily.

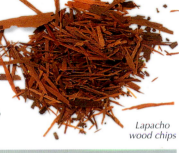

Lapacho wood chips

Tanacetum parthenium
FEVERFEW

WHY IT'S USED Feverfew is used primarily to help prevent migraine headaches.

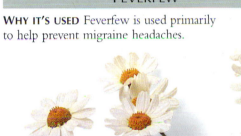

The daisylike flowers bloom throughout the summer

HOW IT WORKS The active ingredient in feverfew is thought to be located in the leaves.

COMMENTS AND CAUTIONS Feverfew works best as a daily preventive measure against migraines. If you take medication for frequent migraines, discuss feverfew with a physician first. Do not take it if you are pregnant; it may cause miscarriage. It can also cause gastrointestinal irritation in children. Do not combine feverfew with blood-thinning drugs such as warfarin (p. 195).

DOSAGE 80–100 mg powdered whole leaves in capsule form.

The leaves contain parthenolide, a substance that helps prevent migraine

Taraxacum officinale
DANDELION

WHY IT'S USED Dandelion root is used to treat minor digestive problems and to support the digestive and metabolic functions of the liver. Dandelion leaf is used as a diuretic and to treat edema (fluid retention).

HOW IT WORKS Dandelion contains substances that stimulate the flow of digestive juices. Because dandelion leaf is high in potassium, it is a useful diuretic – it replaces some of the potassium lost by increased urination.

COMMENTS AND CAUTIONS If you have ulcers, gastritis, gallstones, gallbladder disease, or biliary duct disease, use dandelion only under a physician's supervision. Dandelion may cause dehydration in children.

DOSAGE •Tea: Steep 1–2 teaspoons of dried leaves in 1 cup of boiling water for 10 minutes; drink up to 1 cup before mealtimes. Steep ½ teaspoon of dried root in 1 cup of boiling water for 10 minutes; drink up to 1 cup before mealtimes. **•Liquid extract or tincture:** See package directions.

The leaves contain high levels of potassium, and can be eaten raw in salads

Thymus vulgaris
THYME

WHY IT'S USED Thyme is used to relieve coughs related to upper respiratory infections and minor digestive disorders.

HOW IT WORKS Substances in thyme leaves help relax the bronchial tubes and intestinal tract.

COMMENTS AND CAUTIONS Do not use thyme oil internally. Avoid toothpaste that contains thyme oil. Large amounts of thyme can cause uterine bleeding and miscarriage in pregnant women.

DOSAGE •Tea: Steep 1 teaspoon of dried leaves in 1 cup of boiling water for 10 minutes. Drink up to 3 cups daily. **•Liquid extract:** ½ teaspoon 1 to 3 times daily or as directed on the package. **•Tincture:** ½ teaspoon 1 to 3 times daily or as directed on the package.

The aromatic, slightly bitter tasting leaves are used to flavor savory dishes

Tilia cordata
LINDEN FLOWER

WHY IT'S USED Linden flower is used to treat colds, flu, and coughs, and promote the sweating that reduces fever.

HOW IT WORKS Compounds present in the flowers promote sweating in the body.

COMMENTS AND CAUTIONS The linden tree is also known as basswood or lime. Do not use linden flowers if you suffer from heart disease: overdoses may damage the heart. They may also have an antianxiety effect, although this has not been proven scientifically.

DOSAGE •Tea: Steep ½ teaspoon of dried flowers in 1 cup of boiling water for 15 minutes. Drink up to 2 cups daily. **•Liquid extract:** ¼ teaspoon up to 2 times daily or see package directions. **•Tincture:** ¼ teaspoon up to 2 times daily or as directed on the package.

The clusters of pale yellow flowers have winglike bracts

Linden flowers and leaves

Trifolium pratense
RED CLOVER

WHY IT'S USED Red clover is used to treat menopausal symptoms, particularly hot flashes. It may also help lower cholesterol levels in postmenopausal women. It is occasionally used to treat eczema and to treat cancer in conjunction with medication.

HOW IT WORKS Red clover contains substances that act as a mild form of estrogen.

COMMENTS AND CAUTIONS Do not use red clover if you are pregnant. Red clover may also cause liver damage in children. If you are on hormone replacement therapy (HRT) or using oral contraceptives, discuss red clover with your physician. Do not combine red clover with blood-thinning drugs such as warfarin (*p. 195*). The benefits of red clover may take up to six weeks to be felt.

DOSAGE •Capsules: 1,000 mg of dried red clover 2 to 3 times daily. **•Concentrated red clover extract:** 1 500-mg tablet daily of a product standardized to contain 40 mg isoflavones. **•Tincture:** ½ teaspoon 3 times a day or as directed on the package.

Red clover is widely grown as a nitrogen-fixing crop

Trigonella foenum-graecum
FENUGREEK SEED

WHY IT'S USED Fenugreek seed is used to treat the symptoms of mild cases of Type 2 diabetes and minor digestive problems such as loss of appetite and constipation.

Fenugreek seeds

WHY IT WORKS How fenugreek helps control symptoms of diabetes is still not fully known. Fenugreek stimulates the flow of saliva and digestive juices, which improves appetite. Fenugreek seeds are high in fiber, which helps relieve constipation.

COMMENTS AND CAUTIONS If you have diabetes, or a child with diabetes, use the seeds only under a physician's supervision; your blood sugar may drop lower than usual. Fenugreek seeds may cause uterine bleeding and miscarriage in pregnant women.

DOSAGE For diabetes, consult a physician about your individual dose. •**Tea:** For indigestion, steep 2 teaspoons of crushed seeds in 1 cup of boiling water for 10 minutes. Sweeten, or add lemon or peppermint, and drink up to 3 cups daily before meals. •**Tincture:** ¾ teaspoon up to 3 times a day or as directed on the package.

Tylophora asthmatica
TYLOPHORA

WHY IT'S USED In Ayurveda (traditional Indian medicine), tylophora is used to treat asthma and hay fever.

HOW IT WORKS Researchers believe that substances contained in the leaves of the tylophora plant are natural antihistamines.

COMMENTS AND CAUTIONS Tylophora is also known as Indian ipecac and Indian lobelia. In Ayurvedic medicine, tylophora is also used to induce vomiting and as an expectorant.

DOSAGE 40 mg powdered extract daily.

AYURVEDIC REMEDY
A twining perennial climber that grows wild on the plains of India, tylophora is valued for its lance-shaped leaves that have anti-inflammatory and antitumor properties.

Ulmus fulva
SLIPPERY ELM

WHY IT'S USED Slippery elm bark is used to relieve sore throat and coughs. It is also used to treat irritable bowel syndrome (IBS) and other intestinal problems.

HOW IT WORKS Slippery elm bark contains complex sugars that soothe mucous membranes such as those in the throat and digestive tract.

COMMENTS AND CAUTIONS The bark is an ingredient in several cough lozenges.

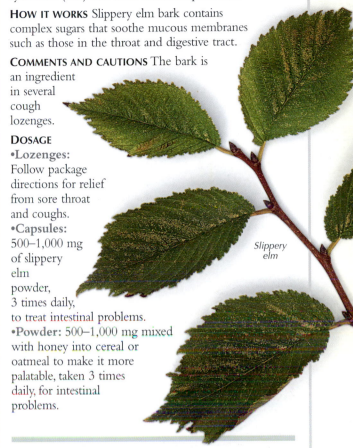

Slippery elm

DOSAGE
•**Lozenges:** Follow package directions for relief from sore throat and coughs.
•**Capsules:** 500–1,000 mg of slippery elm powder, 3 times daily, to treat intestinal problems.
•**Powder:** 500–1,000 mg mixed with honey into cereal or oatmeal to make it more palatable, taken 3 times daily, for intestinal problems.

Uncaria tomentosa
CAT'S CLAW

WHY IT'S USED The bark of cat's claw is traditionally used to relieve inflammation, fight viral illnesses such as herpes, and treat arthritis.

HOW IT WORKS Cat's claw contains complex substances that are not yet completely understood.

COMMENTS AND CAUTIONS Cat's claw is widely used in Europe and Peru, but has been studied less than other popular herbs. If you have an autoimmune illness such as lupus or HIV, discuss cat's claw with a physician before you try it.

DOSAGE Cat's claw products vary considerably in potency; follow the directions on the package.

SHARP HOOKS
The name cat's claw derives from the hooks this climbing vine produces. It grows up to 100 ft (30 m) or more in the tropical rainforests of Central and South America.

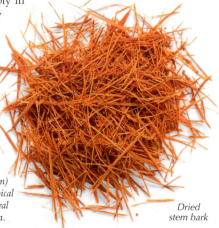

Dried stem bark

57

Urtica dioica
STINGING NETTLE LEAF

WHY IT'S USED Stinging nettle leaf is used to relieve hay fever and seasonal allergies, and treat kidney stones, urinary tract inflammation (UTI), and enlarged prostate (also called benign prostatic hypertrophy, or BPH).

HOW IT WORKS Stinging nettle leaf contains diuretic substances and quercetin, a substance that may prevent allergic responses and relieve symptoms.

COMMENTS AND CAUTIONS To diagnose or treat BPH, consult your physician. Stinging nettle leaves are high in potassium; they are an especially useful diuretic because they replace some of the potassium lost by increased urination. This herb may cause uterine bleeding, contractions, or miscarriage in pregnant women.

Freeze-dried nettle is the most potent form

DOSAGE •Capsules: 300 mg 3 to 4 times daily for allergies. •**Tea:** Steep 2 teaspoons of dried leaves in 1 cup of boiling water for 10 minutes; take ½ cup 3 times daily for allergies. •**Liquid extract:** ½ teaspoon 3 times daily or as directed on the package.

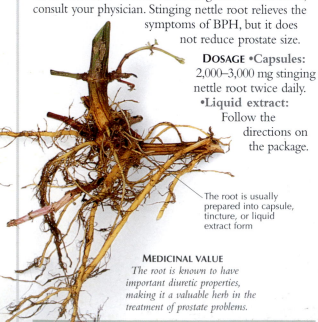

Stinging nettle leaves can be eaten as a tonic vegetable

Urtica dioica
STINGING NETTLE ROOT

WHY IT'S USED Stinging nettle root is used to treat urinary problems such as frequent urination caused by an enlarged prostate gland, also called benign prostatic hypertrophy (BPH).

HOW IT WORKS This herb contains many complex substances, but how they work is not fully known.

COMMENTS AND CAUTIONS To diagnose or treat BPH, consult your physician. Stinging nettle root relieves the symptoms of BPH, but it does not reduce prostate size.

DOSAGE •Capsules: 2,000–3,000 mg stinging nettle root twice daily. •**Liquid extract:** Follow the directions on the package.

The root is usually prepared into capsule, tincture, or liquid extract form

MEDICINAL VALUE
The root is known to have important diuretic properties, making it a valuable herb in the treatment of prostate problems.

Usnea barbata
USNEA

WHY IT'S USED Usnea is used to treat coughs and sore throat, and other mild irritations of the mouth and throat. Some physicians also use usnea to treat certain bacterial and yeast infections.

HOW IT WORKS Usnea contains mucilage, which soothes mucous membranes, and usnic acid, which is antimicrobial.

COMMENTS AND CAUTIONS Usnea is a type of lichen; it is also known as beard moss and old man's beard. Buy usnea only from reputable manufacturers; poor quality products may contain toxic levels of lead.

DOSAGE •Lozenges: 1 lozenge 3 to 6 times daily for coughs and sore throat. •**Capsules:** 100 mg 3 times daily. •**Tincture:** ½ teaspoon 3 times daily or as directed on the package.

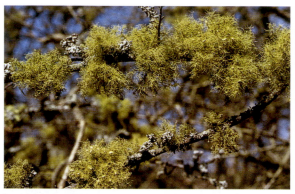

LOOKALIKE HERBS
Many lichen resemble usnea, so only a trained herbalist should gather this plant in the wild.

Vaccinium macrocarpon
CRANBERRY

WHY IT'S USED Cranberry is used to prevent and treat urinary tract infections (UTIs).

HOW IT WORKS A still-unidentified substance in cranberry prevents bacteria from adhering to the wall of the bladder, thus allowing the urinary system to flush it from the body.

COMMENTS AND CAUTIONS When choosing a juice product, look for real cranberry juice, not sweetened cranberry juice cocktail. Dosages 2 to 3 times the preventive dose *(below)* are often used to treat UTIs. Consult your physician if you believe you have a UTI.

DOSAGE •Capsules: 300–400 mg twice daily. •**Juice:** 8–16 ounces of cranberry juice daily.

Cranberries contain tannins, flavonoids, and vitamin C

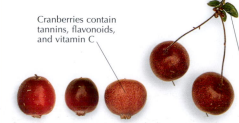

Cranberry thrives in wet, boggy ground and acidic soils

Vaccinium myrtillus
BILBERRY

WHY IT'S USED Bilberry is used to improve night vision and to help prevent age-related macular degeneration (ARMD). It is sometimes used in combination with other medications and herbs to treat ARMD.

HOW IT WORKS Anthocyanadins, blue-colored substances in bilberry, strengthen the tiny blood vessels in the retina and increase the regeneration of rhodopsin, a substance in the retina that is important for vision.

The berries have a strong healing effect on capillaries within the eyes

COMMENTS AND CAUTIONS The effect of bilberry on night vision is almost immediate, but only lasts about two hours, according to some studies.

DOSAGE •Capsule: To improve night vision, 1 50-mg capsule standardized to 25 percent anthocyanosides; to prevent ARMD, 1 80–300 mg capsule standardized to 25 percent anthocyanosides 3 times daily.

Vaccinium spp.
BLUEBERRY

WHY IT'S USED Blueberry juice or extract is used to treat bladder infections, colds, and sore throat. Dried blueberries are used to treat mild diarrhea.

HOW IT WORKS Dried blueberries are rich in astringent substances called tannins and a type of soluble fiber called pectin. Tannins reduce intestinal inflammation and have a mild antimicrobial effect; pectin adds bulk to the stool.

COMMENTS AND CAUTIONS Fresh blueberries could make diarrhea worse. If diarrhea or infection continues for more than 24 hours or gets worse, call your physician.

DOSAGE •Dried berries: For diarrhea, soak ½ cup of dried blueberries in boiling water to cover until softened. Eat the berries and drink the liquid up to 3 times daily. •**Tea:** Steep 1 teaspoon of dried leaves in 1 cup of boiling water for 15 minutes. Drink up to 3 cups daily. •**Tincture:** 1 teaspoon up to 3 times daily, or as directed on the package.

Blueberry

Valeriana officinalis
VALERIAN

WHY IT'S USED Valerian root is used to treat insomnia.

HOW IT WORKS Researchers are still not sure which are the active ingredients in valerian.

COMMENTS AND CAUTIONS Valerian has a sedative effect; take appropriate precautions. It may also cause excessive drowsiness in children. Do not combine with alcohol or other sedative herbs, supplements, or medications. It appears to work best when taken regularly; the sedative effect increases over several weeks, then levels off. Taking capsules helps reduce valerian's unpleasant taste and odor.

DOSAGE •Capsules: 1–2 150-mg capsules containing valerian standardized to 1 percent valerenic acid, taken 1 hour before bedtime. •**Liquid extract:** ½–1 teaspoon, taken 1 hour before bedtime or as directed on the package. •**Tincture:** ¾ teaspoon taken 1 hour before bedtime or as directed on the package.

The root contains properties that induce sleep

Verbascum thapsus
MULLEIN

WHY IT'S USED Mullein flower is used to treat coughs and sore throat related to upper respiratory infections such as colds and flu. Mullein oil is used to relieve the pain associated with ear infections.

HOW IT WORKS Mullein flowers contain mucilage, a substance that soothes mucous membranes such as those in the mouth and throat, and soapy substances, called saponins, that have an expectorant effect.

COMMENTS AND CAUTIONS Use mullein oil for an ear infection only if you are certain that the eardrum is not punctured.

DOSAGE •Tea: Steep 1 teaspoon of dried mullein flowers in 1 cup of boiling water for 10 minutes. Drink up to 2 cups daily. •**Liquid extract:** ½ teaspoon 2 times daily or as directed on the package. •**Tincture:** ¼–½ teaspoon 2 to 3 times daily. •**Oil:** Place 1–3 drops in the ear canal up to 3 times daily.

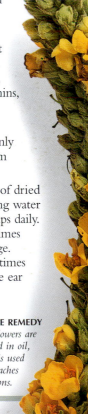

EARACHE REMEDY
Mullein flowers are often soaked in oil, and the oil is used to treat earaches and infections.

VERVAIN
Verbena hastata, V. officinalis

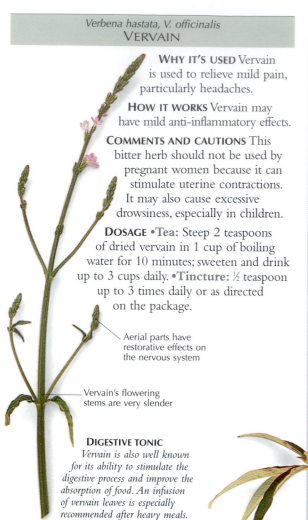

WHY IT'S USED Vervain is used to relieve mild pain, particularly headaches.

HOW IT WORKS Vervain may have mild anti-inflammatory effects.

COMMENTS AND CAUTIONS This bitter herb should not be used by pregnant women because it can stimulate uterine contractions. It may also cause excessive drowsiness, especially in children.

DOSAGE •**Tea:** Steep 2 teaspoons of dried vervain in 1 cup of boiling water for 10 minutes; sweeten and drink up to 3 cups daily. •**Tincture:** ½ teaspoon up to 3 times daily or as directed on the package.

Aerial parts have restorative effects on the nervous system

Vervain's flowering stems are very slender

DIGESTIVE TONIC
Vervain is also well known for its ability to stimulate the digestive process and improve the absorption of food. An infusion of vervain leaves is especially recommended after heavy meals.

CHASTEBERRY
Vitex agnus-castus

WHY IT'S USED Chasteberry, also called agnes castus or chaste tree, is used to relieve symptoms of premenstrual syndrome (PMS), especially breast tenderness. It is also used to treat irregular menstruation and menopausal symptoms.

HOW IT WORKS Substances in chasteberry suppress the pituitary gland's release of prolactin, a hormone linked to breast tenderness during the menstrual cycle.

COMMENTS AND CAUTIONS The benefits of this herb may not be noticed for several months. Do not use chasteberry if you are pregnant or nursing, since it can cause hormonal changes and uterine bleeding. Chasteberry may also cause hormonal imbalance in children.

DOSAGE •**Capsules:** 20–40 mg once daily, preferably in the morning. •**Liquid extract and tincture:** Follow package directions.

CHASTE TREE
In ancient times, chasteberry was believed to suppress the libido and reduce sexual desire.

The yellow-red berries have a hormonal action on the body

CRAMP BARK
Viburnum opulus

WHY IT'S USED Cramp bark, as its name suggests, is used primarily to treat muscle cramps and spasms, including menstrual cramps.

HOW IT WORKS The active ingredient in cramp bark has not yet been identified.

COMMENTS AND CAUTIONS Do not confuse cramp bark with black haw (*Viburnum prunifolium*), which sometimes goes by the same common name. Do not use cramp bark if you are pregnant.

DOSAGE •**Capsules:** 1,000 mg 3 times daily. •**Liquid extract:** ½ teaspoon 3 times daily or as directed on the package. •**Tincture:** ½ teaspoon 3 times daily or as directed on the package.

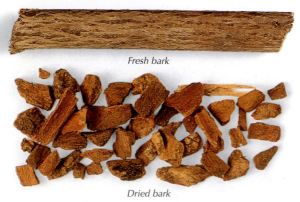

Fresh bark

Dried bark

GRAPESEED EXTRACT
Vitis vinifera

WHY IT'S USED Grapeseed extract is used to treat varicose veins and poor circulation to the legs. It may also help prevent diabetic neuropathy (a painful nerve condition), eye problems such as diabetic retinopathy and macular degeneration, and heart disease.

HOW IT WORKS Grapeseed extract contains powerful antioxidants – substances that limit free radical damage – and it is a rich source of oligomeric proanthocyanins (OPCs). These substances strengthen blood vessel walls, reduce swelling, and help prevent bleeding and bruising.

COMMENTS AND CAUTIONS Do not combine grapeseed extract with blood-thinning drugs such as warfarin (*p. 195*), unless your physician advises it.

DOSAGE •**Capsules:** 75–150 mg, twice daily, of a product standardized to contain 92–95 percent OPCs.

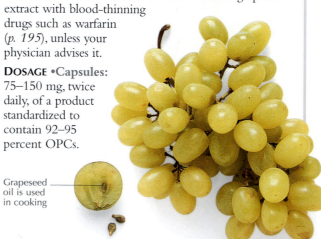

Grapeseed oil is used in cooking

Withania somniferum
ASHWAGANDHA

WHY IT'S USED In traditional Indian medicine, ashwagandha is used to improve overall health, energy, and immunity, improve fertility, lower cholesterol, as a mild sedative, improve mental function, relieve stress, and treat Alzheimer's disease.

HOW IT WORKS How ashwagandha works is not fully understood.

COMMENTS AND CAUTIONS Ashwagandha may have a mild sedative effect; take appropriate precautions. Do not combine it with alcohol or other sedative herbs, supplements, or medications. It may cause miscarriage in pregnant women and hormonal imbalance in children.

DOSAGE •Tea: Stir 1 teaspoon of ashwagandha powder into ½ cup of boiling water. Let cool before drinking; take up to 2 times daily. **•Capsules:** 500–1,000 mg twice daily.

Ashwagandha

Yucca spp.
YUCCA

WHY IT'S USED Yucca is sometimes used to treat pain and inflammation from arthritis.

HOW IT WORKS Yucca contains soapy substances called saponins that are believed to decrease the absorption of toxins that can aggravate the symptoms of arthritis.

COMMENTS AND CAUTIONS Yucca is used as an ingredient in natural shampoos and soaps. High doses of yucca may cause diarrhea, especially in children. Do not use yucca continuously for more than three months; it can block your absorption of fat-soluble vitamins including vitamins A and E.

DOSAGE •Tablets: 2–4 tablets daily of concentrated yucca saponins or as directed on the package.

Yucca flower

DESERT EVERGREEN
In addition to its medicinal uses, yucca is an ingredient in many soaps, shampoos, and other cosmetics.

Yucca leaf

Zea mays
CORN SILK

WHY IT'S USED Corn silk is used to help treat bladder problems.

HOW IT WORKS Corn silk contains mild diuretics and anti-inflammatory substances.

COMMENTS AND CAUTIONS Do not use corn silk if you take a diuretic drug, a blood-thinning drug such as warfarin (*p. 195*), or medications to treat high blood pressure or diabetes. Corn silk may cause dehydration in children.

Leafy husk

Fresh corn silk

Corn

DOSAGE •Capsules: 2–4 grams 3 times daily. **•Tea:** Steep 1 teaspoon of corn silk in 1 cup of boiling water for 10 minutes; drink up to 3 cups daily. **•Liquid extract:** 1 teaspoon 3 times daily or as directed on the package. **•Tincture:** 1 teaspoon 3 times daily or as directed on the package.

Corn silk

Zingiber officinale
GINGER ROOT

WHY IT'S USED Ginger is used to treat nausea and motion sickness, and may be helpful for treating rheumatoid arthritis and migraine headaches.

HOW IT WORKS Researchers believe that gingerol and shogol, two pungent substances present in ginger, help prevent nausea. Ginger may also act as a mild analgesic.

COMMENTS AND CAUTIONS Small amounts of dietary ginger are generally safe for pregnant women, but avoid it if the risk of miscarriage is high. If you want to treat morning sickness with ginger, discuss it with a physician first. Medicinal use may cause stomach upset in children.

DOSAGE •Powdered ginger: 250–500 mg 4 times daily to treat nausea; use the same amount for motion sickness, taking the first dose 1 hour before your trip. 1,000–2,000 mg twice daily for rheumatoid arthritis. Consult your physician for the proper dose for migraine. **•Tincture:** ½ teaspoon 2 to 3 times daily.

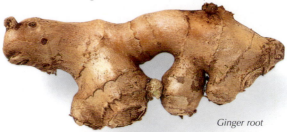

Ginger root

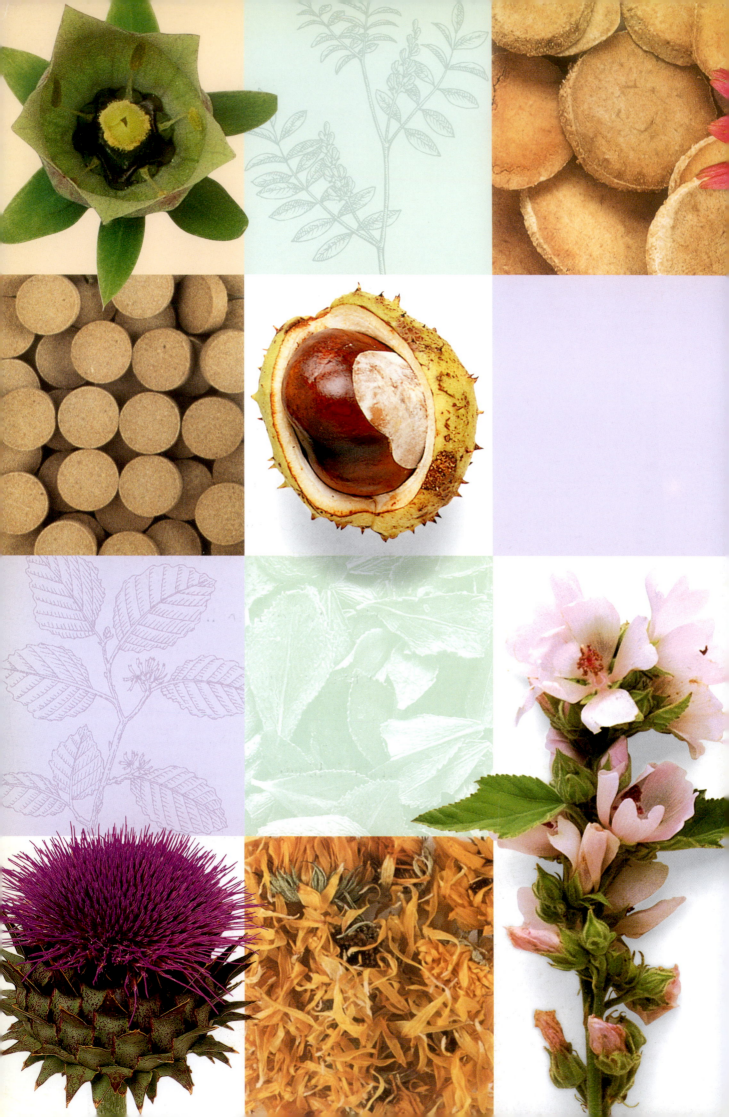

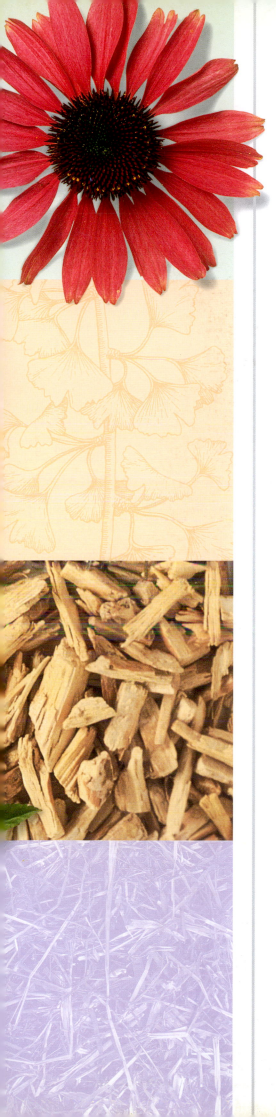

SAFE AND EFFECTIVE MULTIHERB FORMULAS

Premixed formulas, when used correctly, can be particularly effective at treating common health problems. Two or more herbs in combination can act synergistically: each herb contributes a benefit that adds up to more than either one can give individually. The effects of herbal combinations are generally stronger and are usually felt more quickly than individual herbs; therefore, use the formulas with caution.

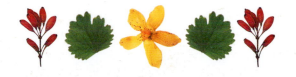

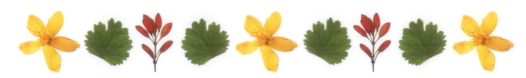

UNDERSTANDING MULTIHERB FORMULAS

IF ONE HERB is good for you, are two or more herbs even better? Very often, the answer is yes, but only when the right herbs are combined. Based upon years of experience and thousands of scientific studies, modern herbal practitioners have developed a number of premixed formulas that are generally considered to be safe and effective.

❖ BOTTLED FOR YOUR ❖ CONVENIENCE – AND SAFETY

Many premixed herbal formulas are now available in natural product stores. Some of these multiherb formulas can be used to help relieve common ailments such as coughs, colds, and minor digestive conditions, while others can be taken to nourish and assist a particular organ or system of the body, such as the eyes, liver, or immune system. Still other

COMPLEMENTARY MEDICINES
Licorice, echinacea, and ligustrum are all individually known for their ability to fight infection and enhance the immune system; when combined in a multiherb formula, their powerful effectiveness increases to help treat particular conditions (see p. 71).

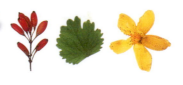

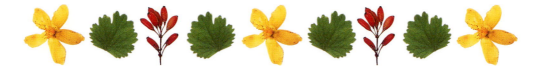

WORDS OF CAUTION

MULTIHERB formulas are often more powerful and fast-acting than individual herbs. Consequently, they should be used with even greater caution. Always start with the smallest possible dose, increasing it gradually if necessary, but never exceeding the recommended dosage unless your physician specifically advises it. Stop using the product immediately if you experience nausea, dizziness, headache, skin rash, or any other symptoms after taking it.

Contact your physician if any of the following conditions apply:

• you wish to use a combination formula for longer than two weeks, or to treat a serious illness

• you have a chronic health problem such as diabetes, heart disease, high blood pressure, or asthma

• you are experiencing a severe or sudden illness

• the condition you are treating does not improve (or becomes worse) within 48 hours of treatment

• you are treating vomiting or diarrhea that shows no signs of improvement within 24 hours.

multiherb formulas can be used to help treat chronic health problems such as arthritis, migraines, menopause, and enlarged prostate.

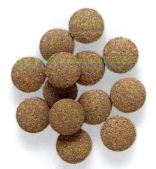

PRESCRIBED DRUGS
Some medications and herbs can interact negatively with one another. If you want to try an herbal remedy and already take medication, consult your physician before taking it.

❖ CHECK THE INGREDIENTS ❖

When looking for an appropriate multiherb formula to treat your condition, always read the package label carefully before you buy it to check the ingredients. If you're considering using a formula that is included in this chapter, look up the individually listed herbs in Chapter 1, *Safe Herbs Catalog*; there, you'll find a detailed explanation of what each herb does and how it works, along with reasons why some people should avoid them. If you take any medications, refer to Chapter 5, *Drug Catalog*, to find out if the herbs you're considering using might interact negatively with your prescribed drugs.

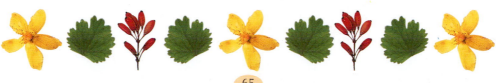

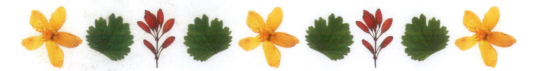

If you purchase a premixed formula that doesn't exactly match one of the formulas discussed in this chapter, find the entry that is closest to your chosen formula and refer back to Chapter 1 to check the safety of any additional herbs the formula contains. Sometimes you'll have a choice of several different formulas for the same health problem; find the formula that most closely matches your particular condition. If you are in still doubt, don't guess – call your physician and ask for advice.

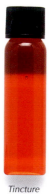

Tincture

❖ DOSAGE GUIDELINES ❖

Premixed multiherb formulas are available in a variety of forms, including tablets, capsules, teas, and tinctures. Naturopathic practitioners most often recommend tinctures because they allow for variable dosages. Always

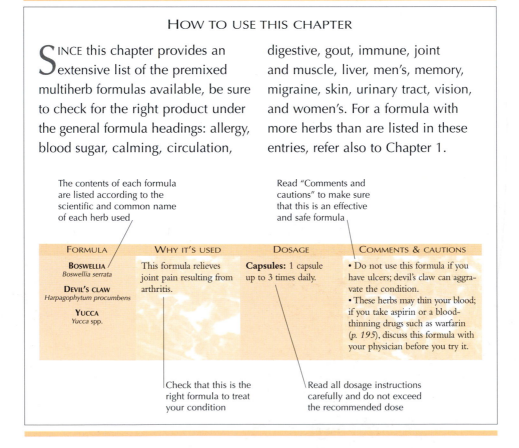

HOW TO USE THIS CHAPTER

SINCE this chapter provides an extensive list of the premixed multiherb formulas available, be sure to check for the right product under the general formula headings: allergy, blood sugar, calming, circulation, digestive, gout, immune, joint and muscle, liver, men's, memory, migraine, skin, urinary tract, vision, and women's. For a formula with more herbs than are listed in these entries, refer also to Chapter 1.

The contents of each formula are listed according to the scientific and common name of each herb used

Read "Comments and cautions" to make sure that this is an effective and safe formula

FORMULA	WHY IT'S USED	DOSAGE	COMMENTS & CAUTIONS
BOSWELLIA *Boswellia serrata* **DEVIL'S CLAW** *Harpagophytum procumbens* **YUCCA** *Yucca spp.*	This formula relieves joint pain resulting from arthritis.	**Capsules:** 1 capsule up to 3 times daily.	• Do not use this formula if you have ulcers; devil's claw can aggravate the condition. • These herbs may thin your blood; if you take aspirin or a blood-thinning drugs such as warfarin (*p. 195*), discuss this formula with your physician before you try it.

Check that this is the right formula to treat your condition

Read all dosage instructions carefully and do not exceed the recommended dose

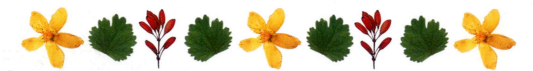

read the dosage instructions on the product packaging, or refer to the dosages recommended in this chapter. Remember that although herbs are gentler on the body than drugs, they often take longer to become fully effective. You may be advised to take a multiherb formula for several days, or even a few weeks, to feel the full benefits. Be patient, but not too patient: in general, if the premixed formula you are taking doesn't help you within a few days, or if the condition you're treating doesn't improve (or worsens), make sure that you see your physician as soon as possible.

❖ DON'T MIX AND MATCH ❖

It is generally best to stick to the premixed multiherb formulas prepared by reliable manufacturers, since the combination of herbal ingredients they use are known to be safe and have beneficial interactions. Creating your own multiherb formulas can cause potentially dangerous interactions, as explained in Chapter 3 on pages 91–93.

MULTIHERB FORMULAS

ALLERGY FORMULAS
These formulas relieve symptoms of hay fever and other allergies.

FORMULA	WHY IT'S USED	DOSAGE	COMMENTS & CAUTIONS
CAYENNE PEPPER *Capsicum annuum, C. frutescens* **HORSERADISH** *Armoracia rusticana* **ROSE HIPS** *Rosa rugosa, R. canina, R. centifolia* **STINGING NETTLE LEAF** *Urtica dioica*	This formula may relieve the symptoms of upper respiratory allergies such as runny nose, sneezing, and chest congestions and wheeziness.	**Tincture or capsules:** Follow the directions on the package.	• The herbs used in this formula can upset your stomach. Do not take this formula if you have ulcers, gastritis, or esophagitis. *Cayenne*
COLEUS *Coleus forskohlii* **LICORICE** *Glycyrrhiza glabra* **INDIAN IPECAC** *Tylophora asthmatica*	This formula may reduce the symptoms of hay fever and mild asthma caused by allergies.	**Capsules:** 1 capsule up to 4 times daily.	• If you take prescription medication for asthma, discuss this formula with your physician before you try it. Do not use it as a substitute for asthma medication. • Use only formulas containing deglycyrrhizinated licorice (DGL).

BLOOD SUGAR FORMULAS

These formulas can help people with mild cases of Type 2 diabetes and those with hypoglycemia (low blood sugar) to control their blood sugar levels. Use these formulas only under a physician's supervision.

FORMULA	WHY IT'S USED	DOSAGE	COMMENTS & CAUTIONS
BITTER MELON *Momordica charantia* **GYMNEMA** *Gymnema sylvestre*	The herbs in this formula stimulate the pancreas to release insulin and reduce insulin resistance.	When deciding the right dose for you, your physician will consider many factors, such as the severity of the condition, your weight, and any medications you take.	• Use this formula with caution. Check your blood sugar level frequently to make sure it does not drop too low.
ALOE VERA JUICE *Aloe vera* **FENUGREEK SEED** *Trigonella foenum-graecum* **GINKGO** *Ginkgo biloba*	This formula may be helpful in controlling the symptoms of hypoglycemia (low blood sugar) and mild cases of Type 2 diabetes.	When deciding the right dose for you, your physician will consider many factors, such as the severity of the condition, your weight, and any medications you take.	• The herbs in this formula appear to reduce blood sugar levels. Check frequently to make sure your blood sugar level does not drop too low.
FENUGREEK SEED *Trigonella foenum-graecum* **GUM KINO** *Pterocarpus marsupium* **SALT BUSH** *Atriplex halimus*	This formula is used to treat the symptoms of mild cases of Type 2 diabetes.	When deciding the right dose for you, your physician will consider many factors.	• Salt bush contains chromium – check your supplements to make sure you take no more than 200 mcg chromium daily. • Use this formula with caution and check your blood sugar level.

CALMING FORMULAS

These formulas contain mild sedatives that relieve anxiety and encourage sleep. Since these formulas may cause drowsiness, take appropriate precautions.

FORMULA	WHY IT'S USED	DOSAGE	COMMENTS & CAUTIONS
CALIFORNIA POPPY *Eschscholzia californica* **CATNIP** *Nepeta cataria* **LEMON BALM** *Melissa officinalis* **PASSIONFLOWER** *Passiflora incarnata*	This formula is used as a stress reliever and a mild sedative.	**Tincture or capsules:** Take as directed on the package.	• Do not combine this formula with alcohol or other sedative herbs, drugs, or supplements.
CALIFORNIA POPPY *Eschscholzia californica* **CATNIP** *Nepeta cataria* **KAVA KAVA** *Piper methysticum* **PASSIONFLOWER** *Passiflora incarnata*	This formula is used as a stress reliever and a mild sedative.	**Tincture or capsules:** Take as directed on the package.	• Do not combine this formula with alcohol or other sedative herbs, drugs, or supplements. • Do not combine this formula with antianxiety or MAOI antidepressant drugs such as phenelzine (*p. 180*); excessive drowsiness can occur when these drugs are combined with passionflower.
KAVA KAVA *Piper methysticum* **ST. JOHN'S WORT** *Hypericum perforatum*	This formula relieves mild depression, reduces anxiety, and aids sleep.	**Tincture or capsules:** Follow the directions on the package.	• St. John's wort can interact dangerously with several prescription drugs, and should be used with caution.

California poppy

CIRCULATION FORMULAS

These formulas are designed to strengthen the cardiovascular system, reduce blood pressure, and lower cholesterol. Use them only under your physician's supervision to ensure that they are appropriate for your condition and will not interfere with any medications you are taking.

FORMULA	WHY IT'S USED	DOSAGE	COMMENTS & CAUTIONS
DANDELION LEAF *Taraxacum officinale* **GINKGO** *Ginkgo biloba* **HAWTHORN** *Crataegus oxyacantha* **PARSLEY** *Petroselinum crispum*	This formula is used to support the heart, especially in cases of mild heart failure. It is also used as a mild diuretic, which helps reduce blood pressure.	Consult your physician for individualized dosage instructions.	• Heart failure is a serious medical condition. If you have symptoms of heart failure, such as fatigue, shortness of breath, or leg swelling, see your physician at once. Treatment should always be coordinated by your physician, who needs to know about all the herbs, supplements, and drugs you may be taking.
GINKGO *Ginkgo biloba* **GINGER ROOT** *Zingiber officinale* **GOTU KOLA** *Centella asiatica* **HORSE CHESTNUT** *Aesculus hippocastanum*	This formula improves circulation to the extremities, which can be helpful in treating hemorrhoids, erectile dysfunction, varicose veins, and intermittent claudication (a circulatory problem in the legs).	**Tincture or capsules:** Follow the package directions or take as directed by your physician.	• Some herbs in this formula work by thinning your blood. If you take aspirin or a blood-thinning drug such as warfarin (p. 195), discuss this formula with your physician before you try it.
BILBERRY *Vaccinium myrtillus* **BLUEBERRY** *Vaccinium* spp. **GINKGO** *Ginkgo biloba* **GOTU KOLA** *Centella asiatica* **GRAPESEED EXTRACT** *Vitis vinifera* **HORSE CHESTNUT** *Aesculus hippocastanum*	This formula is used to treat varicose veins and hemorrhoids.	**Capsules:** Follow the package directions, or take as directed by your physician.	• Many of the herbs in this formula strengthen the walls of veins and small blood vessels. 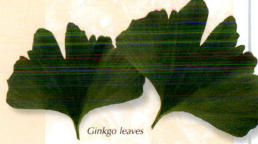 *Ginkgo leaves*
COLEUS *Coleus forskohlii* **GINKGO** *Ginkgo biloba* **HAWTHORN** *Crataegus oxyacantha*	This formula is used to lower high blood pressure.	**Tincture or capsules:** Follow the package directions or take as directed by your physician.	• Coleus is a powerful herb; use this formula only under a physician's supervision. • If you take blood-thinning drugs such as warfarin (p. 195) or medication for high blood pressure, discuss ginkgo with your physician before you try it.
GARLIC *Allium sativum* **GUGGUL** *Commiphora mukul* **PSYLLIUM SEED** *Plantago ovata, P. afra*	This formula is used to lower cholesterol.	**Capsules:** Follow the package directions or take as directed by your physician.	• The cholesterol-lowering effect of this formula may take up to eight weeks to become apparent. • The fiber in this formula may block your absorption of other herbs, supplements, and medications; take it two hours before or after them.

DIGESTIVE FORMULAS

These formulas contain herbs noted for their ability to relieve digestive problems.

FORMULA	WHY IT'S USED	DOSAGE	COMMENTS & CAUTIONS
GENTIAN ROOT *Gentiana lutea* **GINGER ROOT** *Zingiber officinale*	In combination, gentian and ginger root are used to treat loss of appetite and nausea, especially nausea resulting from motion sickness or stress.	**Tincture:** Follow package directions, or add ½ teaspoon to 1 cup of warm water. Sweeten lightly to disguise gentian's bitter taste; sip with your meal.	• These herbs are most effective when taken as a tea.
CHAMOMILE *Matricaria recutita* (German) **LICORICE** *Glycyrrhiza glabra* **MARSHMALLOW LEAF** *Althaea officinalis* **SLIPPERY ELM** *Ulmus fulva*	This formula is used to treat minor digestive problems including cramps, stomach pain, and diarrhea, and may also relieve ulcers and irritable bowel syndrome.	**Tincture:** ¼–½ teaspoon in 1 cup of warm water, or as directed on the package.	• These herbs are soothing to the digestive tract. • Use only a formula containing deglycyrrhizinated licorice (DGL).
LICORICE *Glycyrrhiza glabra* **MINT** *Mentha arvensis* **SLIPPERY ELM** *Ulmus fulva*	This formula is helpful for stomach cramps, diarrhea with cramping, and irritable bowel syndrome.	**Tincture:** ¼ teaspoon in 1 cup of warm water, or as directed on the package.	• Mint has a relaxing effect on the intestinal tract. • Use only deglycyrrhizinated licorice (DGL).
LICORICE *Glycyrrhiza glabra* **OAT BRAN** *Avena sativa* **PSYLLIUM SEED** *Plantago ovata, P. afra* **SLIPPERY ELM** *Ulmus rubra, U. fulva*	This formula is a safe, gentle treatment for constipation. It can also relieve the symptoms of mild diarrhea.	**Capsules:** 4–6 capsules in the morning (for evening results) or at bedtime (for morning results) with 8 ounces of water, or as directed on the package.	• Oat bran and psyllium provide soluble fiber that relieves constipation; this fiber absorbs excess fluid to relieve mild diarrhea. In both cases, slippery elm and licorice are anti-inflammatory and soothing to the digestive tract. • Use only formulas containing deglycyrrhizinated licorice (DGL).

Slippery elm

GOUT FORMULA

This formula is used to reduce the inflammation and pain associated with gout.

FORMULA	WHY IT'S USED	DOSAGE	COMMENTS & CAUTIONS
BROMELAIN *Ananas comosus* **DEVIL'S CLAW** *Harpagophytum procumbens*	This formula helps relieve the symptoms of gout, a painful joint condition.	**Capsules:** 1 capsule 2 to 3 times daily.	• Do not attempt to diagnose or treat gout on your own; see your physician. • Do not combine this formula with any gout medication unless your physician advises it. This formula should be taken only during a gout attack, not as a preventive measure.

IMMUNE FORMULAS

These formulas contain herbs noted for their immune-enhancing and infection-fighting abilities. Do not use for more than 10 days; if your symptoms do not improve within 48 hours (or if they get worse) discontinue use and call your physician. If you have HIV/AIDS or an autoimmune disease, rheumatoid arthritis or lupus, discuss these formulas with your physician before you try them.

FORMULA	WHY IT'S USED	DOSAGE	COMMENTS & CAUTIONS
ECHINACEA *Echinacea purpurea, E. angustifolia* **GOLDENSEAL** *Hydrastis canadensis*	The herbs in this formula stimulate immunity and help treat mild bacterial and viral infections, including colds.	**Tincture:** ¼ teaspoon 2 to 3 times daily or as directed on the package.	• Liquid forms of echinacea sometimes cause a harmless tingling sensation or temporary numbness of the tongue.
ECHINACEA *Echinacea purpurea, E. angustifolia* **LICORICE** *Glycyrrhiza glabra* **LIGUSTRUM** *Ligustrum lucidum*	The herbs in this formula stimulate immunity and help treat mild bacterial and viral infections including colds, especially those related to stress or exhaustion.	**Tincture:** ¼ teaspoon 2 to 3 times daily or as directed on the package.	• Liquid forms of echinacea sometimes cause a harmless tingling sensation or temporary numbness of the tongue. • Licorice and ligustrum stimulate the immune system and can relieve stress-related illnesses. • Deglycyrrhizinated licorice (DGL), used primarily to treat ulcers, does not improve immunity, so do not use licorice in DGL form. • Do not use licorice if you have cardiovascular, liver, or kidney disease.
ASTRAGALUS *Astragalus membranaceus* **ECHINACEA** *Echinacea purpurea, E. angustifolia* **LICORICE** *Glycyrrhiza glabra* **LIGUSTRUM** *Ligustrum lucidum* **REISHI** *Ganoderma lucidum*	The herbs in this formula stimulate immunity and help treat mild bacterial and viral infections including colds, especially those related to stress or exhaustion. This formula may also be used to prevent illness during the flu season.	**Tincture:** ⅛–¼ teaspoon 2 to 3 times daily or as directed on the package.	• Liquid forms of echinacea sometimes cause a harmless tingling sensation or temporary numbness of the tongue. • Licorice and ligustrum stimulate the immune system and relieve stress-related illnesses. • Deglycyrrhizinated licorice (DGL), used primarily to treat ulcers, does not improve immunity, so do not use licorice in DGL form. • Do not use licorice if you have cardiovascular, liver, or kidney disease.
ECHINACEA *Echinacea purpurea, E. angustifolia* **GOLDENSEAL** *Hydrastis canadensis* **WILD CHERRY** *Prunus serotina* **YERBA SANTA** *Eriodictyon californicum*	The herbs in this formula stimulate immunity and treat mild bacterial and viral infections including colds, especially those accompanied by a cough.	**Tincture:** ¼ teaspoon 2 to 3 times daily or as directed on the package.	• Liquid forms of echinacea sometimes cause a harmless tingling sensation or temporary numbness of the tongue. • Wild cherry relieves spasms in the respiratory tract, and yerba santa is an expectorant.

Echinacea

CHAPTER 2 SAFE AND EFFECTIVE MULTIHERB FORMULAS

IMMUNE FORMULAS, CONTINUED

FORMULA	WHY IT'S USED	DOSAGE	COMMENTS & CAUTIONS
ELDERBERRY *Sambucus nigra* **SPILANTHES** *Spilanthes oleracea* **ST. JOHN'S WORT** *Hypericum perforatum*	The herbs in this formula stimulate immunity and treat mild bacterial and viral infections including colds, especially those accompanied by nausea, coughing, or loss of appetite. This formula may also relieve intestinal flu.	**Tincture:** ⅛–¼ teaspoon 2 to 3 times daily or as directed on the package.	• St. John's wort has mild antiviral properties; in combination with elderberry, it inhibits the flu virus. • Spilanthes stimulates immune and digestive activity.
GARLIC *Allium sativum* **GOLDENSEAL** *Hydrastis canadensis* **LICORICE** *Glycyrrhiza glabra* **MYRRH** *Commiphora molmol* **OREGON GRAPE** *Berberis acquifolium,* *Mahonia acquifolium*	The herbs in this formula stimulate immunity and treat mild bacterial and viral infections including colds, especially those accompanied by coughs and chest and nasal congestion.	**Tincture:** ¼ teaspoon 2 to 3 times daily or as directed on the package.	• Deglycyrrhizinated licorice (DGL), used primarily to treat ulcers, does not improve immunity, therefore do not use licorice in DGL form. • Do not use licorice if you have cardiovascular, liver, or kidney disease.
ASTRAGALUS *Astragalus membranaceus* **CODONOPSIS** *Codonopsis* spp. **GINSENG** *Panax ginseng,* *Panax quinquefolium* **SCHISANDRA** *Schisandra chinensis*	This formula is used to stimulate immunity, particularly for patients with viral illnesses and those resulting from severe stress. It is sometimes used in conjunction with chemotherapy, radiation therapy, and traditional treatments for hepatitis.	**Tincture:** Consult your physician for an individualized dosage.	• This formula is designed for seriously ill patients and should be used only under a physician's supervision.

Schisandra

72

JOINT AND MUSCLE FORMULAS

These formulas are used to relieve joint and muscle pain, including arthritis, tendinitis, bursitis, gout, and overexertion.

FORMULA	WHY IT'S USED	DOSAGE	COMMENTS & CAUTIONS
BOSWELLIA *Boswellia serrata* **DEVIL'S CLAW** *Harpagophytum procumbens* **YUCCA** *Yucca* spp.	This formula relieves joint pain resulting from arthritis.	**Capsules:** 1 capsule up to 3 times daily.	• Do not use this formula if you have ulcers; devil's claw can aggravate the condition. • These herbs may thin your blood; if you take aspirin or a blood-thinning drugs such as warfarin (*p. 195*), discuss this formula with your physician before you try it.
CRAMP BARK *Viburnum opulus* **LICORICE** *Glycyrrhiza glabra* **PASSIONFLOWER** *Passiflora incarnata* **TURMERIC ROOT** *Curcuma longa* **VALERIAN** *Valeriana officinalis* **WILLOW BARK** *Salix* spp.	This formula relieves pain and swelling from arthritis, particularly rheumatoid arthritis. It also eases muscle pain and tension.	**Capsules:** 1 capsule up to 3 times daily.	• Do not use willow bark if you are allergic to salicylates or aspirin. • Use only deglycyrrhizinated licorice (DGL). • Passionflower and valerian are mild sedatives and may cause drowsiness; take appropriate precautions. • Do not combine this formula with alcohol or other sedative herbs, supplements, or medications.

LIVER FORMULAS

These formulas are designed to relieve the symptoms of hepatitis, jaundice, and other liver problems.

FORMULA	WHY IT'S USED	DOSAGE	COMMENTS & CAUTIONS
ARTICHOKE LEAF *Cynara scolymus* **BEET LEAF** *Beta vulgaris* **DANDELION** *Taraxacum officinale* **LICORICE ROOT** *Glycyrrhiza glabra* **MILK THISTLE** *Silybum marianum*	The herbs in this formula protect the liver, treat symptoms of mild hepatitis and jaundice, and encourage the flow of bile. This formula may interfere with other medications; discuss it with your physician.	**Capsules:** 1–2 capsules 2 to 3 times daily or as directed by your physician.	• Because this formula can stimulate the gallbladder, do not use it if you have gallstones, gallbladder disease, or biliary duct disease.
BUPLEURUM *Bupleurum* spp. **DANDELION** *Taraxacum officinale* **MILK THISTLE** *Silybum marianum* **TURMERIC ROOT** *Curcuma longa*	The herbs in this formula protect the liver, treat symptoms of mild hepatitis and jaundice, and encourage the flow of bile. This formula may interfere with other medications; discuss it with your physician.	**Capsules:** 1–2 capsules 2 to 3 times daily or as directed by your physician.	• Because this formula can stimulate the gallbladder, do not use it if you have gallstones, gallbladder disease, or biliary duct disease.

Artichoke leaf

MEN'S FORMULAS

These formulas are designed to treat special health problems faced by men, including benign prostatic hypertrophy, or BPH (also called enlarged prostate) and erectile dysfunction, or ED (impotence). Do not attempt to diagnose or treat these problems on your own; consult your physician to rule out more serious conditions.

FORMULA	WHY IT'S USED	DOSAGE	COMMENTS & CAUTIONS
PYGEUM *Pygeum africanum* **SAW PALMETTO** *Serenoa repens*	This formula is used to relieve the symptoms of mild BPH, especially frequent urination.	**Capsules:** 1 capsule 2 to 3 times daily.	• Although this formula relieves symptoms, it does not reduce prostate size.
PYGEUM *Pygeum africanum* **SAW PALMETTO** *Serenoa repens* **STINGING NETTLE LEAF** *Urtica dioica*	This formula is used to relieve the symptoms of mild to moderate BPH, especially frequent or difficult urination.	**Capsules:** 1 capsule 2 to 3 times daily.	• Although this formula relieves symptoms, it does not reduce prostate size.
GINSENG *Panax ginseng,* *P. quinquefolium* **PUMPKIN SEED** *Curcurbita pepo* **PYGEUM** *Pygeum africanum*	This formula is used to treat male infertility.	**Capsules:** 1 capsule 2 to 3 times daily.	• In addition to its other health benefits, ginseng appears to support male fertility and erectile function. There are many causes of male infertility; use this formula only under your physician's advice, and after serious health problems have been ruled out.
GINSENG *Panax ginseng,* *P. quinquefolium* **MUIRA PUAMA** *Ptychopetalum olacoides,* *P. uncinatum* **PYGEUM** *Pygeum africanum* **SAW PALMETTO** *Serenoa repens* **WILD OATS** *Avena sativa*	This formula is used to treat ED.	**Capsules:** 1 capsule 2 to 3 times daily.	• Although some men report faster results, the benefits of this formula may take a month or more to become apparent.
GINKGO *Ginkgo biloba* **GINSENG** *Panax ginseng,* *P. quinquefolium* **MUIRA PUAMA** *Ptychopetalum olacoides,* *P. uncinatum*	This formula is used to treat ED, particularly when caused by poor circulation to the penis.	**Tincture or capsules:** Follow the package directions, or take as directed by your physician.	• Although some men report faster results, the benefits of this formula may take a month or more to become apparent.

Nettle

MEMORY FORMULA
This formula improves circulation to the brain to improve memory and mental function.

FORMULA	WHY IT'S USED	DOSAGE	COMMENTS & CAUTIONS
GINKGO *Ginkgo biloba* **GINSENG** *Panax ginseng,* *P. quinquefolium*	This formula is used to improve short-term memory and overall mental alertness.	**Capsules:** 1–2 capsules 1 to 2 times daily.	• Do not use this formula if you are taking a blood-thinning drug such as warfarin (*p. 195*) or if you take medication for high blood pressure.

MIGRAINE FORMULA
This formula can reduce the frequency and intensity of migraine attacks.

FORMULA	WHY IT'S USED	DOSAGE	COMMENTS & CAUTIONS
FEVERFEW *Tanacetum parthenium* **WILLOW BARK** *Salix alba, S. spp.*	This formula is used to prevent migraine headaches, and to reduce their severity when they do occur.	**To prevent migraines:** 1 capsule daily, or as directed by your physician. **To treat headaches:** 1 capsule 2 to 3 times daily, or as directed by your physician.	• Feverfew works best when taken as a daily preventive for migraines. • Do not use willow bark if you are allergic to salicylates or aspirin.

SKIN FORMULAS
These formulas are used to treat a variety of minor skin problems; do not use them for severe skin conditions or deep wounds. If there is no improvement in 48 hours, or if the condition becomes worse, consult your physician.

FORMULA	WHY IT'S USED	DOSAGE	COMMENTS & CAUTIONS
BURDOCK ROOT *Arctium lappa* **COLEUS** *Coleus forskohlii* **LICORICE** *Glycyrrhiza glabra*	This formula relieves the symptoms of eczema, including itching and redness.	**Tincture:** Combine ½ teaspoon of the formula in 8 ounces of warm water. Soak a clean cloth in the liquid and apply to the affected area for 10–15 minutes. Repeat up to three times daily.	• For external use only. • Prepare a fresh batch of tincture for each application. • Use licorice root, not deglycyrrhizinated licorice (DGL) in this formula.
GOLDENSEAL *Hydrastis canadensis* **SARSAPARILLA** *Smilax sarsaparilla*	This formula helps relieve the itching, swelling, redness, and flaking caused by psoriasis.	**Capsules:** 1 capsule 2 to 3 times daily.	• If you take medication for psoriasis, discuss this formula with your physician before you try it.
GARLIC *Allium sativum* **GOLDENSEAL** *Hydrastis canadensis* **OREGANO OIL** *Origanum vulgare*	This formula is used to treat fungal infections of the skin, such as athlete's foot.	**Tincture:** Follow the package directions.	

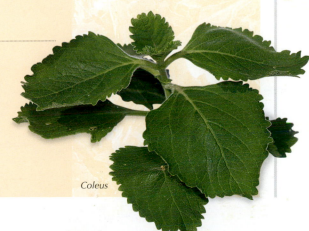

Coleus

URINARY TRACT FORMULAS

These formulas contain herbs noted for their effect on the urinary tract; most of them also contain diuretic herbs that increase the flow of urine. Consult your physician if you suspect a urinary tract infection (UTI); serious health problems can result if a UTI is improperly treated.

FORMULA	WHY IT'S USED	DOSAGE	COMMENTS & CAUTIONS
BUCHU *Barosma betulina, B. crenulata, B. serratifolia* **CRANBERRY** *Vaccinium macrocarpon*	This formula is helpful for treating mild urinary tract infections (UTIs).	**Tincture:** ½ teaspoon up to 3 times daily or as directed on the package. **Capsules:** 1 capsule 3 times daily or as directed on the package.	• Cranberry prevents bacteria from attaching to the bladder wall. • Buchu is both antibacterial and diuretic, and helps to flush bacteria from the body.
BUCHU *Barosma betulina, B. crenulata, B. serratifolia* **GOLDENSEAL** *Hydrastis canadensis* **UVA URSI** *Arctostaphylos uva-ursi*	Physicians sometimes recommend this formula to treat stubborn urinary tract infections (UTIs).	**Tincture:** ½ teaspoon up to 3 times daily or as directed on the package. **Capsules:** 1 capsule 3 times daily or as directed on the package.	• Goldenseal and uva ursi are antiseptics; buchu is antibacterial and diuretic, and helps to flush bacteria out of the body.
BUCHU *Barosma betulina, B. crenulata, B. serratifolia* **CORN SILK** *Zea mays* **ECHINACEA** *Echinacea purpurea, E. angustifolia* **USNEA** *Usnea barbata, U. florida, U. hirta, U plicata* **UVA URSI** *Arctostaphylos uva-ursi*	This formula is used to treat urinary tract infections (UTIs) accompanied by vaginal yeast infection.	**Tincture:** ½ teaspoon up to 3 times daily or as directed on the package. **Capsules:** 1 capsule 3 times daily or as directed on the package.	• Usnea contains antimicrobial substances that are helpful for treating yeast infections.
CRANBERRY *Vaccinium macrocarpon* **MARSHMALLOW LEAF** *Althaea officinalis* **STINGING NETTLE LEAF** *Urtica dioica* **UVA URSI** *Arctostaphylos uva-ursi*	This formula is used to treat urinary tract infections (UTIs) and kidney stones.	**Tincture:** ½ teaspoon up to 3 times daily or as directed on the package. **Capsules:** 1 capsule 3 times daily or as directed on the package.	• Marshmallow soothes urinary discomfort.
ALOE VERA JUICE *Aloe vera, A. barbadensis* **CRANBERRY** *Vaccinium macrocarpon* **KHELLA** *Ammi visnaga*	This formula is used to ease discomfort from kidney stones, and to encourage the stones to pass.	**Tincture:** ½ teaspoon up to 3 times daily or as directed on the package. **Capsules:** 1 capsule 3 times daily or as directed on the package.	• Khella relaxes the smooth muscles of the urinary tract.

Cranberry

VISION FORMULAS

These formulas contain herbs known to help maintain
eye health and preserve vision.

FORMULA	WHY IT'S USED	DOSAGE	COMMENTS & CAUTIONS
BILBERRY *Vaccinium myrtillus* **GRAPE SEED EXTRACT** *Vitis vinifera* **PINE BARK EXTRACT** *Pinus maritima*	This formula is used to maintain eye health.	**Capsules:** 1 capsule 2 to 3 times daily.	• The herbs in this formula support the health of the tiny blood vessels that nourish the eye.
BILBERRY *Vaccinium myrtillus* **GINKGO** *Ginkgo biloba*	This formula is used to treat glaucoma, a condition caused by high pressure within the eye.	**Capsules:** 1 capsule 2 to 3 times daily.	• These herbs are not a substitute for glaucoma medication; if you have glaucoma, discuss this formula with your physician.
BILBERRY *Vaccinium myrtillus* **GINKGO** *Ginkgo biloba* **GRAPESEED EXTRACT** *Vitis vinifera*	This formula is used to treat age-related macular degeneration (ARMD). It is usually taken in conjunction with the dietary supplements lutein and zeaxanthin.	**Capsules:** 1 capsule 2 to 3 times daily.	• These herbs support the health of the tiny blood vessels of the retina, the light-sensitive portion of the eye.

WOMEN'S FORMULAS

The formulas below are designed to treat special health
problems faced by women, including premenstrual
syndrome (PMS) and the symptoms of menopause.

FORMULA	WHY IT'S USED	DOSAGE	COMMENTS & CAUTIONS
BLACK COHOSH ROOT *Cimicifuga racemosa rhizoma* **DONG QUAI** *Angelica sinensis* **LICORICE ROOT** *Glycyrrhiza glabra* **MOTHERWORT** *Leonurus cardiaca* **SARSAPARILLA** *Smilax sarsaparilla*	This formula is used to treat menopausal symptoms, especially hot flashes and uterine cramps.	**Capsules:** 1 capsule 1 to 3 times daily or as directed on the package.	• If you have a history of or are at high risk for breast cancer, do not use this formula. • Use only deglycyrrhizinated licorice (DGL).
ARTICHOKE LEAF *Cynara scolymus* **CHASTEBERRY** *Vitex agnus-castus* **DANDELION** *Taraxacum officinale* **DONG QUAI** *Angelica sinensis* **VALERIAN** *Valeriana officinalis*	This formula is used to relieve the symptoms of PMS, especially breast tenderness, bloating and fluid retention, irritability, and insomnia.	**Capsules:** 1 capsule 1 to 3 times daily or as directed on the package.	• For best results, begin using this formula 10 days before menstruation, stopping when menstruation ends. The benefits of this formula may take several cycles to begin. • Do not use this formula if you are considering becoming pregnant. *Dandelion leaves*

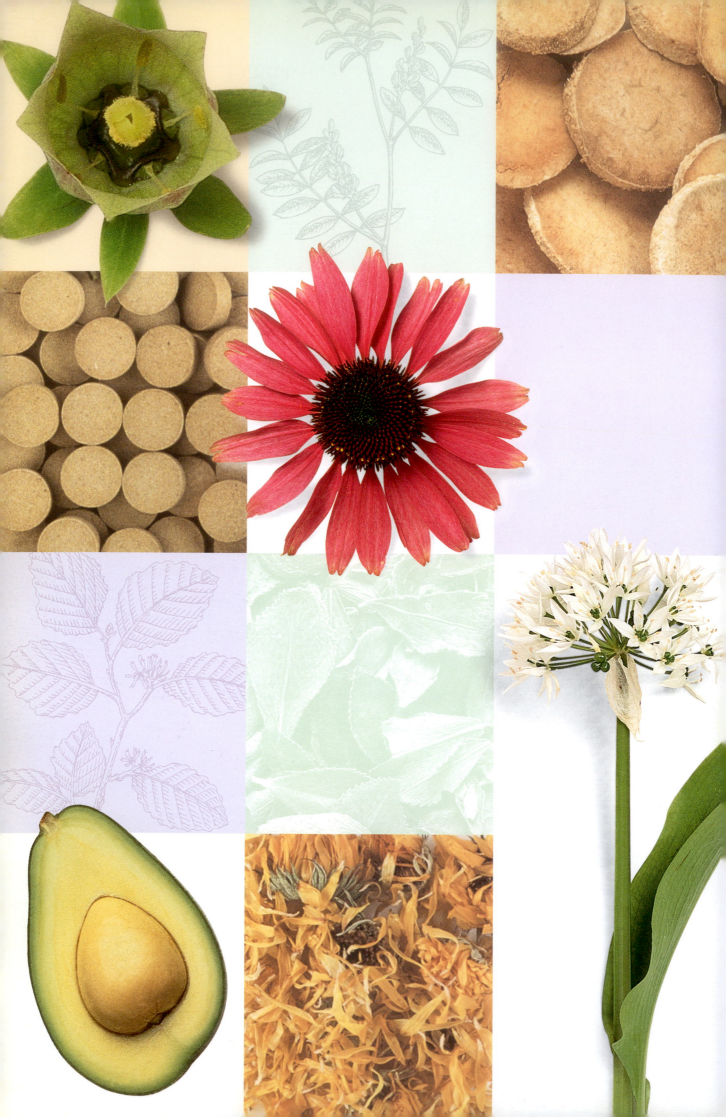

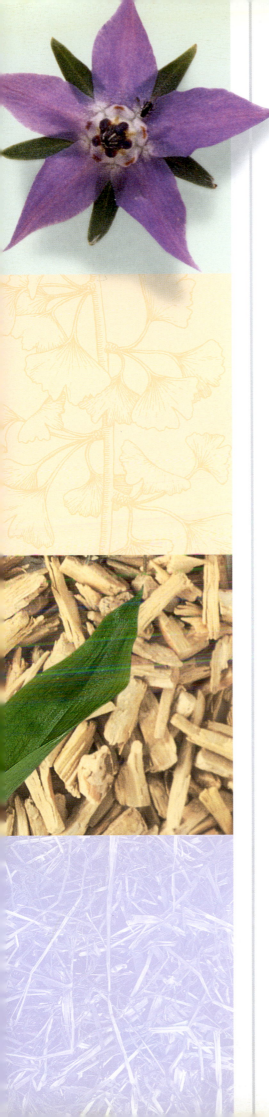

CHAPTER 3

HERB-HERB AND HERB-FOOD INTERACTIONS

USING TWO HERBS TOGETHER, or combining an herb with the right food, can be quite effective at relieving many common health problems. Because every herb or food acts in a slightly different way, combining them can either enhance their effects or result in dangerous interactions. Extra caution is needed, too, because two herbs are often more powerful together than one alone.

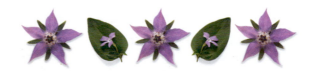

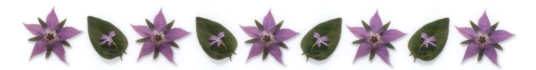

UNDERSTANDING HERB-HERB INTERACTIONS

Bilberry

W HEN THE RIGHT two herbs are combined, the overall effect is synergistic; it conveys a greater benefit than either herb alone.

After years of experience and many careful studies, herbal practitioners have learned which herbs can be safely combined to treat a variety of minor health problems. For example, the herbs horse chestnut *(Aesculus hippocastanum, p. 18)* and bilberry *(Vaccinium myrtillus, p. 59)* both help to strengthen the tiny blood vessels called capillaries, but they work in slightly different ways. When these herbs are combined, they complement one another, working together to build up the blood vessels more effectively than each of them could alone.

Horse chestnut

❖ FOOD-HERB INTERACTIONS ❖

What you eat can interact surprisingly powerfully with the herbs you take. In general, herbal practitioners advise their patients to eat a healthy, well-balanced diet that is low in fat and rich in fresh fruits, vegetables, and whole grains. However, that advice may require a little modification when you take herbs for specific health problems.

Although the tiny amount of alcohol used in herbal tinctures has no impact on their effectiveness, the benefits of many herbs are altered when you drink alcoholic beverages. For example, sedative herbs such as valerian *(Valeriana officinalis, p. 59)* can become dangerous if combined with alcohol. When taking herbs to treat a health

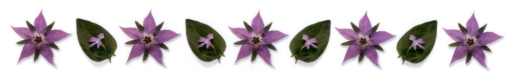

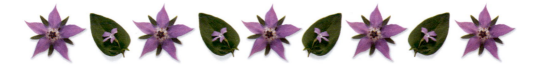

WORDS OF CAUTION

WHILE many herbs work safely and effectively together, others can lead to dangerous interactions. Avoid experimenting with two herbs; stick with well-tested herbal combinations. Two herbs with similar actions can sometimes be too powerful in combination, as is the case with kola nut *(Cola acuminata, C. nitida, p. 31)* and ginseng *(Panax ginseng, Panax quinquefolium, p. 44)*, which can raise blood pressure to dangerously high levels. On the other hand, two herbs with opposing actions can cancel out each other's benefits: maté *(Ilex paraguariensis, p. 39)* contains a stimulant that counteracts the sedative effect of passionflower *(Passiflora incarnata, p. 45)*. Before using two herbs together, check each herb in Chapter 1 for complete information, including actions, cautions, and standardization information. The dosages given are safe guidelines for the relief of minor problems; to use herbs for more than two weeks, or to treat a chronic health problem, talk to your physician. Be especially alert for side effects such as digestive upsets or skin rashes within a few hours of taking the herbs and stop taking them immediately if these occur.

problem, it is generally best to avoid liquor, wine, beer, and over-the-counter medications that contain alcohol. Caffeine can reduce the effectiveness of herbal remedies by causing the body to excrete the active ingredients in herbs too quickly. It also counteracts the effect of sedative herbs and intensifies the effect of stimulant herbs, so if you take herbs avoid caffeine and drink water, mild herbal teas, or decaffeinated drinks. Also read the labels of all drugs and supplements carefully to check for any hidden caffeine.

Foods that are high in fiber can block your absorption of herbs, supplements, and medications, so take herbs two hours before or after you eat high-fiber foods such as beans, whole grains, or large amounts of fruit and vegetables — or a fiber supplement such as flaxseed or psyllium. If you need to take an herb with meals, avoid large amounts of fiber. Check individual entries in Chapter 1 to see if an herb works best when taken with meals or on an empty stomach. Also check to see if you should avoid certain foods while taking it, or if it is high in fiber and should be taken before or after other herbs.

ALCOHOL AVOIDANCE
Alcohol can interfere with the absorption of herbs or create a dangerous interaction with them.

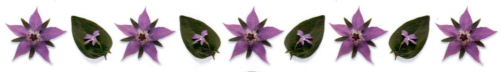

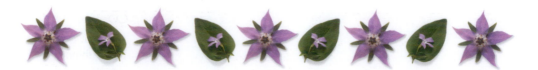

HOW TO USE THIS CHAPTER

THIS chapter contains three sections: beneficial herb–herb interactions, then potentially harmful herb–herb interactions, and finally food–herb interactions. To check an herb–herb interaction, find the Latin name that comes first alphabetically.

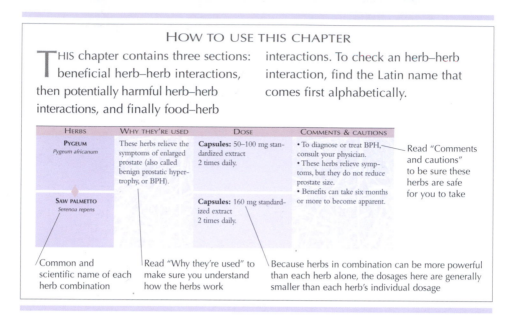

HERBS	WHY THEY'RE USED	DOSE	COMMENTS & CAUTIONS
PYGEUM *Pygeum africanum*	These herbs relieve the symptoms of enlarged prostate (also called benign prostatic hypertrophy, or BPH).	**Capsules:** 50–100 mg standardized extract 2 times daily.	• To diagnose or treat BPH, consult your physician. • These herbs relieve symptoms, but they do not reduce prostate size. • Benefits can take six months or more to become apparent.
SAW PALMETTO *Serenoa repens*		**Capsules:** 160 mg standardized extract 2 times daily.	

Read "Comments and cautions" to be sure these herbs are safe for you to take

Common and scientific name of each herb combination

Read "Why they're used" to make sure you understand how the herbs work

Because herbs in combination can be more powerful than each herb alone, the dosages here are generally smaller than each herb's individual dosage

BENEFICIAL HERB-HERB INTERACTIONS

HERBS	WHY THEY'RE USED	DOSE	COMMENTS & CAUTIONS
HORSE CHESTNUT *Aesculus hippocastanum*	These herbs are used to improve circulation and to strengthen veins and capillaries.	**Capsules:** 50–75 mg 2 times daily.	• These herbs may be helpful for treating hemorrhoids, varicose veins, and poor circulation in the legs. • If you have liver or kidney disease, discuss these herbs with your physician before trying them.
BILBERRY *Vaccinium myrtillus*		**Capsules:** 100–300 mg standardized extract 1 to 2 times daily.	

HERBS	WHY THEY'RE USED	DOSE	COMMENTS & CAUTIONS
GARLIC *Allium sativum*	These herbs are used to lower high cholesterol.	**Capsules:** 300 mg standardized extract 3 times daily.	• Do not combine with blood-thinning drugs such as warfarin (*p. 195*). •Benefits may take up to four weeks to be felt.
GUGGUL *Commiphora mukul*		**Capsules:** 25 mg of guggulsterone extract 3 times daily.	

HERBS	WHY THEY'RE USED	DOSE	COMMENTS & CAUTIONS
GARLIC *Allium sativum*	These herbs are used to improve circulation and support the immune system.	**Capsules:** 600 mg standardized extract 3 times daily.	• Do not combine with blood-thinning drugs such as warfarin (*p. 195*). • Do not use if you are pregnant.
GINGER ROOT *Zingiber officinale*		**Capsules:** 1,000–2,000 mg of powdered ginger twice daily. **Tincture:** ⅛–¼ teaspoon 2 to 3 times daily or as directed on the package.	

Garlic

HERBS	WHY THEY'RE USED	DOSE	COMMENTS & CAUTIONS
MARSHMALLOW LEAF *Althaea officinalis*	These herbs are used to relieve the symptoms of ulcers, Crohn's disease, and irritable bowel syndrome (IBS).	**Capsules:** 1,000–1,500 mg twice daily. **Liquid extract or tincture:** See package directions.	• People with diabetes should use these herbs only under the supervision of their physician. • These herbs may block the absorption of other substances; take two hours before or after other drugs, herbs, and supplements.
SLIPPERY ELM *Ulmus fulva, U. rubra*		**Capsules:** 500–1,000 mg 3 times daily.	

HERBS	WHY THEY'RE USED	DOSE	COMMENTS & CAUTIONS
BROMELAIN *Ananas comosus*	These herbs are used to treat minor digestive problems such as loss of appetite, nausea, and gas.	**Capsules:** Bromelain is measured in units called MCU or GDU. Take 1800 MCU or 1200 GDU 3 to 4 times daily.	• Do not combine with antibiotics, high blood pressure medication, or blood-thinning drugs such as warfarin (*p. 195*). • Do not take use these herbs if you have gastritis, ulcers, esophagitis, gallstones, gallbladder disease, or biliary duct disease.
TURMERIC ROOT *Curcuma longa*		**Capsules:** 400–600 mg of curcumin (the active ingredient in turmeric) up to 3 times daily. **Liquid extract or tincture:** See package directions.	

HERBS	WHY THEY'RE USED	DOSE	COMMENTS & CAUTIONS
DONG QUAI *Angelica sinensis*	These herbs can be helpful for treating menopausal symptoms, especially hot flashes.	**Capsules:** 250–500 mg 3 times daily. **Tincture:** ½–1 teaspoon 3 times daily or as directed on the package.	• Do not use these herbs if you are pregnant, nursing, using oral contraceptives, or on hormone replacement therapy. • Do not use for longer than six months unless your physician recommends it.
BLACK COHOSH ROOT *Cimicifuga racemosa rhizoma*		**Capsules:** 150–750 mg twice daily. **Tincture:** ½–1 teaspoon 3 times daily or as directed on the package.	

HERBS	WHY THEY'RE USED	DOSE	COMMENTS & CAUTIONS
DONG QUAI *Angelica sinensis*	These herbs are used to treat the symptoms of premenstrual syndrome (PMS), especially breast tenderness, and menopausal symptoms, especially hot flashes.	**Capsules:** 250–500 mg 3 times daily. **Tincture:** ½–1 teaspoon 3 times daily or as directed on the package.	• For unknown reasons, only about half of the women who try these herbs find them helpful. • Do not use these herbs if you are pregnant, nursing, using oral contraceptives, or on hormone replacement therapy.
CHASTEBERRY *Vitex agnus-castus*		**Capsules:** 20–40 mg once a day. **Liquid extract and tincture:** Follow package directions.	

HERBS	WHY THEY'RE USED	DOSE	COMMENTS & CAUTIONS
ASTRAGALUS *Astragalus membranaceus*	These herbs are used to support the immune system and prevent illness, especially during times of stress and fatigue.	**Capsules:** 250–500 mg 1 to 3 times daily, or as directed by your physician. **Liquid extract:** As directed by your physician.	• If you have diabetes or take any prescription medication, consult your physician before trying these herbs. • Do not use these herbs for more than 30 days without your physician's supervision.
GINSENG *Panax ginseng, P. quinquefolium*		**Tablets or capsules:** 100 mg twice daily. **Powdered root (nonstandardized):** 1,000–2,000 mg twice daily. **Tincture:** ½ teaspoon up to 3 times daily or as directed on the package.	

HERBS	WHY THEY'RE USED	DOSE	COMMENTS & CAUTIONS
ASTRAGALUS *Astragalus membranaceus*	These herbs are used to support the immune system and to prevent illness, especially colds and flu.	**Capsules:** 250–500 mg 1 to 3 times daily for up to 30 days, or as directed by your physician. **Fluid extract:** 1–3 teaspoons daily, or as directed by your physician.	• If you are already taking prescription medication, check with your physician before using these herbs.
ELDERBERRY *Sambucus nigra*		**Liquid extract or tincture:** Follow package directions.	

HERBS	WHY THEY'RE USED	DOSE	COMMENTS & CAUTIONS
GOTU KOLA *Centella asiatica*	These herbs are used to improve circulation and to strengthen veins and capillaries.	**Capsules:** 30–60 mg standardized extract twice daily.	• These herbs may help hemorrhoids, varicose veins, and poor circulation in the legs. • Benefits may take several weeks to become apparent.
BILBERRY *Vaccinium myrtillus*		**Capsules:** 100–300 mg standardized extract up to 2 times daily.	

Bilberry

HERBS	WHY THEY'RE USED	DOSE	COMMENTS & CAUTIONS
CHAMOMILE *Chamaemelum nobile* (Roman), *Matricaria recutita* (German)	These herbs are used to relieve intestinal cramps and bronchial spasms.	**Capsules and tablets:** As directed by your physician.	• Use these herbs only under the supervision of your physician. • Avoid chamomile if you are severely allergic to ragweed or plants in the daisy family such as cornflower (*Centaurea cyanus*) or mugwort (*Artemisia vulgaris, p. 22*).
COLEUS *Coleus forskohlii*		**Capsules:** As directed by your physician.	

HERBS	WHY THEY'RE USED	DOSE	COMMENTS & CAUTIONS
CHAMOMILE *Chamaemelum nobile* (Roman), *Matricaria recutita* (German)	These herbs are used to treat minor digestive problems such as loss of appetite, mild nausea, stomach cramps, bloating, and gas.	**Capsules and tablets:** 1,000 mg 2 to 3 times daily.	• Peppermint can aggravate heartburn, liver disease, and biliary duct disease. • Avoid chamomile if you are severely allergic to ragweed or plants in the daisy family such as cornflower (*Centaurea cyanus*) or mugwort (*Artemisia vulgaris, p. 22*).
PEPPERMINT LEAF *Mentha piperita*		**Enteric-coated capsules:** 0.2 ml 2 to 3 times daily. **Liquid extract or tincture:** Follow package directions.	

Chamomile

HERBS	WHY THEY'RE USED	DOSE	COMMENTS & CAUTIONS
CHAMOMILE *Chamaemelum nobile* (Roman), *Matricaria recutita* (German)	These herbs are used to relieve anxiety and insomnia.	**Capsules and tablets:** 1,000 mg 2 to 3 times daily.	• These herbs are sedatives; exercise appropriate caution when using them. • Do not use in combination with alcohol or other sedative substances, or with MAOI antidepressants such as phenelzine (*p. 180*). • Avoid chamomile if you are severely allergic to ragweed or plants in the daisy family such as cornflower or mugwort (*Artemisia vulgaris, p. 22*).
PASSIONFLOWER *Passiflora incarnata*		**Capsules:** 1,000 mg up to 3 times daily for up to 7 days or as directed by your physician.	

HERBS	WHY THEY'RE USED	DOSE	COMMENTS & CAUTIONS
CHAMOMILE *Chamaemelum nobile* (Roman), *Matricaria recutita* (German)	These herbs are used to relieve anxiety and insomnia.	**Capsules and tablets:** 1,000 mg 2 to 3 times daily.	• These herbs are sedatives; use with caution and do not combine with alcohol or other sedative substances. • Avoid chamomile if you are severely allergic to ragweed or plants in the daisy family such as cornflower or mugwort (*Artemisia vulgaris, p. 22*). • These herbs are most effective when taken regularly. • The sedative effect levels off after about two weeks.
VALERIAN *Valeriana officinalis*		**Capsules:** 250–500 mg standardized extract per day. **Liquid extract or tincture:** Follow package directions.	

HERBS	WHY THEY'RE USED	DOSE	COMMENTS & CAUTIONS
COLEUS *Coleus forskohlii*	These herbs are used to reduce high blood pressure.	**Capsules:** As directed by your physician.	• Use these herbs only under the supervision of your physician. • Do not combine with blood-thinning drugs such as warfarin (*p. 195*).
GINKGO *Ginkgo biloba*		**Capsules or tablets:** 60–120 mg standardized extract twice daily.	

HERBS	WHY THEY'RE USED	DOSE	COMMENTS & CAUTIONS
COLEUS *Coleus forskohlii*	These herbs are used to relieve the symptoms of irritable bowel syndrome (IBS).	**Capsules:** As directed by your physician.	• Use these herbs only under the supervision of your physician.
PEPPERMINT LEAF *Mentha piperita*		**Enteric-coated capsules, liquid extract, or tincture:** As directed by your physician.	
Peppermint leaf			

HERBS	WHY THEY'RE USED	DOSE	COMMENTS & CAUTIONS
HAWTHORN *Crataegus oxyacantha*	These herbs are used to strengthen blood vessels and connective tissues.	**Capsules:** 100–300 mg standardized extract 2 to 3 times daily. **Tincture:** 1 teaspoon 3 times daily or as directed on the package.	• Do not use these herbs if you are also taking digitalis-type drugs such as digoxin (*p. 147*).
HORSETAIL *Equisetum arvense*		**Capsules:** 1,000 mg up to 3 times daily. **Liquid extract or tincture:** Follow package directions.	

HERBS	WHY THEY'RE USED	DOSE	COMMENTS & CAUTIONS
HAWTHORN *Crataegus oxyacantha*	These herbs are used to support heart function, to reduce blood pressure, and to relieve mild angina symptoms and benign heart palpitations.	**Capsules:** 100–300 mg standardized extract 2 to 3 times daily. **Tincture:** 1 teaspoon 3 times daily or as directed on the package.	• Do not combine with blood-thinning drugs such as warfarin (*p. 195*). • If you have heart disease and want to try these herbs, discuss them with your physician first, even if you do not take any medication.
GINKGO *Ginkgo biloba*		**Capsules or tablets:** 60–120 mg of standardized extract twice daily.	

HERBS	WHY THEY'RE USED	DOSE	COMMENTS & CAUTIONS
TURMERIC ROOT *Curcuma longa*	These herbs are used to treat arthritis and improve vascular health.	**Capsules:** 400–600 mg of curcumin (the active ingredient in turmeric) 3 times daily. **Liquid extract or tincture:** As directed on the package.	• Do not use these herbs if you have ulcers, gallstones, gallbladder disease, or biliary duct disease. • Do not combine with blood-thinning drugs such as warfarin (*p. 195*) without the supervision of your physician.
GRAPESEED EXTRACT *Vitis vinifera*		**Capsules:** 75–150 mg standardized extract twice daily.	

HERBS	WHY THEY'RE USED	DOSE	COMMENTS & CAUTIONS
ECHINACEA *Echinacea angustifolia, E. purpurea*	These herbs are used to improve immunity, and to help prevent and treat minor illnesses and infections.	**Capsules:** 200–300 mg 3 times daily. **Liquid extract or tincture:** Follow package directions.	• Do not use if you are pregnant, have an autoimmune disease such as lupus or multiple sclerosis, are the recipient of an organ transplant, or are allergic to plants in the daisy family such as cornflower (*Centaurea cyanus*) or mugwort (*Artemisia vulgaris, p. 22*).
GOLDENSEAL *Hydrastis canadensis*		**Capsules:** 250–500 mg standardized extract 3 times daily. **Tincture:** ¼–½ teaspoon up to 3 times daily or as directed on the package.	

HERBS	WHY THEY'RE USED	DOSE	COMMENTS & CAUTIONS
ECHINACEA *Echinacea angustifolia, E. purpurea*	These herbs are used improve immunity and to help prevent and treat minor illnesses and infections.	**Capsules:** 200–300 mg 3 times daily. **Liquid extract or tincture:** Follow package directions.	• Do not use if you have kidney disease, an autoimmune disease such as lupus or multiple sclerosis, are the recipient of an organ transplant, or are allergic to plants in the daisy family such as cornflower (*Centaurea cyanus*) or mugwort (*Artemisia vulgaris, p. 22*). • Do not use for more than 10 days without your physician's supervision.
LARCH *Larix occidentalis*		**Powder:** Mix 1–3 teaspoons with 8 ounces of juice or water and take 2 to 3 times daily until symptoms improve.	*Larch*

HERBS	WHY THEY'RE USED	DOSE	COMMENTS & CAUTIONS
ECHINACEA *Echinacea angustifolia, E. purpurea*	These herbs are used improve immunity and to help prevent and treat minor illnesses and infections.	**Capsules:** 200–300 mg 3 times daily. **Liquid extract or tincture:** Follow package directions.	• Do not use if you have an autoimmune disease such as lupus or multiple sclerosis, are the recipient of an organ transplant, or are allergic to plants in the daisy family such as cornflower (*Centaurea cyanus*) or mugwort (*Artemisia vulgaris, p. 22*).
OREGON GRAPE *Berberis acquifolium, Mahonia acquifolium*		**Capsules or tablets:** 250 mg 2 to 3 times daily. **Tincture:** ½ teaspoon up to 3 times daily or as directed on the package.	

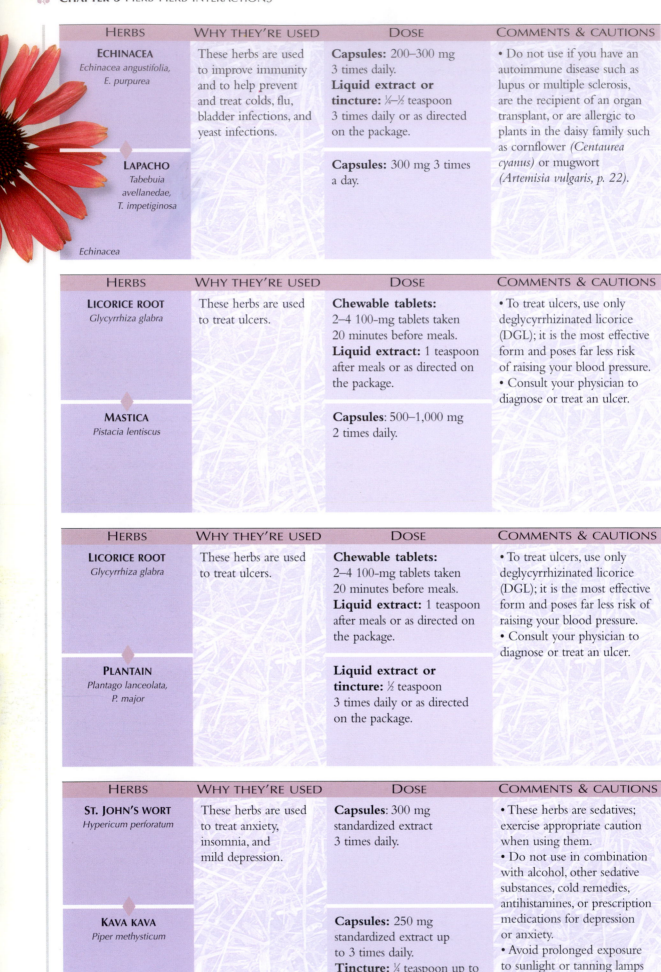

HERBS	WHY THEY'RE USED	DOSE	COMMENTS & CAUTIONS
ECHINACEA *Echinacea angustifolia, E. purpurea*	These herbs are used to improve immunity and to help prevent and treat colds, flu, bladder infections, and yeast infections.	**Capsules:** 200–300 mg 3 times daily. **Liquid extract or tincture:** ¼–½ teaspoon 3 times daily or as directed on the package.	• Do not use if you have an autoimmune disease such as lupus or multiple sclerosis, are the recipient of an organ transplant, or are allergic to plants in the daisy family such as cornflower *(Centaurea cyanus)* or mugwort *(Artemisia vulgaris, p. 22).*
LAPACHO *Tabebuia avellanedae, T. impetiginosa*		**Capsules:** 300 mg 3 times a day.	

Echinacea

HERBS	WHY THEY'RE USED	DOSE	COMMENTS & CAUTIONS
LICORICE ROOT *Glycyrrhiza glabra*	These herbs are used to treat ulcers.	**Chewable tablets:** 2–4 100-mg tablets taken 20 minutes before meals. **Liquid extract:** 1 teaspoon after meals or as directed on the package.	• To treat ulcers, use only deglycyrrhizinated licorice (DGL); it is the most effective form and poses far less risk of raising your blood pressure. • Consult your physician to diagnose or treat an ulcer.
MASTICA *Pistacia lentiscus*		**Capsules:** 500–1,000 mg 2 times daily.	

HERBS	WHY THEY'RE USED	DOSE	COMMENTS & CAUTIONS
LICORICE ROOT *Glycyrrhiza glabra*	These herbs are used to treat ulcers.	**Chewable tablets:** 2–4 100-mg tablets taken 20 minutes before meals. **Liquid extract:** 1 teaspoon after meals or as directed on the package.	• To treat ulcers, use only deglycyrrhizinated licorice (DGL); it is the most effective form and poses far less risk of raising your blood pressure. • Consult your physician to diagnose or treat an ulcer.
PLANTAIN *Plantago lanceolata, P. major*		**Liquid extract or tincture:** ½ teaspoon 3 times daily or as directed on the package.	

HERBS	WHY THEY'RE USED	DOSE	COMMENTS & CAUTIONS
ST. JOHN'S WORT *Hypericum perforatum*	These herbs are used to treat anxiety, insomnia, and mild depression.	**Capsules:** 300 mg standardized extract 3 times daily.	• These herbs are sedatives; exercise appropriate caution when using them. • Do not use in combination with alcohol, other sedative substances, cold remedies, antihistamines, or prescription medications for depression or anxiety. • Avoid prolonged exposure to sunlight or tanning lamps while using St. John's wort.
KAVA KAVA *Piper methysticum*		**Capsules:** 250 mg standardized extract up to 3 times daily. **Tincture:** ¼ teaspoon up to 3 times daily or as directed on the package.	

HERBS	WHY THEY'RE USED	DOSE	COMMENTS & CAUTIONS
CATNIP *Nepeta cataria*	These herbs are used to relieve anxiety and insomnia.	**Tincture:** 1 teaspoon up to 3 times daily or as directed on the package.	• These herbs act as sedatives; exercise appropriate caution when using them. • Do not use in combination with alcohol, other sedative substances, or antidepressants, including MAOI antidepressant drugs such as phenelzine *(p. 180)*.
PASSIONFLOWER *Passiflora incarnata*		**Capsules:** 1,000 mg up to 3 times daily for up to 7 days or as directed by your physician.	

HERBS	WHY THEY'RE USED	DOSE	COMMENTS & CAUTIONS
PASSIONFLOWER *Passiflora incarnata*	These herbs are used to relieve anxiety and insomnia.	**Capsules:** 1,000 mg up to 3 times daily for up to 7 days or as directed by your physician.	• These herbs act as sedatives; exercise appropriate caution when using them. • Do not use in combination with alcohol, other sedative substances, or antidepressants, including MAOI antidepressant drugs such as phenelzine *(p. 180)*. • These herbs are most effective when taken regularly. The sedative effect levels off after about two weeks.
VALERIAN *Valeriana officinalis*		**Capsules:** 150–300 mg standardized extract taken 1 hour before bedtime. **Liquid extract or tincture:** Follow package directions.	

HERBS	WHY THEY'RE USED	DOSE	COMMENTS & CAUTIONS
PARSLEY *Petroselinum crispum*	These diuretic herbs are often helpful in treating urinary tract infections (UTIs) and kidney stones.	**Liquid extract:** ½ teaspoon 3 times daily or as directed on the package.	• Do not use these herbs if you have ulcers, gastritis, or kidney disease. • If you have heart disease, discuss these herbs with your physician before trying them.
DANDELION *Taraxacum officinale*		**Liquid extract or tincture:** ½ teaspoon 3 times daily before meals or as directed on the package.	

Parsley

HERBS	WHY THEY'RE USED	DOSE	COMMENTS & CAUTIONS
MUIRA PUAMA *Ptychopetalum olacoides, P. uncinatum*	These herbs are used to improve male sexual function.	**Capsules or tablets:** 250 mg up to 3 times daily.	• Do not use these herbs if you have gastritis, ulcers, or kidney disease. • Do not use in combination with the medication digoxin *(p. 147)*.
SARSAPARILLA *Smilax sarsaparilla*		**Capsules:** 250–500 mg 2 to 3 times daily. **Tincture:** ½ teaspoon 3 times daily or as directed on the package.	

HERBS	WHY THEY'RE USED	DOSE	COMMENTS & CAUTIONS
PYGEUM *Pygeum africanum*	These herbs relieve the symptoms of enlarged prostate (also called benign prostatic hypertrophy, or BPH).	**Capsules:** 50–100 mg standardized extract 2 times daily.	• To diagnose or treat BPH, consult your physician. • These herbs relieve symptoms, but they do not reduce prostate size. • Benefits can take six months or more to become apparent.
SAW PALMETTO *Serenoa repens*		**Capsules:** 160 mg standardized extract 2 times daily.	

HERBS	WHY THEY'RE USED	DOSE	COMMENTS & CAUTIONS
BUTCHER'S BROOM *Ruscus aculeatus*	These herbs improve circulation and strengthen veins and capillaries, particularly those nourishing that the eyes.	**Capsules:** 25–50 mg ruscogenins twice daily.	• These herbs may be helpful for treating hemorrhoids and varicose veins.
BILBERRY *Vaccinium myrtillus*		**Capsules:** 100–300 mg standardized extract up to 2 times daily.	

HERBS	WHY THEY'RE USED	DOSE	COMMENTS & CAUTIONS
WILLOW BARK *Salix* spp.	These herbs are used to prevent and treat migraine headaches.	**Capsules:** 500–1,000 mg standardized extract up to 3 times daily. **Liquid extract or tincture:** ¼ teaspoon up to 3 times daily or as directed on the package.	• These herbs work together best as a daily preventive against migraines. • If you take migraine medication, discuss these herbs with your physician before you try them. • These herbs should not be taken by children or teenagers, pregnant women, people with ulcers or gastritis, or those people allergic to aspirin or salicylates.
FEVERFEW *Tanacetum parthenium*		**Capsules:** 80–100 mg daily or 250 mcg parthenolides daily.	

HERBS	WHY THEY'RE USED	DOSE	COMMENTS & CAUTIONS
MILK THISTLE *Silybum marianum*	These herbs are used to support the liver, especially in cases of jaundice and hepatitis.	**Capsules:** 250 mg standardized extract 2 times daily.	• Do not use these herbs if you have ulcers, gastritis, gallstones, gallbladder disease, or biliary duct disease.
DANDELION *Taraxacum officinale*		**Liquid extract or tincture:** ½ teaspoon 3 times daily before meals or as directed on the package.	

Dandelion

POTENTIALLY HARMFUL HERB-HERB INTERACTIONS

CHAMOMILE *Chamaemelum nobile* (Roman), *Matricaria recutita* (German)

DO NOT USE WITH	INTERACTION	COMMENTS & CAUTIONS
KOLA NUT *Cola acuminata, C. nitida*	Kola nut contains caffeine, which counteracts the sedative effect of chamomile.	• Do not use kola nut if you have high blood pressure or should avoid caffeine.
EPHEDRA *Ephedra sinica*	Ephedra is a powerful stimulant that counteracts the sedative effect of chamomile.	• Ephedra, also known as ma huang, is a potentially dangerous stimulant herb.
MATÉ *Ilex paraguariensis*	Maté contains caffeine, which counteracts the sedative effect of chamomile.	• Do not use maté if you have high blood pressure or should avoid caffeine.
GUARANA *Paullinia cupana*	Guarana contains caffeine, which counteracts the sedative effect of chamomile.	• Do not use guarana if you have high blood pressure or should avoid caffeine.

KOLA NUT *Cola acuminata, C. nitida*

DO NOT USE WITH	INTERACTION	COMMENTS & CAUTIONS
CHAMOMILE *Chamaemelum nobile* (Roman), *Matricaria recutita* (German)	Kola nut contains caffeine, which counteracts the sedative effect of chamomile.	• Do not use kola nut if you have high blood pressure or should avoid caffeine.
GINSENG *Panax ginseng,* *P. quinquefolium*	Both kola nut and ginseng can raise your blood pressure; in combination, they can raise it to dangerous levels. Combining these two stimulants can also cause headaches and insomnia.	• Do not use kola nut or ginseng if you have high blood pressure. Do not use kola nut if you should avoid caffeine.
PASSIONFLOWER *Passiflora incarnata*	Kola nut contains caffeine, which counteracts the sedative effect of passionflower.	• Do not use kola nut if you have high blood pressure or should avoid caffeine.
KAVA KAVA *Piper methysticum*	Kola nut contains caffeine, a stimulant that counteracts the sedative effect of kava.	• Do not use kola nut if you have high blood pressure or should avoid caffeine.
VALERIAN *Valeriana officinalis*	Kola nut contains caffeine, which counteracts the sedative effect of valerian.	• Do not use kola nut if you have high blood pressure or should avoid caffeine.

EPHEDRA *Ephedra sinica*

DO NOT USE WITH	INTERACTION	COMMENTS & CAUTIONS
CHAMOMILE *Chamaemelum nobile* (Roman), *Matricaria recutita* (German)	Ephedra counteracts the sedative effect of chamomile.	• Ephedra, also known as ma huang, is a potentially dangerous stimulant herb.
PASSIONFLOWER *Passiflora incarnata*	Ephedra counteracts the sedative effect of passionflower.	• Ephedra, also known as ma huang, is a potentially dangerous stimulant herb.
KAVA KAVA *Piper methysticum*	Ephedra counteracts the sedative effect of kava.	• Ephedra, also known as ma huang, is a potentially dangerous stimulant herb.
VALERIAN *Valeriana officinalis*	Ephedra counteracts the sedative effect of valerian.	• Ephedra, also known as ma huang, is a potentially dangerous stimulant herb.

MATÉ *Ilex paraguariensis*

DO NOT USE WITH	INTERACTION	COMMENTS & CAUTIONS
CHAMOMILE *Chamaemelum nobile* (Roman), *Matricaria recutita* (German)	Maté contains caffeine, which counteracts the sedative effect of chamomile.	• Do not use maté if you have high blood pressure or should avoid caffeine.
GINSENG *Panax ginseng,* *P. quinquefolium*	In combination, these stimulants can raise your blood pressure and cause headaches and insomnia.	• Do not use ginseng or maté if you take medication for high blood pressure. Do not use maté if you should avoid caffeine.
PASSIONFLOWER *Passiflora incarnata*	Maté contains caffeine, which counteracts the sedative effect of passionflower.	• Do not use maté if you have high blood pressure or should avoid caffeine.
KAVA KAVA *Piper methysticum*	Maté contains caffeine, which counteracts the sedative effect of kava.	• Do not use maté if you have high blood pressure or should avoid caffeine.
VALERIAN *Valeriana officinalis*	Maté contains caffeine, which counteracts the sedative effect of valerian.	• Do not use maté if you have high blood pressure or should avoid caffeine.

GINSENG *Panax ginseng, P. quinquefolium*

DO NOT USE WITH	INTERACTION	COMMENTS & CAUTIONS
KOLA NUT *Cola acuminata, C. nitida*	Both ginseng and kola nut can raise your blood pressure; in combination they can raise it to dangerous levels. Combining these two stimulants can also cause headaches and insomnia.	• Do not use ginseng or kola nut if you have high blood pressure. Do not use kola nut of you should should avoid caffeine.
MATÉ *Ilex paraguariensis*	In combination, these stimulants can raise your blood pressure and cause headaches and insomnia.	• Do not use ginseng or maté if you have high blood pressure. • Do not use maté if you should avoid caffeine.
GUARANA *Paullinia cupana*	In combination, these stimulants can raise your blood pressure and cause headaches and insomnia.	• Do not use ginseng if you have high blood pressure. • Do not use guarana if you should avoid caffeine.

PASSIONFLOWER *Passiflora incarnata*

DO NOT USE WITH	INTERACTION	COMMENTS & CAUTIONS
KOLA NUT *Cola acuminata, C. nitida*	Kola nut contains caffeine, which counteracts the sedative effect of passionflower.	• Do not use kola nut if you have high blood pressure or should avoid caffeine.
EPHEDRA *Ephedra sinica*	Ephedra is a powerful stimulant that counteracts the sedative effect of passionflower.	• Ephedra, also known as ma huang, is a potentially dangerous stimulant herb.
MATÉ *Ilex paraguariensis*	Maté contains caffeine, which counteracts the sedative effect of passionflower.	• Do not use maté if you have high blood pressure or should avoid caffeine.
GUARANA *Paullinia cupana*	Guarana contains caffeine, which counteracts the sedative effect of passionflower.	• Do not use guarana if you have high blood pressure or should avoid caffeine.

GUARANA *Paullinia cupana*

DO NOT USE WITH	INTERACTION	COMMENTS & CAUTIONS
CHAMOMILE *Chamaemelum nobile* (Roman), *Matricaria recutita* (German)	Guarana contains caffeine, which counteracts the sedative effect of chamomile.	• Do not use guarana if you have high blood pressure or should avoid caffeine.
GINSENG *Panax ginseng, P. quinquefolium*	In combination, these stimulants can raise your blood pressure and cause headaches and insomnia.	• Do not use ginseng or guarana if you have high blood pressure. • Do not take guarana if you should avoid caffeine.
PASSIONFLOWER *Passiflora incarnata*	Guarana contains caffeine, which counteracts the sedative effect of passionflower.	• Do not use guarana if you have high blood pressure or should avoid caffeine.
KAVA KAVA *Piper methysticum*	Guarana contains caffeine, which counteracts the sedative effect of kava.	• Do not use guarana if you have high blood pressure or should avoid caffeine.
VALERIAN *Valeriana officinalis*	Guarana contains caffeine, which counteracts the sedative effect of valerian.	• Do not use guarana if you have high blood pressure or should avoid caffeine.

KAVA *Piper methysticum*

DO NOT USE WITH	INTERACTION	COMMENTS & CAUTIONS
KOLA NUT *Cola acuminata, C. nitida*	Kola nut is a stimulant that counteracts the sedative effect of kava.	• Do not use kola nut if you have high blood pressure or should avoid caffeine.
EPHEDRA *Ephedra sinica*	Ephedra is a powerful stimulant that counteracts the sedative effect of kava.	• Ephedra, also known as ma huang, is a potentially dangerous stimulant herb.
MATÉ *Ilex paraguariensis*	Maté contains caffeine, which counteracts the sedative effect of kava.	• Do not use maté if you have high blood pressure or should avoid caffeine.
GUARANA *Paullinia cupana*	Guarana contains caffeine, which counteracts the sedative effect of kava.	• Do not use guarana if you have high blood pressure or should avoid caffeine.

VALERIAN *Valeriana officinalis*

DO NOT USE WITH	INTERACTION	COMMENTS & CAUTIONS
KOLA NUT *Cola acuminata, C. nitida*	Kola nut contains caffeine, which counteracts the sedative effect of valerian.	• Do not use kola nut if you have high blood pressure or should avoid caffeine.
EPHEDRA *Ephedra sinica*	Ephedra is a powerful stimulant that counteracts the sedative effect of valerian.	• Ephedra, also known as ma huang, is a potentially dangerous stimulant herb.
MATÉ *Ilex paraguariensis*	Maté contains caffeine, which counteracts the sedative effect of valerian.	• Do not use maté if you have high blood pressure or should avoid caffeine.
GUARANA *Paullinia cupana*	Guarana contains caffeine, which counteracts the sedative effect of valerian.	• Do not use guarana if you have high blood pressure or should avoid caffeine.

Valerian

FOOD-HERB INTERACTIONS

ALCOHOL

Never combine herbs and alcohol. Alcohol can prevent many herbs from working effectively in the body, and can be extremely dangerous if used in combination with sedative or antidepressant herbs that affect the central nervous system, such as kava *(Piper methysticum, p. 46)*, valerian *(Valeriana officinalis, p. 59)*, St. John's wort *(Hypericum perforatum, p. 39)*, and passionflower *(Passiflora incarnata, p. 45)*. Alcohol can also negate the liver-protecting effect of herbs such as milk thistle.

Alcohol, present in beer, wine, and liquor, is also an ingredient in some prescription and nonprescription medications, including cough syrups. To avoid alcohol in medications, look for alcohol-free formulations. Very small amounts of alcohol can also be found in many herbal tinctures. Although the amount is unlikely to cause problems, use alcohol-free preparations whenever possible.

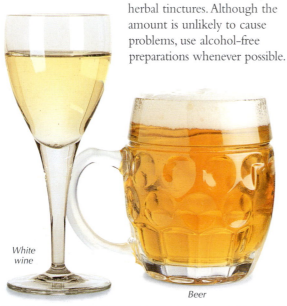

White wine

Beer

CAFFEINE

Caffeine – the stimulant found in guarana *(Paullinia cupana, p. 45)*, maté *(Ilex paraguariensis, p. 39)*, coffee, tea, chocolate, and caffeine supplements – can increase the activity of liver enzymes that break down and remove various chemicals, hormones, drugs, and toxic substances from your body. Thus taking caffeine lessens the effectiveness of certain herbs and drugs.

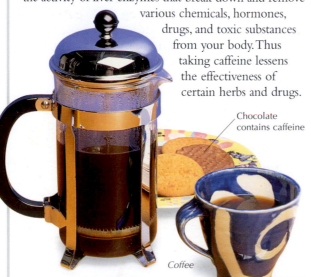

Chocolate contains caffeine

Coffee

CHARBROILED FOODS

Like caffeine, charbroiled foods speed up your body's metabolism of certain herbs and drugs. If an herb is removed from your body too quickly the treatment will be less effective, so avoid charbroiled foods.

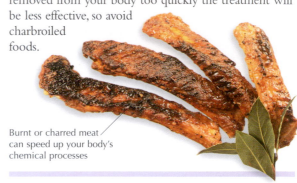

Burnt or charred meat can speed up your body's chemical processes

HIGH-FIBER FOODS

Foods that are high in fiber, such as beans, whole grains, and large amounts of fresh fruits and vegetables, can decrease the effectiveness of herbs. Fiber can prevent your body from absorbing enough of an herb's active ingredient. Be sure to take herbal remedies two hours before eating high-fiber foods or taking fiber supplements.

Apple

Kidney beans

MIGRAINE TRIGGERS

When taking herbs such as feverfew *(Tanacetum parthenium, p. 55)* to treat migraines, avoid foods that are known to trigger migraines. Such foods include:

- red wine
- beer
- chocolate
- aged cheeses
- caffeine
- some food additives such as MSG and nitrates
- smoked and cured foods
- overripe produce.

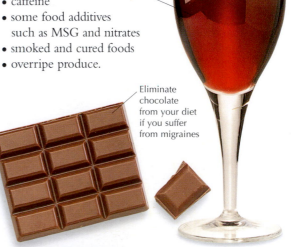

Prevent migraines by avoiding red wine

Eliminate chocolate from your diet if you suffer from migraines

TYRAMINE-CONTAINING FOODS

The amino acid tyramine, which is present in many foods, can cause a dangerous interaction with St. John's wort *(Hypericum perforatum, p. 39)*. This is because St. John's wort may work in the same way as the antidepressant drugs known as monoamine oxidase inhibitors (MAOIs), which include phenelzine, isocarboxazid, and tranylcypromine. When people who take these drugs eat foods high in tyramine, they may become nauseated or dizzy. The same effect can occur in people who take St. John's wort.

If you are taking St. John's wort, avoid foods high in tyramine, which include:

• alcohol in any form, including beer, wine, and liquor
• cheese, yogurt, and other cultured or aged dairy foods
• fermented and pickled foods, including sauerkraut, pickles, olives, pickled herring, and soy sauce
• smoked and preserved meats, including bacon, bologna, salami, and pepperoni
• organ meats such as liver or kidneys
• some fruits and vegetables, including bananas, avocados, figs, and pineapples
• all dried fruits such as prunes and raisins
• nuts and seeds, including peanuts
• caffeine
• chocolate.

Your physician can provide you with a comprehensive list of tyramine-containing foods.

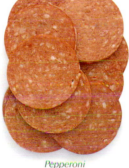

Olives   *Pepperoni*

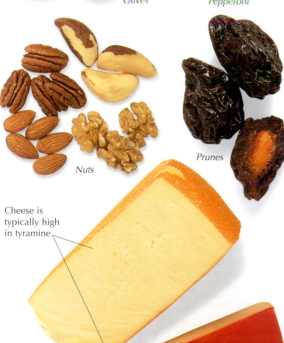

Nuts   *Prunes*

Cheese is typically high in tyramine

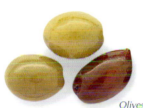

POTASSIUM-RICH FOODS

Potassium, an essential mineral, can be reduced to dangerously low levels if you use herbal diuretics such as buchu *(Barosma betulina, p. 24)*, dandelion *(Taraxacum officinale, p. 56)*, or uva ursi *(Arcostaphylos uva-ursi, p. 21)*. To make sure you get enough potassium while using these herbs, eat at least one serving a day of potassium-rich fruits and vegetables such as:

• avocados
• bananas
• beans
• kiwi fruits
• orange juice
• potatoes
• tomatoes

Bananas are high in potassium

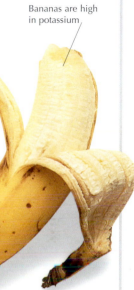

Avocado

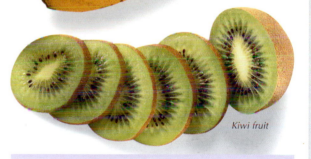

Kiwi fruit

WHOLE GRAINS

Whole grains are important for your diet, but they contain natural substances known as phytates that can block your absorption of herbs (and some minerals). To avoid this problem, take your herbs and mineral supplements two hours before eating whole grain foods (such as whole wheat bread, brown rice, bulgur, oat bran, wheat bran, wheat berries, cracked wheat, wild rice, buckwheat, and barley).

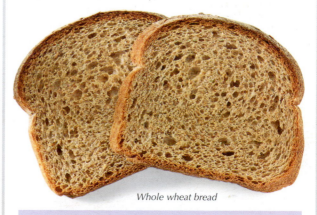

Whole wheat bread

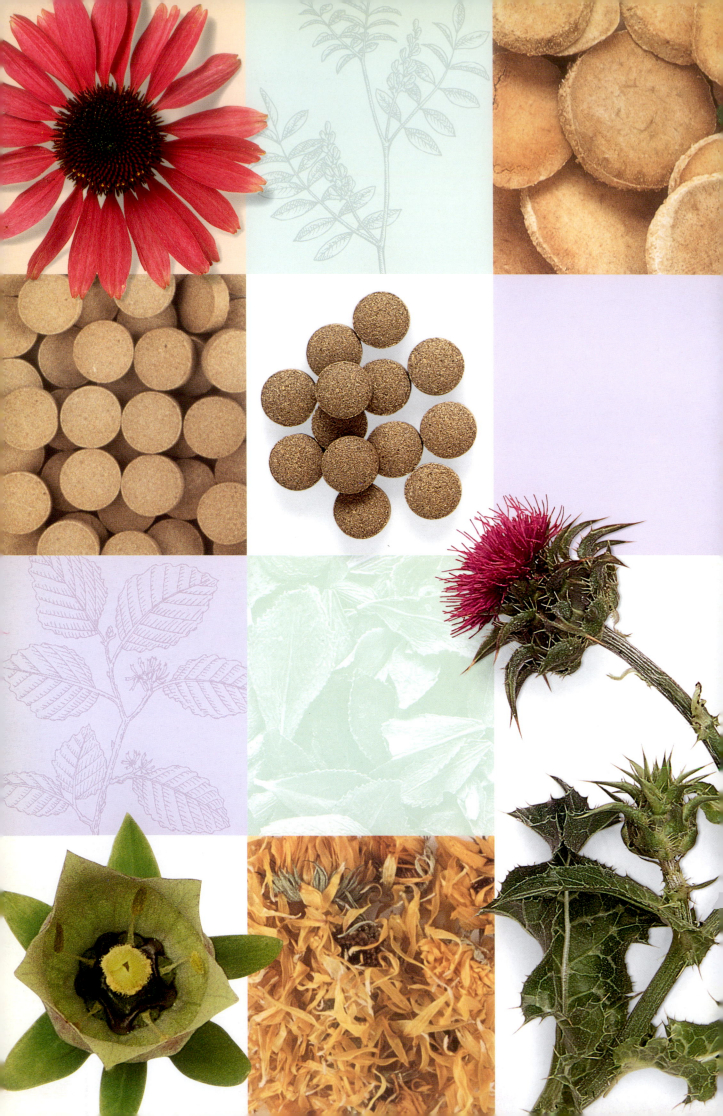

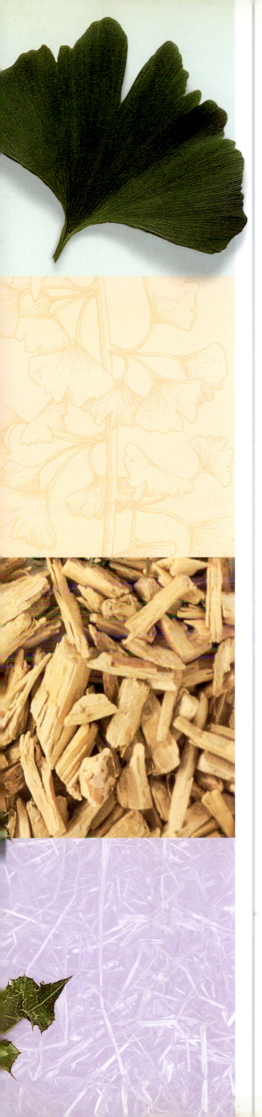

CHAPTER 4

DIETARY SUPPLEMENT -HERB INTERACTIONS

DIETARY SUPPLEMENTS SUCH as vitamins, minerals, and other substances can have powerful beneficial effects on your health. The right dietary supplement in combination with the right herb can be even more beneficial – but the wrong combination may have no effect, and could even be harmful. Here you'll learn about the supplements and herbs that work together to improve your health, and those combinations that you should avoid.

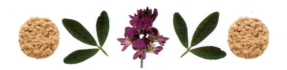

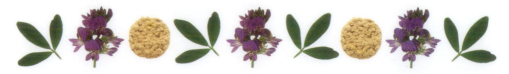

UNDERSTANDING DIETARY SUPPLEMENT-HERB INTERACTIONS

MANY COMMON health problems can be treated effectively with a combination of herbs and supplements – nutrients, vitamins, and minerals, some of which occur naturally in our bodies. For example, vitamin C and echinacea *(Echinacea angustifolia, p. 33)* can both help shorten the duration of a common cold; when taken together, they work to get you back on your feet even faster.

Over the years, herbal practitioners have learned which herbs and dietary supplements work safely in combination to treat many health problems. When used properly, these herb–supplement combinations can be gentler and safer than drugs. They are also usually slower to act; you may have to take the combination for several days or longer to feel the benefits.

BENEFICIAL COMBINATIONS
Echinacea and vitamin C tablets can work powerfully to beat minor illnesses if you take them together.

❖ AVOIDING NEGATIVE INTERACTIONS ❖

This chapter contains beneficial herb–supplement combinations and potentially harmful interactions. It is best not to experiment with supplements and herbs; you may combine two substances that work well together, but it is equally likely they won't have any positive effect – and they may even interact negatively.

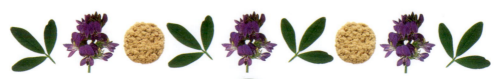

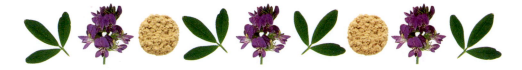

WORDS OF CAUTION

BEFORE you take a supplement and an herb together, first read the herb's full entry in Chapter 1. There you will find more information, including actions, cautions, and standardization information. Be certain you understand how the herb works and make sure that it is safe for you to take.

Like herbs, dietary supplements must be used with caution. In particular, it is important to avoid large doses of vitamins and minerals. For example, many people find that large amounts of vitamin C (usually in dosages of more than 1,000 mg daily) can cause diarrhea; large amounts of trace minerals such as selenium can be toxic. Always start with the smallest recommended dosage, increasing it gradually if needed. Do not exceed the maximum recommended dosage unless your physician specifically advises it.

If you would like to continue taking your usual supplements and medications while also taking an herbal product on a short-term basis, talk to your physician to be sure the combination is safe. If you have a chronic health problem such as diabetes or heart disease, discuss herbs and dietary supplements with your physician before you try them.

Pay attention to any side effects; if you experience dizziness, nausea, skin rashes, or other unpleasant symptoms within a few hours of using a dietary supplement–herb combination, stop taking it.

❖ SEDATIVE EFFECTS ❖

When herbs and dietary supplements that both have a sedative effect are combined, such as calcium and passionflower (*Passiflora incarnata, p. 45*), they tend to reinforce each other. Herbal practitioners often recommend these combinations to treat anxiety or insomnia. But other combinations, such as melatonin and St. John's wort (*Hypericum perforatum, p. 39*) can be dangerous, so do not combine sedative supplements and herbs unless they are recognized as safe.

ST. JOHN'S WORT
The popular sedative herbal remedy St. John's wort should not be taken in combination with certain herbs, dietary supplements or prescribed drugs.

Take appropriate precautions when using safe sedative supplement–herb combinations: make sure you are in a safe place and that you won't have to drive, supervise small children, operate machinery, or do anything else that requires alertness. Do not

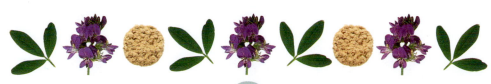

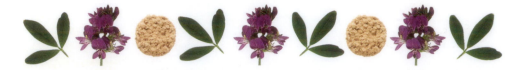

combine sedative supplements and herbs with alcohol, other types of sedatives, or other substances that cause drowsiness – a dangerous interaction could occur.

❖ CHOOSING SUPPLEMENTS WISELY ❖

When selecting supplements, look for high-quality products from well-known, reliable manufacturers; these companies follow good manufacturing practices similar to those required by the FDA for drug companies. Avoid products that claim to give "miraculous" or "instant" results. If you don't know what a supplement does, don't buy it, or if you need help in selecting supplements, ask your pharmacist. To ensure that your supplements will be fresh and effective, buy only enough to last a month to six weeks. Store them in a cool, dry place away from light and out of the reach of children.

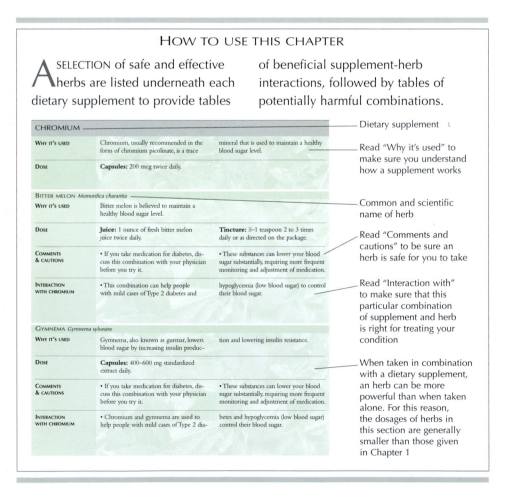

HOW TO USE THIS CHAPTER

A SELECTION of safe and effective herbs are listed underneath each dietary supplement to provide tables of beneficial supplement-herb interactions, followed by tables of potentially harmful combinations.

Dietary supplement

Read "Why it's used" to make sure you understand how a supplement works

Common and scientific name of herb

Read "Comments and cautions" to be sure an herb is safe for you to take

Read "Interaction with" to make sure that this particular combination of supplement and herb is right for treating your condition

When taken in combination with a dietary supplement, an herb can be more powerful than when taken alone. For this reason, the dosages of herbs in this section are generally smaller than those given in Chapter 1

CHROMIUM

WHY IT'S USED	Chromium, usually recommended in the form of chromium picolinate, is a trace	mineral that is used to maintain a healthy blood sugar level.
DOSE	**Capsules:** 200 mcg twice daily.	

BITTER MELON *Momordica charantia*

WHY IT'S USED	Bitter melon is believed to maintain a healthy blood sugar level.	
DOSE	**Juice:** 1 ounce of fresh bitter melon juice twice daily.	**Tincture:** ½–1 teaspoon 2 to 3 times daily or as directed on the package.
COMMENTS & CAUTIONS	• If you take medication for diabetes, discuss this combination with your physician before you try it.	• These substances can lower your blood sugar substantially, requiring more frequent monitoring and adjustment of medication.
INTERACTION WITH CHROMIUM	• This combination can help people with mild cases of Type 2 diabetes and	hypoglycemia (low blood sugar) to control their blood sugar.

GYMNEMA *Gymnema sylvestre*

WHY IT'S USED	Gymnema, also known as gurmar, lowers blood sugar by increasing insulin produc-	tion and lowering insulin resistance.
DOSE	**Capsules:** 400–600 mg standardized extract daily.	
COMMENTS & CAUTIONS	• If you take medication for diabetes, discuss this combination with your physician before you try it.	• These substances can lower your blood sugar substantially, requiring more frequent monitoring and adjustment of medication.
INTERACTION WITH CHROMIUM	• Chromium and gymnema are used to help people with mild cases of Type 2 dia-	betes and hypoglycemia (low blood sugar) control their blood sugar.

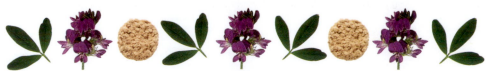

BENEFICIAL DIETARY SUPPLEMENT-HERB INTERACTIONS

BORON

WHY IT'S USED	Boron, a trace mineral necessary for good health, helps maintain strong bones and	may stimulate estrogen production.
DOSE	**Tablets:** 1–3 mg daily.	
COMMENTS & CAUTIONS	• Boron is found in many multivitamin and mineral formulations. Good dietary sources of boron include apples, beans, grapes, nuts, pears, peaches, and raisins.	• Do not use boron if you take oral contraceptives, are on hormone replacement therapy, or have a history of breast or reproductive cancer.

BLACK COHOSH ROOT *Cimicifuga racemosa rhizoma*

WHY IT'S USED	Black cohosh is used to help relieve symptoms of premenstrual syndrome (PMS) and menopause, especially hot flashes.
DOSE	**Capsules:** 150–500 mg twice daily. **Tincture:** ½–1 teaspoon 3 times daily or as directed on the package.
COMMENTS & CAUTIONS	• Do not use black cohosh root if you are pregnant. • Do not take for more than six months without the supervision of your physician.
INTERACTION WITH BORON	• Together boron and black cohosh can help relieve menopausal symptoms, especially hot flashes.

Black cohosh

DONG QUAI *Angelica sinensis*

WHY IT'S USED	Dong quai is used for variety of women's health problems such as premenstrual syndrome (PMS), menstrual cramps, and	irregular menstruation, and menopausal symptoms, especially hot flashes.
DOSE	**Capsules:** 250–500 mg 3 times daily. **Tincture:** ½–1 teaspoon 3 times daily or as directed on the package.	
COMMENTS & CAUTIONS	• Do not take dong quai if you are pregnant.	• Avoid prolonged exposure to sunlight and tanning lamps while taking dong quai.
INTERACTION WITH BORON	• Together boron and dong quai relieve premenstrual syndrome (PMS), painful	menstruation, fibrocystic breast disease, and menopausal symptoms, especially hot flashes.

CALCIUM

WHY IT'S USED	Calcium is a mineral that promotes bone, muscle, and nerve health and relieves	insomnia and irritability.
DOSE	**Tablets:** 600 mg twice daily, or 1,200 mg at bedtime.	

CHAMOMILE *Chamaemelum nobile* (Roman), *Matricaria recutita* (German)

WHY IT'S USED	Chamomile is used to relieve anxiety.	
DOSE	**Capsules and tablets:** Follow package directions.	**Tincture:** ¼–½ teaspoon 2 to 3 times daily or as directed on the package.
COMMENTS & CAUTIONS	• Do not use chamomile if you are severely allergic to ragweed or plants	in the daisy family such as cornflower or mugwort *(Artemisia vulgaris, p. 22)*.
INTERACTION WITH CALCIUM	• Calcium and chamomile are used together to relieve stress and insomnia.	

HORSETAIL *Equisetum arvense*

WHY IT'S USED	Horsetail contains silicon, which is used to promote bone and joint health.	
DOSE	**Capsules:** 1,000 mg up to 3 times daily. **Liquid extract:** ½ teaspoon up to 3 times daily or as directed on the package.	**Tincture:** ½ teaspoon up to 3 times daily or as directed on the package.
COMMENTS & CAUTIONS	• Do not use horsetail if you are also taking digitalis-type drugs such as digoxin *(p. 147)*; a dangerous loss of potassium might occur.	• Buy only from a reputable manufacturer and purchase a product that has been treated to remove the enzyme thiaminase.
INTERACTION WITH CALCIUM	• Used together, calcium and horsetail help maintain healthy bones and prevent	osteoporosis (thin, brittle bones that break easily).

PASSIONFLOWER *Passiflora incarnata*

WHY IT'S USED	Passionflower is a mild sedative that is used to treat insomnia.	
DOSE	**Capsules:** 1,000 mg up to 3 times daily for up to 7 days, or as directed by your physician.	**Tincture:** ¼ teaspoon twice daily or as directed on the package.
COMMENTS & CAUTIONS	• Do not use in combination with alcohol or other sedative herbs, supplements, or drugs; MAOI antidepressant drugs such as	phenelzine *(p. 180)*; or any prescription or nonprescription sleep aids. Excessive drowsiness may occur.
INTERACTION WITH CALCIUM	• Calcium and passionflower act as a mild sedative to help relieve stress and insomnia.	

VALERIAN *Valeriana officinalis*

WHY IT'S USED	Valerian is helpful for treating insomnia.	
DOSE	**Capsules:** 150–300 mg standardized extract 1 hour before bedtime. **Liquid extract:** ½–1 teaspoon 1 hour before	bedtime or as directed on the package. **Tincture:** ¾ teaspoon 1 hour before bedtime or as directed on the package.
COMMENTS & CAUTIONS	• Valerian appears to work best if it is taken regularly. The sedative effect increases over several weeks and then levels off.	• Because valerian has an unpleasant aroma and taste, many people prefer to use capsules.
INTERACTION WITH CALCIUM	• Calcium and valerian are used together to treat insomnia.	

CARNITINE

WHY IT'S USED	Carnitine is an amino acid, one of the building blocks that makes up protein. It strengthens the heart.
DOSE	**Capsules or tablets:** 500–1,500 mg twice daily 2 hours before or after meals.

HAWTHORN *Crataegus oxyacantha*

WHY IT'S USED	Hawthorn helps to strengthen the heart and circulatory system. It is also used to treat early-stage congestive heart failure.	
DOSE	**Capsules:** 100–300 mg standardized extract 2 to 3 times daily.	**Tincture:** 1 teaspoon up to 3 times daily or as directed on the package.
COMMENTS & CAUTIONS	• If you have heart disease and want to try this combination, discuss it with a physician	first, even if you do not take medication. • Benefits may take 4 to 12 weeks to be felt.
INTERACTION WITH CARNITINE	• Carnitine and hawthorn are used together to improve heart function in early-stage congestive heart failure.	

Hawthorn

CHOLINE

WHY IT'S USED	Choline is a vitamin that helps to metabolize fats in the liver.	
DOSE	**Capsules:** 250–500 mg twice daily.	
COMMENTS & CAUTIONS	• Because pure choline can cause an unpleasant body odor, many patients	prefer to use it in the form of phosphatidyl choline (PC).

BEET LEAF *Beta vulgaris*

WHY IT'S USED	Beet leaf supports the metabolic and digestive functions of the liver.
DOSE	**Capsules:** 2,500–5,000 mg twice daily.
COMMENTS & CAUTIONS	• Do not use this combination if you have gallstones, gallbladder disease, or biliary duct disease.
INTERACTION WITH CHOLINE	• Choline and beet leaf are used together to provide liver support.

DANDELION ROOT *Taraxacum officinale*

WHY IT'S USED	Dandelion root contains substances that support the metabolic and digestive	functions of the liver, stimulate the flow of digestive juices, and act as a diuretic.
DOSE	**Liquid extract:** 1–2 teaspoons 3 times daily before meals or as directed on the	package. **Tincture:** ½ teaspoon 3 times daily before meals or as directed on the package.
COMMENTS & CAUTIONS	• If you have gallstones, gallbladder disease, or biliary duct disease, discuss this	combination with your physician before you try it.
INTERACTION WITH CHOLINE	• Together this combination nourishes and supports the liver.	

CHOLINE, CONTINUED

MILK THISTLE *Silybum marianum*

WHY IT'S USED	Milk thistle contains silymarin, a compound that protects liver cells against damage and stimulates regeneration.
DOSE	**Capsules:** 250 mg standardized extract 2 times daily.
COMMENTS & CAUTIONS	If you have gallstones, gallbladder disease, or biliary duct disease, discuss this combination with your physician first.
INTERACTION WITH CHOLINE	• Together choline and milk thistle provide liver support, especially in cases of hepatitis, jaundice, and cirrhosis.

Milk thistle

CHROMIUM

WHY IT'S USED	Chromium, usually recommended in the form of chromium picolinate, is a trace	mineral that is used to maintain a healthy blood sugar level.
DOSE	**Capsules:** 200 mcg twice daily.	

BITTER MELON *Momordica charantia*

WHY IT'S USED	Bitter melon is believed to maintain a healthy blood sugar level.	
DOSE	**Juice:** 1 ounce of fresh bitter melon juice twice daily.	**Tincture:** ½–1 teaspoon 2 to 3 times daily or as directed on the package.
COMMENTS & CAUTIONS	• If you take medication for diabetes, discuss this combination with your physician before you try it.	• These substances can lower blood sugar levels substantially, requiring more frequent monitoring and adjustment of medication.
INTERACTION WITH CHROMIUM	• This combination can help people with mild cases of Type 2 diabetes and	hypoglycemia (low blood sugar) to control their blood sugar.

GYMNEMA *Gymnema sylvestre*

WHY IT'S USED	Gymnema, also known as gurmar, lowers blood sugar levels by increasing insulin	production and lowering insulin resistance.
DOSE	**Capsules:** 400–600 mg standardized extract daily.	
COMMENTS & CAUTIONS	• If you take medication for diabetes, discuss this combination with your physician before you try it.	• These substances can lower blood sugar levels substantially, requiring more frequent monitoring and adjustment of medication.
INTERACTION WITH CHROMIUM	• Chromium and gymnema are used to help people with mild cases of Type 2	diabetes and hypoglycemia (low blood sugar) control their blood sugar levels.

COENZYME Q_{10}

WHY IT'S USED	Coenzyme Q_{10}, also known as CoQ_{10} or ubiquinone, is found naturally in the body and converts food into energy.	
DOSE	**Tablets:** 25–75 mg twice daily.	

HAWTHORN *Crataegus oxyacantha*

WHY IT'S USED	Hawthorn is used to support cardiovascular health. It is also used to	treat early-stage congestive heart failure.
DOSE	**Capsules:** 100–300 mg standardized extract 2 to 3 times daily.	**Tincture:** 1 teaspoon 3 times daily or as directed on the package.
COMMENTS & CAUTIONS	• Do not use if you take a blood-thinning drug such as warfarin (*p. 195*). • If you have heart disease and want to try	this combination, discuss it with a physician, even if you do not take any medication. • Benefits may take several months.
INTERACTION WITH COENZYME Q_{10}	• Together, CoQ_{10} and hawthorn are used to improve heart function for conditions	that involve a weakening of the heart such as early-stage congestive heart failure.

GLUTATHIONE

WHY IT'S USED	Glutathione is one of the body's most abundant natural antioxidants (substances that reduce the damage of free radicals);	it is critical for normal liver and kidney function.
DOSE	**Capsules:** 250 mg 1–2 times daily or as directed by your physician.	

DANDELION ROOT *Taraxacum officinale*

WHY IT'S USED	Dandelion root contains substances that support the metabolic and digestive	functions of the liver, stimulate the flow of digestive juices, and act as a diuretic.
DOSE	**Liquid extract:** 1–2 teaspoons 3 times daily before meals or as directed on the package.	**Tincture:** ½ teaspoon 3 times daily before meals or as directed on the package.
COMMENTS & CAUTIONS	• If you have gallstones, gallbladder disease, or biliary duct disease, discuss dandelion root with your physician before you try it.	
INTERACTION WITH GLUTATHIONE	• This combination is used to support liver and kidney function.	

Dandelion

MILK THISTLE *Silybum marianum*

WHY IT'S USED	Milk thistle contains silymarin, a compound that protects liver cells against damage and stimulates regeneration.	
DOSE	**Capsules:** 250 mg standardized extract 2 times daily.	
COMMENTS & CAUTIONS	• If you have gallstones, gallbladder disease, or biliary duct disease, discuss this	combination with your physician before you try it.
INTERACTION WITH GLUTATHIONE	• Glutathione and milk thistle support liver function. This combination is	especially helpful in cases of hepatitis, jaundice, and cirrhosis.

INOSITOL

WHY IT'S USED	Inositol is a vitamin that aids in the metabolism of fat and cholesterol, and	helps remove fats from the liver.
DOSE	**Capsules:** 500 mg 1–2 times daily.	

DANDELION ROOT *Taraxacum officinale*

WHY IT'S USED	Dandelion root contains substances that support the metabolic and digestive	functions of the liver, stimulate the flow of digestive juices, and act as a diuretic.
DOSE	**Liquid extract:** 1–2 teaspoons 3 times daily before meals or as directed on the package.	**Tincture:** ½ teaspoon 3 times daily before meals or as directed on the package.
COMMENTS & CAUTIONS	• If you have gallstones, gallbladder disease, or biliary duct disease, discuss this	combination with your physician before you try it.
INTERACTION WITH INOSITOL	• This combination provides liver support.	

MILK THISTLE *Silybum marianum*

WHY IT'S USED	Milk thistle contains silymarin, a compound that protects liver cells against damage and stimulates regeneration.
DOSE	**Capsules:** 250 mg standardized extract 2 times daily.
COMMENTS & CAUTIONS	• Especially helpful in cases of hepatitis, jaundice, and cirrhosis. • If you have gallstones, gallbladder disease, or biliary duct disease, discuss this combination with your physician first.
INTERACTION WITH INOSITOL	• Inositol and milk thistle provide liver support.

Milk thistle

MAGNESIUM

WHY IT'S USED	Magnesium, an essential trace mineral, helps maintain normal blood pressure.
DOSE	**Tablets:** 125–175 mg twice daily.
COMMENTS & CAUTIONS	• Large doses of magnesium can cause diarrhea.

COLEUS *Coleus forskohlii*

WHY IT'S USED	Coleus is used to treat high blood pressure and angina (a condition causing chest pain).	
DOSE	**Capsules:** 50 mg standardized extract 2 to 3 times daily.	
COMMENTS & CAUTIONS	• Use only under a physician's supervision. • Extra precautions may be necessary if you	take blood-thinning drugs such as warfarin (*p. 195*), or drugs for high blood pressure.
INTERACTION WITH MAGNESIUM	• This combination helps to reduce high blood pressure.	

MAGNESIUM, CONTINUED

GINKGO *Ginkgo biloba*

WHY IT'S USED	Ginkgo extract contains compounds that are believed to keep blood vessels opened.
DOSE	**Tablets:** 60–120 mg standardized extract twice daily.
COMMENTS & CAUTIONS	• Use only under a physician's supervision. • Extra precautions may be necessary if you take blood-thinning drugs such as warfarin (*p. 195*) or medication for high blood pressure.
INTERACTION WITH MAGNESIUM	• This combination can help reduce high blood pressure, especially if caused by arteriosclerosis (hardening of arterial walls).

Ginkgo

METHIONINE

WHY IT'S USED	Methionine is an amino acid, one of the building blocks that makes up protein. It metabolizes fats in the liver.
DOSE	**Capsules:** 500 mg twice daily.
COMMENTS & CAUTIONS	• Take a daily vitamin B complex supplement while using methionine, since methionine can increase the risk of atherosclerosis and heart disease in those people with a deficiency in B vitamins.

BEET LEAF *Beta vulgaris*

WHY IT'S USED	Beet leaf supports the metabolic and digestive functions of the liver.
DOSE	**Capsules:** 2,500–5,000 mg twice daily.
COMMENTS & CAUTIONS	• Do not use if you have gallstones, gall-bladder disease, or biliary duct disease.
INTERACTION WITH METHIONINE	This combination is used to provide liver support.

DANDELION ROOT *Taraxacum officinale*

WHY IT'S USED	Dandelion root contains substances that support the metabolic and digestive	functions of the liver, stimulate the flow of digestive juices, and act as a diuretic.
DOSE	**Liquid extract:** 1–2 teaspoons 3 times daily before meals or as directed on the package.	**Tincture:** ½ teaspoon 3 times daily before meals or as directed on the package.
COMMENTS & CAUTIONS	• If you have gallstones, gallbladder disease, or biliary duct disease, discuss this combination with a physician before you try it.	
INTERACTION WITH METHIONINE	• This combination is used to provide liver support.	

METHIONINE, CONTINUED
MILK THISTLE *Silybum marianum*

WHY IT'S USED	Milk thistle contains silymarin, a compound that protects liver cells against damage and stimulates regeneration.
DOSE	**Capsules:** 250 mg standardized extract 2 times daily.
COMMENTS & CAUTIONS	• If you have gallstones, gallbladder disease, or biliary duct disease, discuss this combination with your physician before you try it.
INTERACTION WITH METHIONINE	• This combination is helpful for supporting the liver, especially in cases of hepatitis, jaundice, and cirrhosis.

N-ACETYLCYSTEINE (NAC)

WHY IT'S USED	N-acetylcysteine increases your body's levels of glutathione, a substance that is important for healthy liver and lung function.
DOSE	**Capsules:** 125–750 mg twice daily.
COMMENTS & CAUTIONS	• When taken for more than two weeks, NAC may cause the loss of trace minerals such as zinc from the body; be sure to discuss a daily mineral supplement with your physician.

BEET LEAF *Beta vulgaris*

WHY IT'S USED	Beet leaf supports the metabolic and digestive functions of the liver.
DOSE	**Capsules:** 2,500–5,000 mg twice daily.
COMMENTS & CAUTIONS	• If you have gallstones, gallbladder disease, or biliary duct disease, discuss this combination with your physician before you try it.
INTERACTION WITH N-ACETYLCYSTEINE (NAC)	• This combination is used to provide liver support.

DANDELION ROOT *Taraxacum officinale*

WHY IT'S USED	Dandelion root contains substances that support the metabolic and digestive functions of the liver, stimulate the flow of digestive juices, and act as a diuretic.
DOSE	**Capsules:** 2,500–5,000 mg twice daily.
COMMENTS & CAUTIONS	• If you have gallstones, gallbladder disease, or biliary duct disease, discuss this combination with your physician first.
INTERACTION WITH N-ACETYLCYSTEINE (NAC)	• This combination is used to support liver function.

Dandelion

N-ACETYLCYSTEINE (NAC), CONTINUED

MILK THISTLE *Silybum marianum*

WHY IT'S USED	Milk thistle contains silymarin, a compound that protects liver cells against damage and stimulates regeneration.
DOSE	**Capsules:** 250 mg standardized extract 2 times daily.
COMMENTS & CAUTIONS	• If you have gallstones, gallbladder disease, or biliary duct disease, discuss this combination with your physician first.
INTERACTION WITH N-ACETYLCYSTEINE (NAC)	• This combination is helpful for treating liver problems caused by exposure to drugs, industrial chemicals, and other toxins.

Milk thistle

WILD CHERRY *Prunus serotina*

WHY IT'S USED	Wild cherry relieves coughs.	
DOSE	**Tincture:** ½ teaspoon up to 3 times daily or as directed on the package.	
COMMENTS & CAUTIONS	• Pregnant and nursing women should not use this combination.	• This herb has a sedative effect; use with caution.
INTERACTION WITH N-ACETYLCYSTEINE (NAC)	• NAC and wild cherry are used together to treat coughs resulting from upper respiratory infections such as colds, flu,	and bronchitis. This combination is most useful for treating coughing accompanied by mucus.

TAURINE

WHY IT'S USED	Taurine is an amino acid, one of the building blocks that makes up protein. It is used to help regulate the heartbeat.
DOSE	**Capsules or tablets:** 2,000 mg 3 times daily 2 hours before or after food.

HAWTHORN *Crataegus oxyacantha*

WHY IT'S USED	Hawthorn is used to support heart function and blood vessel integrity. It is also used to treat early-stage congestive heart failure.	
DOSE	**Capsules:** 100–300 mg standardized extract 2 to 3 times daily. **Tincture:** 1 teaspoon 3 times daily or as directed on the package.	
COMMENTS & CAUTIONS	• If you have heart disease and want to try this combination, discuss it with a physician	even if you do not take any medication. • Benefits may take 4 to 12 weeks to be felt.
INTERACTION WITH TAURINE	• This combination is used to strengthen the heart and regulate the heartbeat,	especially in early-stage congestive heart failure.

Hawthorn

VITAMIN B COMPLEX

WHY IT'S USED	All the B vitamins are important for proper nerve function and for releasing energy within your body's cells.
DOSE	**Tablets:** 1 B–50 or B–100 tablet daily.
COMMENTS & CAUTIONS	• Select a vitamin B formula that contains at least 400 mcg of biotin, folic acid, and B$_{12}$, and 50 or 100 mg of the other B vitamins.

GINSENG *Panax ginseng, P. quinquefolium*

WHY IT'S USED	Ginseng is helpful for improving overall energy and concentration.	
DOSE	**Tablets or capsules:** 100 mg standardized extract 2 times daily. **Powdered root** (nonstandardized): 1,000–2,000 mg 2 times daily.	**Tincture:** ½ teaspoon up to 3 times daily or as directed on the package.
COMMENTS & CAUTIONS	• If you have diabetes or take medication for a seizure disorder, discuss this combination with your physician. • Ginseng may raise your blood pressure; do not use it if you also take medication for high blood pressure.	• Because ginseng has a mildly stimulating effect, do not combine it with caffeine-containing herbs such as coffee or tea. • Do not use this combination for more than two weeks in a row without the supervision of your physician.
INTERACTION WITH VITAMIN B COMPLEX	• This combination improves general energy and vitality, especially during times of stress or fatigue.	

VITAMIN B$_6$ (PYRIDOXINE)

WHY IT'S USED	Vitamin B$_6$ is important for normal brain function and mood; supplemental vitamin B$_6$ is used to treat anxiety and depression.
DOSE	**Tablets:** 100 mg daily.

KAVA KAVA *Piper methysticum*

WHY IT'S USED	Kava is a mild sedative that relieves anxiety.
DOSE	**Capsules:** 250 mg standardized extract 3 times daily. **Tincture:** ¼ teaspoon up to 3 times daily or as directed on the package.
COMMENTS & CAUTIONS	• Do not take use this combination for longer than three months without medical supervision. • Do not use in combination with alcohol, other sedative substances, cold remedies, antihistamines, or prescription medications for depression or anxiety. • The antianxiety effects of this combination may take several weeks.
INTERACTION WITH VITAMIN B$_6$	• This combination works synergistically to relieve anxiety.

Kava

VITAMIN B₆ (PYRIDOXINE), CONTINUED

ST. JOHN'S WORT *Hypericum perforatum*

WHY IT'S USED	St. John's wort is used to relieve mild anxiety and depression.	
DOSE	**Capsules:** 300 mg standardized extract 3 times daily.	
COMMENTS & CAUTIONS	• Discuss this combination with your physician before you try it. Do not use prescription medications for depression or anxiety while taking this combination. • St. John's wort *(Hypericum perforatum, p. 39)* can interact negatively with a number of prescription drugs.	• The antianxiety effects of this combination may take a month or more to be felt.
INTERACTION WITH VITAMIN B₆	• Vitamin B₆ and St. John's wort are used together to treat anxiety and depression.	

St. John's wort

VITAMIN C

WHY IT'S USED	Vitamin C is used to prevent colds and flu, and to prevent allergic responses.	
DOSE	**Tablets:** 500 mg 3 to 4 times daily.	
COMMENTS & CAUTIONS	• Single large doses of vitamin C (more than 1,500 mg daily) can cause diarrhea.	

ECHINACEA *Echinacea angustifolia, E. purpurea*

WHY IT'S USED	Echinacea supports the immune system and helps prevent and treat colds,	flu, and infections.
DOSE	**Capsules:** 200–300 mg 3 times daily. **Liquid extract:** ¼–½ teaspoon 3 times daily or as directed on the package.	**Tincture:** ¾–1 teaspoon 3 times daily or as directed on the package.
COMMENTS & CAUTIONS	• Echinacea should not be used if you have an autoimmune disease such as lupus or multiple sclerosis.	• Do not use echinacea if you are allergic to plants in the daisy family such as cornflower *(Centaurea cyanus)* or mugwort *(Artemisia vulgaris, p. 22).*
INTERACTION WITH VITAMIN C	• This combination is used to provide immune support and help prevent and	treat colds, flu, and infections.

STINGING NETTLE LEAF *Urtica dioica*

WHY IT'S USED	Stinging nettle leaves are high in a substance called quercetin, which can help	block allergic responses.
DOSE	**Capsules:** 300 mg of freeze-dried leaf 2 to 3 times daily.	**Liquid extract:** ½ teaspoon 3 times daily or as directed on the package.
COMMENTS & CAUTIONS	• May cause digestive upset in sensitive individuals.	
INTERACTION WITH VITAMIN C	• This combination is helpful for relieving allergy symptoms, especially those	resulting from hay fever and seasonal pollen allergies.

ZINC

WHY IT'S USED	Zinc is an essential mineral that is important for immune and prostate function.	
DOSE	**Lozenges:** Up to 6 daily. **Tablets:** 30 mg daily.	
COMMENTS & CAUTIONS	• To treat colds, use lozenges made from zinc gluconate with glycine; let the lozenge dissolve slowly in your mouth. •To reduce the chances of nausea, take the lozenges after a meal or snack. • Zinc lozenges may leave a metallic aftertaste; frequent use of zinc lozenges may affect your senses of taste and smell;	they will quickly return to normal after use is discontinued. • As a dietary supplement, zinc is absorbed best in the form of zinc gluconate or zinc citrate. • To avoid a copper deficiency, take 1–3 mg daily supplemental copper when taking zinc.

ECHINACEA *Echinacea angustifolia, E. purpurea*

WHY IT'S USED	Echinacea supports the immune system and helps prevent and treat colds,	flu, and infections.
DOSE	**Capsules:** 200–300 mg 3 times daily. **Liquid extract:** ¼–½ teaspoon 3 times daily or as directed on the package.	**Tincture:** ¾–1 teaspoon 3 times daily or as directed on the package.
COMMENTS & CAUTIONS	• A tingling or numbing sensation on the tongue is normal when using echinacea in liquid form. • Echinacea should not be used if you have an autoimmune disease such as lupus	or multiple sclerosis. • Do not use echinacea if you are allergic to plants in the daisy family such as cornflower (*Centaurea cyanus*) or mugwort (*Artemisia vulgaris, p. 22*).
INTERACTION WITH ZINC	• This combination is used to support immune function and to help prevent	infections. It is also helpful for shortening the duration of colds.

PYGEUM *Pygeum africanum*

WHY IT'S USED	Pygeum is used to treat benign prostatic hypertrophy (BPH) by reducing prostate	inflammation and inhibiting prostate growth.
DOSE	**Capsules:** 50–100 mg standardized extract 2 times daily.	
COMMENTS & CAUTIONS	• Do not diagnose BPH on your own; see your physician to rule out a more serious condition.	• The full effects of this combination may take six months or longer to be felt.
INTERACTION WITH ZINC	• This combination is helpful for treating male urinary problems, particularly frequent urination caused by enlarged	prostate (also called benign prostatic hypertrophy, or BPH).

SAW PALMETTO *Serenoa repens*

WHY IT'S USED	Saw palmetto berries contain substances that are helpful in the treatment of	enlarged prostate (also called benign prostatic hypertrophy, or BPH).
DOSE	**Capsules:** 160 mg standardized extract 2 times daily.	
COMMENTS & CAUTIONS	• Do not diagnose BPH on your own; see your physician to rule out a more serious condition.	• The full effects of this combination may take six months or longer to be felt.
INTERACTION WITH ZINC	• This combination is helpful for treating male urinary problems, particularly	frequent urination caused by an enlarged prostate.

POTENTIALLY HARMFUL DIETARY SUPPLEMENT-HERB INTERACTIONS

5-HTP

WHY IT'S USED	5-HTP, a form of the amino acid tryptophan, is used to relieve depression,	anxiety, and insomnia.
COMMENTS & CAUTIONS	• Do not use in combination with alcohol or other sedative herbs, supplements, or medications, or with antidepressants,	particularly selective serotonin reuptake inhibitors (SSRIs) such as fluoxetine *(p. 155)*.

ST. JOHN'S WORT *Hypericum perforatum*

WHY IT'S USED	St. John's wort is used to treat insomnia, anxiety, and mild depression.	
COMMENTS & CAUTIONS	• Do not use in combination with alcohol or other sedative herbs, supplements, or medications, or with antidepressants, particularly selective serotonin reuptake inhibitors (SSRIs) such as fluoxetine *(p. 155)*.	• Avoid prolonged exposure to sunlight or tanning lamps while taking St. John's wort.
INTERACTION WITH 5-HTP	• Together, these substances can cause excessive drowsiness.	

KAVA KAVA *Piper methysticum*

WHY IT'S USED	Kava is used to treat anxiety and insomnia.	
COMMENTS & CAUTIONS	• Do not use in combination with alcohol or other sedative herbs, supplements, or medications, or with antidepressants, particularly selective serotonin reuptake	inhibitors (SSRIs) such as fluoxetine *(p. 155)*.
INTERACTION WITH 5-HTP	• Together, these substances can cause excessive drowsiness.	

VALERIAN *Valeriana officinalis*

WHY IT'S USED	Valerian is commonly used to help treat insomnia and mild anxiety.	
COMMENTS & CAUTIONS	• Do not use in combination with alcohol or other sedative herbs, supplements, or medications, or with antidepressants,	particularly selective serotonin reuptake inhibitors (SSRIs) such as fluoxetine *(p. 155)*.
INTERACTION WITH 5-HTP	• Together, these two substances can cause excessive drowsiness.	

MELATONIN

WHY IT'S USED	Melatonin is a hormone that helps to regulate your body's sleep/wake cycle. It is	commonly used to treat insomnia and jet lag.
COMMENTS & CAUTIONS	• Do not use in combination with alcohol or other sedative herbs, supplements, or medications, or with antidepressants,	particularly selective serotonin reuptake inhibitors (SSRIs) such as fluoxetine *(p. 155)*.

ST. JOHN'S WORT *Hypericum perforatum*

WHY IT'S USED	St. John's wort is used to treat insomnia, anxiety, and mild depression.	
COMMENTS & CAUTIONS	• Do not use in combination with alcohol or other sedative herbs, supplements, or medications, or with antidepressants, particularly selective serotonin reuptake inhibitors (SSRIs) such as fluoxetine *(p. 155)*.	• Avoid prolonged exposure to sunlight or tanning lamps while taking St. John's wort.
INTERACTION WITH MELATONIN	• Together, these two substances can cause excessive drowsiness.	

KAVA KAVA *Piper methysticum*

WHY IT'S USED	Kava is used to treat anxiety and insomnia.	
COMMENTS & CAUTIONS	• Do not use in combination with alcohol or other sedative herbs, supplements, or medications, or with	antidepressants, particularly selective serotonin reuptake inhibitors (SSRIs) such as fluoxetine *(p. 155)*.
INTERACTION WITH MELATONIN	• Together, these two substances can cause excessive drowsiness.	

VALERIAN *Valeriana officinalis*

WHY IT'S USED	Valerian is used to help treat insomnia and mild anxiety.
COMMENTS & CAUTIONS	• Do not use in combination with alcohol or other sedative herbs, supplements, or medications, or with antidepressants, particularly selective serotonin reuptake inhibitors (SSRIs) such as fluoxetine *(p. 155)*.
INTERACTION WITH MELATONIN	• Together, these two substances can cause excessive drowsiness.

Valerian

SAME (S-ADENOSYLMETHIONINE)

WHY IT'S USED	SAMe (S-adenosylmethionine) is compound that is produced naturally in	your body; it relieves mild depression, anxiety, and insomnia.
COMMENTS & CAUTIONS	• Do not use in combination with alcohol or other sedative herbs, supplements, or medications, or with antidepressants,	particularly selective serotonin reuptake inhibitors (SSRIs) such as fluoxetine *(p. 155).*

ST. JOHN'S WORT *Hypericum perforatum*

WHY IT'S USED	St. John's wort is used to treat insomnia, anxiety, and mild depression.
COMMENTS & CAUTIONS	• Do not use in combination with alcohol or other sedative herbs, supplements, or medications, or with antidepressants, particularly selective serotonin reuptake inhibitors (SSRIs) such as fluoxetine *(p. 155).* • Avoid prolonged exposure to sunlight or tanning lamps while taking St. John's wort.
INTERACTION WITH SAME	• Because there isn't enough research on potential interactions between these two substances, and because both affect brain chemistry, this combination should be avoided.

St. John's wort

KAVA KAVA *Piper methysticum*

WHY IT'S USED	Kava is used to treat anxiety and insomnia.	
COMMENTS & CAUTIONS	• Do not combine either of these substances with alcohol or other sedative herbs, supplements, or medications, or	with antidepressants, particularly selective serotonin reuptake inhibitors (SSRIs) such as fluoxetine *(p. 155).*
INTERACTION WITH SAME	• In combination, these substances can cause excessive drowsiness.	

VALERIAN *Valeriana officinalis*

WHY IT'S USED	Valerian is used to help treat insomnia and mild anxiety.	
COMMENTS & CAUTIONS	• Do not use in combination with alcohol or other sedative herbs, supplements, or medications, or with antidepressants,	particularly selective serotonin reuptake inhibitors (SSRIs) such as fluoxetine *(p. 155).*
INTERACTION WITH SAME	• In combination, these two substances can cause excessive drowsiness.	

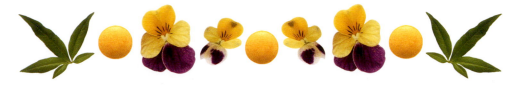

HOW TO USE THIS CHAPTER

ALL the prescription and non-prescription drugs mentioned in this chapter are listed alphabetically according to their generic name. Each drug entry contains the brand name or names, alongside the generic name, and lists the type of drug. A general description of the medication is also included, as well as the conditions or diseases for which it might be prescribed by physicians. Each entry contains a "Don't mix with" section that explains which herbs are known to interact negatively with a particular drug, and a "Do take with" section of beneficial herbs that can be taken together with a drug to enhance the effects of the drug on the body.

If you are taking a medication that is not listed in this section, consult your physician before you begin to take an herb. Never take an herb in combination with a prescription drug without checking this chapter first and making an appointment to see your physician.

Generic drug name

The intended action of the drug in the body

A drug may be known by more than one brand name

Each entry carries a full description of what a drug does, the effect it has on the body, and any dangerous side effects

ASPIRIN		BRAND NAMES Anacin, Bayer, Bufferin, Ecotrin, Empirin, others
TYPE OF DRUG	Pain reliever, fever reducer, and nonsteroidal anti-inflammatory drug	
DESCRIPTION	Aspirin, also known as acetylsalicylic acid, is one of the most commonly used non-prescription drugs throughout the world. Studies have shown that the long-term use of low-dose aspirin can reduce your risk of heart disease and stroke, and may also protect against developing Alzheimer's disease and some forms of cancer. Aspirin must be used with caution. Long-term use of aspirin can cause stomach irrita-	tion, gastrointestinal bleeding, and ulcers. It can also cause bleeding problems, particularly in people who also take blood-thinning medications. Do not give aspirin to children and teenagers. Reye syndrome, a rare but serious childhood illness, is associated with aspirin use.
DON'T MIX WITH	**Garlic** *(Allium sativum)*. Large amounts of garlic combined with aspirin may increase your risk of internal bleeding.	**Ginkgo** *(Ginkgo biloba)*. Taking this herb with aspirin may increase your risk of internal bleeding.
DO TAKE WITH	**Deglycyrrhizinated licorice** (also called DGL, derived from *Glycyrrhiza glabra*). DGL can help prevent stomach	irritation from aspirin. Consider taking licorice supplements (250 mg 2 to 3 times daily).
KEEP IN MIND	• Taking aspirin with vitamin E or bromelain may increase the risk of internal bleeding. • Mixing alcohol and aspirin can increase the risk of stomach irritation and ulcers. • Long-term use of aspirin can lower your folic acid and vitamin C levels. Consider taking supplements (400–800 mcg folate and 500 mg vitamin C daily).	• High doses of aspirin (more than 3 grams a day) can reduce zinc levels. Consider taking supplements (10 mg daily, taken with food to avoid stomach upset).

Always read "Don't mix with" to ensure that you will not have a negative interaction with a particular herb.

Read "Do take with" to check which herbs are safe to take with a drug, or which may benefit the action of the drug in the body.

Read "Keep in mind" to check for possible cautions or comments about the drug.

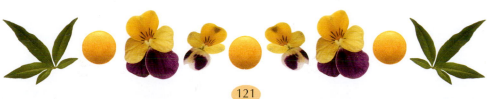

DRUG CATALOG

ACEBUTOLOL		BRAND NAME *Sectral*
TYPE OF DRUG	Beta blocker	
DESCRIPTION	Acebutolol is used to treat high blood pressure and abnormal heart rhythms. It is a powerful drug that can interact adversely with a number of prescription drugs; it must be used with caution. Be certain to tell your physician about any other prescription and nonprescription drugs and dietary supplements you are taking.	The antacid cimetidine *(p. 137)* and related antacids (known as H2-antagonists) such as famotidine *(p. 155)* and ranitidine *(p. 186)*, increase the amount of acebutolol absorbed from the gut into the bloodstream, thus increasing blood levels of this drug. Ask your physician or pharmacist to help you choose a different type of antacid.
DON'T MIX WITH	No known herbal interactions. However, because acebutolol has so many potential drug interactions, avoid taking any herbal	supplements unless they are recommended by your physician.
KEEP IN MIND	• Beta blockers impede your body's use of coenzyme Q_{10} (also known as CoQ_{10} or ubiquinone), which is needed for energy	production within your body's cells. Consider taking CoQ_{10} supplements (20–50 mg daily).

ACETAMINOPHEN	BRAND NAMES *Anacin 3, Aspirin-Free Excedrin, Bayer Select, Excedrin PM, Panadol, Tylenol, others*	
TYPE OF DRUG	Pain reliever and fever reducer	
DESCRIPTION	Acetaminophen is used to relieve fever and pain. It does not relieve inflammation. Acetaminophen is sold as a nonprescription drug, and is also used in many non-prescription drug combinations for treating pain, fever, and the symptoms of colds and flu. As a prescription drug for pain it is	usually used in combination with powerful narcotics. Note, however, that although acetaminophen is very widely used, there is a risk of liver damage if this drug is taken in large doses for long periods of time (a year or longer).
DON'T MIX WITH	No known herbal interactions.	
DO TAKE WITH	**Milk thistle** *(Silybum marianum)*. Silymarin, an active compound in milk thistle, may help prevent liver damage from long-term use of acetaminophen. Consider taking 150 mg 3 to 4 times daily.	**Schisandra** *(Schisandra chinensis)*. Animal studies show that a compound in this herb may help prevent liver damage caused by long-term use of acetaminophen. Consider taking 250 mg once or twice daily.
KEEP IN MIND	• To avoid the possibility of liver damage, do not drink alcohol while you are taking acetaminophen. According to a 1976 study, very large doses of vitamin C (over 3 grams a day) may increase the level of acetaminophen in your bloodstream by reducing the rate at which your body excretes the drug. As a	result, you could take less of the drug, but you may take too much accidentally. Both coenzyme Q_{10} (CoQ_{10} or ubiquinone) and the amino acid methionine may help prevent liver damage from the long-term use of acetaminophen. Consider taking 20–50 mg of CoQ_{10} or 250 mg of methionine daily.

Milk thistle

ACETAZOLAMIDE

TYPE OF DRUG	Carbonic anhydrase inhibitor diuretic
DESCRIPTION	Acetazolamide is prescribed for some people with glaucoma because it helps reduce pressure inside the eye. It is sometimes used to treat certain forms of epilepsy, altitude sickness, and heart disease.

DON'T MIX WITH

Herbal diuretics. Avoid herbal diuretics, including: bilberry leaf *(Vaccinium myrtillus)*, buchu *(Barosma betulina)*, burdock *(Arctium lappa)*, couch grass *(Agropyron repens)*, damiana *(Turnera diffusa)*, dandelion *(Taraxacum officinale)*, fennel seed *(Foeniculum vulgare)*, goldenrod *(Solidago virgaurea)*, horsetail *(Equisetum arvense)*, kava kava *(Piper methysticum)*, kola nut *(Cola* spp.*)*, marshmallow *(Althaea officinalis)*, maté *(Ilex paraguariensis)*, parsley *(Petroselinum* spp.*)*, sarsaparilla *(Smilax* spp.*)*, saw palmetto *(Serenoa repens)*, uva ursi *(Arctostaphylos uva-ursi)*, vervain *(Verbena* spp. and *V. hastata)*, and yarrow *(Achillea millefolium)*. Any other prescription or nonprescription diuretics should also be avoided, except on medical advice.

Herbal stimulants. Because stimulants can make glaucoma worse, avoid caffeine, ephedra *(Ephedra* spp.*)*, ginseng *(Panax ginseng)*, guarana *(Paullinia cupana)*, kola nut *(Cola* spp.*)*, maté *(Ilex paraguariensis)*, sarsaparilla *(Smilax* spp.*)*, yohimbe *(Pausinystalia yohimbe)*, and all other herbal stimulants. **Salicylate-containing herbs.** The herbs white willow bark *(Salix* spp.*)* and meadowsweet *(Filipendula ulmaria)* interact adversely with acetazolamide. Note that aspirin is a salicylate-containing drug; discuss alternatives to aspirin and aspirin-like drugs with your physician.

Bilberry

KEEP IN MIND

• Acetazolamide can decrease the potassium in your body. Eating two servings a day of potassium-rich foods (bananas, kiwis, oranges and other citrus fruits, and tomatoes) helps replace the lost potassium; your physician may also prescribe a potassium supplement.

ACYCLOVIR

TYPE OF DRUG	Antiviral
DESCRIPTION	Acyclovir is used to treat herpes simplex, shingles, chickenpox, and some other viral infections. It is usually used as an ointment applied to the skin; pills are generally prescribed only for patients who have frequent flare-ups of herpes blisters.
DON'T MIX WITH	No known herbal interactions.

KEEP IN MIND

• The amino acid arginine seems to encourage the growth of the herpes virus. Avoiding foods high in arginine, such as chocolate, wheat, oats, peanuts, nuts, and beer, may help prevent a flare-up.

• The amino acid lysine seems to inhibit the growth of the herpes virus. Eating foods rich in lysine, such as fish, chicken, lean meat, milk, and cheese, may help reduce the severity of a herpes flare-up. Consider taking lysine supplements (2,000–3,000 mg daily).

ALBUTEROL
BRAND NAMES *Proventil, Ventolin, Volmax*

TYPE OF DRUG	Bronchodilator
DESCRIPTION	Albuterol is used to treat and prevent asthma attacks. It is usually inhaled, but it can also be taken in tablet form.
DON'T MIX WITH	**Digitalis** (*Digitalis* spp., also known as foxglove, and *D. lanata*). This dangerous herb is very similar to the heart drug digoxin, which was originally derived from the plant. One study showed that albuterol reduces digoxin levels. Until more is known, do not take digitalis and albuterol concurrently.
KEEP IN MIND	• Several reports suggest that albuterol can lower your levels of calcium, magnesium, and potassium. The reports all involved albuterol that was given intravenously by injection or orally; none involved inhaled albuterol. However, whatever form you're taking, be sure you're getting enough of these minerals by eating foods rich in calcium (such as dairy products and fortified soy products), magnesium (such as nuts, beans, and dark-green leafy vegetables), and potassium (such as bananas, citrus fruits, beans, potatoes, and tomatoes).

Foxglove

ALENDRONATE
BRAND NAME *Fosamax*

TYPE OF DRUG	Bisphosphonate
DESCRIPTION	Alendronate is used to treat and prevent osteoporosis.
DON'T MIX WITH	No known herbal interactions.
KEEP IN MIND	• Alendronate should be taken on an empty stomach. Food or drink (aside from plain water) sharply reduce the absorption of this drug. • Both calcium supplements and the magnesium found in some antacids, such as Mylanta, may interfere with your absorption of alendronate. To be on the safe side, wait at least two hours after taking alendronate before taking either antacids or supplements. • Alendronate can cause abdominal pain and stomach ulcers. Taking aspirin or other anti-inflammatory drugs in addition to alendronate can increase the chances of developing stomach and intestinal problems. Bromelain, an enzyme derived from pineapple, and betaine HCl, a digestive supplement, can also cause digestive irritation when taken in conjunction with alendronate.

Pineapple

DRUG CATALOG

ALLOPURINOL

BRAND NAMES *Lopurin, Zurinol Purinol, Zyloprim*

TYPE OF DRUG	Antigout medication
DESCRIPTION	Allopurinol is used to treat gout, a very painful form of arthritis caused by too much uric acid in the blood. Taking allopurinol with ACE inhibitor drugs, such as captopril or enalapril, can cause a dangerous interaction. Be certain to tell your physician if you take any medication for high blood pressure.
DON'T MIX WITH	No known herbal interactions.
KEEP IN MIND	• People with gout tend to have much more acidic urine. Taking large doses of vitamin C can make your urine even more acidic, which could lead to an increased risk of kidney stones, according to some studies. The role of vitamin C in causing kidney stones is controversial, however. Discuss supplements with your physician. • Taking large doses of folic acid supplements may help lower uric acid levels. Discuss folic acid supplements with your physician before you try them.

AMANTADINE

BRAND NAME *Symmetrel*

TYPE OF DRUG	Antiparkinson's and antiviral medication
DESCRIPTION	Amantadine is prescribed for several different reasons. It is used to treat and prevent flu, particularly in elderly patients, to treat Parkinson's disease, and sometimes to treat multiple sclerosis.
DON'T MIX WITH	No known herbal interactions.
KEEP IN MIND	• Common side effects of amantadine include nausea, dizziness, and light-headedness. Alcohol worsens these side effects and should be completely avoided when taking amantadine.

AMILORIDE

BRAND NAMES *Midamor, Moduretic*

TYPE OF DRUG	Potassium-sparing diuretic
DESCRIPTION	Amiloride is used primarily to treat high blood pressure and congestive heart failure by reducing the amount of water in the body.

DON'T MIX WITH

Digitalis (*Digitalis* spp., also known as foxglove). This dangerous herb, from which the drug digoxin is derived, interacts with triamterene *(p. 193)* – a drug similar to amiloride – to increase the risk of body fluid imbalance. Until further information is made available, do not use digitalis while taking amiloride.

Herbal diuretics. Avoid herbal diuretics, including bilberry leaf *(Vaccinium myrtillus)*, buchu *(Barosma betulina)*, burdock *(Arctium lappa)*, couch grass *(Agropyron repens)*, damiana *(Turnera diffusa)*, dandelion *(Taraxacum officinale)*, fennel seed *(Foeniculum vulgare)*, goldenrod *(Solidago virgaurea)*, horsetail *(Equisetum arvense)*, kava kava *(Piper methysticum)*, kola nut *(Cola* spp.*)*, marshmallow *(Althaea officinalis)*, maté *(Ilex paraguariensis)*, parsley *(Petroselinum* spp.*)*, sarsaparilla *(Smilax* spp.*)*, saw palmetto *(Serenoa repens)*, uva ursi *(Arctostaphylos uva-ursi)*, vervain *(Verbena* spp. and *V. hastata)*, and yarrow *(Achillea millefolium)*. Any other prescription or non-prescription diuretics should also be avoided, except on medical advice.

Dandelion

KEEP IN MIND

• In animal studies, potassium-sparing diuretics caused an increase in magnesium levels. Although it is unknown if this can happen in humans, magnesium supplements should be avoided.

• Because amiloride is a potassium-sparing diuretic, your potassium level may rise. Do not take potassium supplements, do not use salt substitutes (they are generally high in potassium), and discuss your intake of high-potassium foods, such as bananas and orange juice, with your medical practitioner.

AMIODARONE

BRAND NAMES *Cordarone, Pacerone*

TYPE OF DRUG	Antiarrhythmic
DESCRIPTION	Amiodarone is prescribed for life-threatening abnormal heart rhythms that haven't responded to other treatments. It is a very powerful drug that causes side effects in about 75 percent of the patients who use it. Some of the side effects can be very serious, including potentially fatal lung problems. Amiodarone can also cause dangerous interactions with a long list of drugs.

DON'T MIX WITH

No known herbal interactions. However, because amiodarone has so many potential drug interactions, avoid taking any herbal supplements before discussing them with your physician.

KEEP IN MIND

• Although the research is limited, taking vitamin E could help prevent lung damage caused by amiodarone. Discuss vitamin E supplements with your physician before you try them.

AMITRIPTYLINE

BRAND NAME *Elavil*

TYPE OF DRUG	Tricyclic antidepressant
DESCRIPTION	Amitriptyline is used to treat depression. Like other tricyclic antidepressants, it works by affecting the way chemicals called neurotransmitters, including serotonin and norepinephrine, move in and out of the body's nerve endings.
DON'T MIX WITH	**Ephedra** (*Ephedra* spp., also known as ma huang). Taking ephedra with any tricyclic antidepressant raises your risk of serious high blood pressure and heart arrhythmias. Also avoid the drugs ephedrine and pseudoephedrine, which are similar to ephedra and found in many non-prescription cold and allergy remedies. **Kava kava** (*Piper methysticum*). This herbal relaxant may increase the side effects of amitriptyline. *Ephedra* **St. John's wort** (*Hypericum perforatum*). No interactions have been reported between this herb and amitriptyline, but research suggests that they work in similar ways. To avoid increasing the effects and side effects of the drug, do not take St. John's wort. **Yohimbe** (*Pausinystalia yohimbe*). This dangerous herb, taken to improve male sexual function, can cause a dangerous increase in blood pressure when combined with amitriptyline.
KEEP IN MIND	• Heart problems can be a side effect of tricyclic antidepressants, possibly because these drugs lower the production of coenzyme CoQ_{10}. Consider taking supplements (20–50 mg daily). • Although there are no studies, supplements of both s-adenylmethionine (SAMe) and the amino acid tryptophan (sold as 5-HTP) may increase the side effects of amitriptyline. Until more is known, do not take either concurrently with amitriptyline. • Test-tube studies indicate that tea could interfere with your absorption of amitriptyline. Do not drink tea within two hours of taking the drug.

AMOXICILLIN

BRAND NAMES *Amoxil, Trimox, Wymox*

TYPE OF DRUG	Penicillin antibiotic
DESCRIPTION	Amoxicillin is a form of the antibiotic penicillin. In general, penicillin antibiotics kill the bacteria that cause infections and illness. They do not kill viruses, so they are not helpful for treating colds and flu. Amoxicillin is often prescribed to treat ear infections in children.
DON'T MIX WITH	No known herbal interactions.
KEEP IN MIND	• Amoxicillin kills not only the harmful bacteria that cause illness but also the good bacteria that are normally found in the intestines; this can cause diarrhea. Two recent studies have shown that taking a probiotic supplement that contains *Saccharomyces boulardii* can help prevent or reduce the diarrhea. Consider taking probiotic supplements that contain a mix of organisms including *Lactobacillus acidophilus, Bifidobacterium bifidum,* and *Saccharomyces boulardii* (at least 1.5 billion live organisms daily). • The enzyme found in pineapples, bromelain, increases the absorption of amoxicillin. This may be helpful for people with severe infections, or infections that are not responding to amoxicillin. Discuss taking bromelain with your physician first before you try it.

AMPICILLIN

BRAND NAMES *Marcillin, Omnipen, Principen, Totacillin*

TYPE OF DRUG	Penicillin antibiotic
DESCRIPTION	Ampicillin is similar to amoxicillin in its description and reactions with herbs (*see above for details*); however, it may reduce the effect of the blood pressure-lowering drug atenolol (*p. 128*).

ASPIRIN	BRAND NAMES *Anacin, Bayer, Bufferin, Ecotrin, Empirin, others*
TYPE OF DRUG	Pain reliever, fever reducer, and nonsteroidal anti-inflammatory drug
DESCRIPTION	Aspirin, also known as acetylsalicylic acid, is one of the most commonly used non-prescription drugs throughout the world. Studies have shown that the long-term use of low-dose aspirin can reduce your risk of heart disease and stroke, and may also protect against developing Alzheimer's disease and some forms of cancer. Aspirin must be used with caution. Long-term use of aspirin can cause stomach irritation, gastrointestinal bleeding, and ulcers. It can also cause bleeding problems, particularly in people who also take blood-thinning medications. Do not give aspirin to children and teenagers. Reye syndrome, a rare but serious childhood illness, is associated with aspirin use.
DON'T MIX WITH	**Garlic** *(Allium sativum).* Large amounts of garlic combined with aspirin may increase your risk of internal bleeding. **Ginkgo** *(Ginkgo biloba).* Taking this herb with aspirin may increase your risk of internal bleeding.
DO TAKE WITH	**Deglycyrrhizinated licorice** (also called DGL, derived from *Glycyrrhiza glabra).* DGL can help prevent stomach irritation from aspirin. Consider taking licorice supplements (250 mg 2 to 3 times daily).
KEEP IN MIND	• Taking aspirin with vitamin E or bromelain may increase the risk of internal bleeding. • Mixing alcohol and aspirin can increase the risk of stomach irritation and ulcers. • Long-term use of aspirin can lower your folic acid and vitamin C levels. Consider taking supplements (400–800 mcg folate and 500 mg vitamin C daily). • High doses of aspirin (more than 3 grams a day) can reduce zinc levels. Consider taking supplements (10 mg daily, taken with food to avoid stomach upset).

ATENOLOL	BRAND NAME *Tenormin*
TYPE OF DRUG	Beta blocker
DESCRIPTION	Atenolol is used primarily to treat high blood pressure, abnormal heart rhythms, and angina. It is often prescribed for people who have already had a heart attack, to help prevent another one. Atenolol interacts adversely with a number of prescription drugs. Be certain to tell your physician about any other prescription and nonprescription drugs and dietary supplements you take. The antacid cimetidine *(p. 137)* and related antacids known as H2 antagonists, such as famotidine *(p. 155)* and ranitidine *(p. 193),* increase the amount of atenolol in your bloodstream. Ask your physician or pharmacist to help you choose a different type of antacid.
DON'T MIX WITH	No known herbal interactions.
KEEP IN MIND	• Alcohol can worsen the side effects of atenolol such as drowsiness and dizziness. Beta blockers impede your body's use of coenzyme Q_{10} which is needed for energy production within your cells. Consider taking CoQ_{10} supplements (20–50 mg daily).

ATORVASTATIN

TYPE OF DRUG	Statin cholesterol-lowering agent
DESCRIPTION	Atorvastatin is prescribed to reduce high cholesterol, to slow or prevent hardening of the arteries, and to reduce the risk of heart attack and stroke.
DON'T MIX WITH	No known herbal interactions.
DO TAKE WITH	**Milk thistle** *(Silybum marianum)*. Although there are no studies to date, silymarin, an active compound in the herb milk thistle, may protect against the liver damage that can occur as a side effect of this type of drug. Consider taking supplements (150 mg 3 to 4 times daily).

Milk thistle

KEEP IN MIND	• The dietary supplement red yeast rice, sold as Cholestin, works in a similar way to the statin drugs. Do not use red yeast rice with atorvastatin. • Lovastatin *(see p. 168)*, a drug similar to atorvastatin, interacts adversely with grapefruit juice. There are no studies yet of atorvastatin and grapefruit juice, but similar problems are possible. Until more information is known, do not take atorvastatin with grapefruit juice. • High doses of niacin (2–3 grams daily) can lower cholesterol levels. Combining high-dose niacin with atorvastatin, however, can lead to a serious muscle disorder. The niacin in a daily multivitamin or B vitamin supplement does not cause problems though. • According to one study, statin drugs can gradually raise vitamin A levels. Until more information is known, don't take vitamin A supplements. • Studies show that taking statin drugs can lower your level of coenzyme Q_{10} (CoQ_{10} or ubiquinone), a substance needed for energy production in your cells. Consider taking supplements (100 mg daily).

ATROPINE, HYOSCYAMINE, SCOPALAMINE

TYPE OF DRUG	Anticholinergic combination
DESCRIPTION	Atropine, in combination with other anticholinergic and sedative drugs, is used to relieve stomach and intestinal cramps. It is also used to relieve diarrhea and excessive salivation, and to treat some heart conditions.
DON'T MIX WITH	**Tannin-containing herbs.** Herbs that are high in tannin, including black walnut *(Juglans nigra)*, red raspberry *(Rubus idaeus)*, oak *(Quercus* spp.), uva ursi *(Arctostaphylos uva-ursi)*, and witch hazel *(Hamamelis virginiana)*, can interfere with your absorption of atropine, as can tea.
KEEP IN MIND	• Do not use atropine products to treat diarrhea in babies. Adults who have diarrhea for more than three days should consult a physician.

AZIDOTHYMIDINE (AZT), ZIDOVUDINE — BRAND NAME *Retrovir*

TYPE OF DRUG	Antiviral

DESCRIPTION

AZT is used in combination with the protease inhibitor indinavir *(p. 162)* as part of a "cocktail" of pharmaceuticals to treat HIV infection and AIDS. It is very powerful and can interact badly with a number of other drugs. Be certain to tell your physician about any other prescription and nonprescription drugs and dietary supplements you are taking.

DON'T MIX WITH

St. John's wort *(Hypericum perforatum).* The effectiveness of protease inhibitors is seriously reduced by this herb. Do not take AZT with St. John's wort.

KEEP IN MIND

• Naringinen, a substance found in grapefruit and grapefruit juice, may raise your blood levels of AZT too high. Do not consume grapefruit or grapefruit juice when taking AZT.
• Supplements of the amino acid carnitine may help prevent muscle pain and damage from AZT. Consider taking supplements (250 mg 2 to 4 times daily, or according to your physician's recommendation).
• According to one study, HIV-positive people with low levels of vitamin B_{12} are more likely to develop anemia and other side effects from AZT. Discuss vitamin B_{12} supplements with your physician before you try them (the recommended dosage is 500 mcg daily). Vitamin E may help AZT work better, according to another study. Discuss vitamin E supplements with your physician before you try them (the recommended dosage is 400 IU daily).
• A few studies suggest that AZT lowers your zinc and copper levels. In 1995 a study found that high doses of zinc (200 mg daily) may help prevent respiratory infections in AIDS patients. Discuss zinc supplements with a physician before you try them. When taking large doses of zinc (a minimum of 2–3 mg), additional copper (1–2 mg daily) supplements are necessary.

AZITHROMYCIN — BRAND NAME *Zithromax*

TYPE OF DRUG	Macrolide antibiotic

DESCRIPTION

Azithromycin is used to treat bacterial infections. It is often prescribed for middle ear infections, tonsillitis, pharyngitis, respiratory tract infections, and sexually transmitted diseases. If you take any statin drug such as lovastatin *(p. 168)* or atorvastatin *(p. 129),* do not take azithromycin. The combination could cause a potentially fatal muscle disease.

DON'T MIX WITH

Digitalis *(Digitalis* spp., also known as foxglove). Antibiotics very similar to azithromycin raise your level of both the dangerous herb digitalis and digoxin, a drug with similar effects. No studies show a similar effect from azithromycin, but until more is known, do not combine the two.

Foxglove

KEEP IN MIND

• Azithromycin kills not only the harmful bacteria that cause illness but also the good bacteria that are normally found in your intestines, which can then cause diarrhea. Consider taking probiotic supplements (at least 1.5 billion live organisms daily, including a mixture of *Lactobacillus acidophilus, Bifidobacterium bifidum,* and *Saccharomyces boulardii).*

BENAZEPRIL, CAPTOPRIL, LISINOPRIL, QUINAPRIL, RAMIPRIL

BRAND NAMES *Accupril (quinapril), Altace (ramipril), Capoten (captopril), Lotensin (benazepril), Prinivil (lisinopril), Zestril (lisinopril)*

TYPE OF DRUG	Angiotensin–converting enzyme (ACE) inhibitor
DESCRIPTION	All of these drugs are part of the group known as ACE inhibitors prescribed to treat high blood pressure, some types of heart failure, and kidney disease caused by the condition diabetes.
DON'T MIX WITH	**Cayenne** *(Capsicum frutescens).* Capsaicin, in cayenne pepper capsules, may worsen coughing, a side effect of ACE inhibitors. **Digitalis** *(Digitalis* spp., also known as foxglove). Similar to the heart drug digoxin (derived from the plant), which is excreted more slowly when you use ACE inhibitors, thereby raising the level of digoxin in your blood. Do not take digitalis while taking these drugs. *Cayenne* **Herbal diuretics.** Avoid bilberry leaf *(Vaccinium myrtillus)*, buchu *(Barosma betulina)*, burdock *(Arctium lappa)*, couch grass *(Agropyron repens)*, damiana *(Turnera diffusa)*, dandelion *(Taraxacum officinale)*, fennel seed *(Foeniculum vulgare)*, goldenrod *(Solidago virgaurea)*, horsetail *(Equisetum arvense)*, kava kava *(Piper methysticum)*, kola nut *(Cola* spp.*)*, marshmallow *(Althaea officinalis)*, maté *(Ilex paraguariensis)*, parsley *(Petroselinum* spp.*)*, sarsaparilla *(Smilax* spp.*)*, saw palmetto *(Serenoa repens)*, uva ursi *(Arctostaphylos uva-ursi)*, vervain *(Verbena* spp.*)*, and yarrow *(Achillea millefolium)*, as well as other diuretics.
KEEP IN MIND	• ACE inhibitors may raise blood potassium levels, especially with kidney disease. Do not use potassium supplements or potassium-containing salt substitutes. Discuss high-potassium foods with your physician. • High doses of the amino acid arginine, with an ACE inhibitor, may affect potassium levels unpredictably. Do not take arginine supplements while taking these drugs.

BISMUTH, BISMUTH SUBSALICYLATE

BRAND NAMES *Pepto-Bismol, Bismatrol, others*

TYPE OF DRUG	Antacid and antidiarrheal
DESCRIPTION	Bismuth subsalicylate is a nonprescription drug used to relieve indigestion, nausea, stomach cramps, and diarrhea, especially traveler's diarrhea. It is also often used in combination with prescription drugs to treat ulcers.
DON'T MIX WITH	**Salicylate-containing herbs.** The herbs meadowsweet *(Filipendula ulmaria)*, white willow bark *(Salix alba)*, and wintergreen *(Gaultheria procumbens)* contain salicylates. Taking these herbs with bismuth subsalicylate could, at least in theory, make your salicylate level rise too high. This could cause blood-thinning and bleeding problems, especially if you also take blood-thinning natural substances such as garlic *(Allium sativum)*, ginkgo *(Ginkgo biloba)*, and vitamin E, or a blood-thinning drug such as warfarin *(p. 195)*.

BROMPHENIRAMINE BRAND NAMES *Allent, Bromfed, Dimetapp Allergy, Endafed, DayQuil Allergy Relief, others*

TYPE OF DRUG	Antihistamine
DESCRIPTION	Brompheniramine is a nonprescription drug used to treat symptoms of seasonal allergies, including sneezing, runny nose, and itchy and watering eyes. It is also used to treat the symptoms of colds and upper respiratory infections, including scratchy throat and nasal congestion. In nonprescription allergy and cold formulas, brompheniramine is combined with a decongestant drug such as pseudoephedrine *(p. 185)*. Decongestant drugs should be avoided by people with diabetes, heart disease, high blood pressure, and many other health problems. Read the label carefully.
DON'T MIX WITH	**Henbane** *(Hyoscyamus niger)*. This herb is toxic and should be used only when prescribed and closely monitored by a qualified practitioner. Because brompheniramine and henbane have similar side effects, such as dry mouth, dizziness, and drowsiness, they should never be used in combination with each other.
KEEP IN MIND	• Brompheniramine causes drowsiness. Since alcohol can make the drowsiness worse, and because alcohol may also interact adversely with other ingredients in the formula, do not consume alcohol while taking this drug.

BUPROPION BRAND NAMES *Wellbutrin, Zyban*

TYPE OF DRUG	Antidepressant and smoking-cessation drug
DESCRIPTION	As Wellbutrin, bupropion is used to treat major depression, usually when other drugs haven't helped. As Zyban, bupropion is used to help people stop smoking without gaining weight. Bupropion can cause convulsions, so it should not be used by anyone with a history of seizure disorders. This drug also often causes loss of appetite among other side effects, and can interact adversely with other drugs. Be certain to tell your physician about any other prescription and nonprescription drugs and dietary supplements you are taking.
DON'T MIX WITH	**Sedative herbs.** When combined with bupropion, sedative herbs may cause excessive drowsiness. Avoid sedative herbs such as chamomile *(Matricaria recutita)*, catnip *(Nepeta cataria)*, kava kava *(Piper methysticum)*, passionflower *(Passiflora incarnata)*, St. John's wort *(Hypericum perforatum)*, valerian *(Valeriana officinalis)*, and others, as well as sedative dietary supplements such as 5-HTP, tryptophan, and SAMe.
KEEP IN MIND	• Bupropion causes drowsiness and dizziness. Alcohol can worsen these side effects; do not consume alcohol while taking this drug.

St. John's wort

BUSPIRONE

BRAND NAMES *BuSpar*

TYPE OF DRUG	Antianxiety
DESCRIPTION	Buspirone is prescribed for treating anxiety; it is also sometimes prescribed for treating premenstrual syndrome (PMS).

DON'T MIX WITH

Sedative herbs. When combined with buspirone, sedative herbs may cause excessive drowsiness. Avoid sedative herbs such as chamomile *(Matricaria recutita),* catnip *(Nepeta cataria),* kava kava *(Piper methysticum),* passionflower *(Passiflora incarnata),* St. John's wort *(Hypericum perforatum),* valerian *(Valeriana officinalis),* and others, as well as sedative dietary supplements such as 5-HTP, tryptophan, and SAMe.

KEEP IN MIND

• Buspirone is not a sedative, but it can still cause drowsiness. Alcohol can make this side effect worse; do not consume alcohol while taking this drug.

Chamomile

CAFFEINE

BRAND NAMES *Anacin, Caffedrine, Excedrin, Midol Max-Strength, NoDoz, Vanquish, Vivarin, others*

TYPE OF DRUG	Stimulant

DESCRIPTION

Caffeine stimulates the body's central nervous system and helps you stay awake and alert. As a nonprescription drug (Caffedrine, NoDoz, Vivarin), caffeine is a mild stimulant. In combination with aspirin, it is a nonprescription drug for headaches and pain (Anacin, Excedrin, Midol Max-Strength, Vanquish). Caffeine can also be found in a number of prescription pain drugs.

DON'T MIX WITH

Ephedra *(Ephedra* spp., also known as ma huang). The stimulant herb ephedra is sold to aid weight loss and provide quick energy. It is also used for upper respiratory problems, congestion, and asthma. Use ephedra with caution and do not mix it with caffeine.
Guarana *(Paullinia cupana).* The South American herb guarana is very high in a caffeinelike substance; do not mix with caffeine supplements.

Ephedra

Kola nut *(Cola* spp.). This African nut contains significant amounts of caffeine. It should not be taken in conjunction with other caffeine-containing products.
Maté *(Ilex paraguariensis).* Caffeine is an active ingredient of this South American herb. Do not use it if taking drugs or supplements containing caffeine.

KEEP IN MIND

• Coffee, tea, chocolate, and cola drinks naturally contain caffeine; it is also added to many soft drinks and "energy boosting" products. Limit your intake of these if you take caffeine supplements.

• In 1994, two well-conducted studies suggested that postmenopausal women who drink two or more cups of coffee a day and who also have a low calcium intake are at greater risk for osteoporosis. Another reputable study in 1997, however, found no connection. Until more is known, postmenopausal women should try to limit caffeine intake and take calcium supplements (1,500 mg daily).

CALCIPOTRIENE

BRAND NAME *Dovonex*

TYPE OF DRUG	Topical antipsoriatic
DESCRIPTION	Calcipotriene is prescribed to treat psoriasis. It is applied topically (directly to the skin) in the form of a cream, ointment, or solution.
DON'T MIX WITH	No known herbal interactions.
KEEP IN MIND	• Calcipotriene can cause the body's calcium level to rise, which could lead to kidney stones. Drinking lots of liquids (64 oz a day) may help prevent this. Discuss taking calcium supplements, and your intake of high-calcium foods, with your medical practitioner.

CARBIDOPA, LEVODOPA

BRAND NAMES *Dopar, Larodopa, Lodosyn, Sinemet, Sinemet CR*

TYPE OF DRUG	Antiparkinson's
DESCRIPTION	Levodopa (Dopar, Larodopa) is prescribed for treating Parkinson's disease, restless leg syndrome, and herpes zoster (shingles). Carbidopa (Lodosyn) and the combination of levodopa and carbidopa (Sinemet) are prescribed only for Parkinson's disease. Carbidopa and levodopa are powerful drugs with numerous serious side effects. They can interact adversely with a number of drugs. Tell your physician about any other prescription and nonprescription drugs and dietary supplements you take.
DON'T MIX WITH	**Kava kava** *(Piper methysticum)*. This relaxant herb may worsen the symptoms of Parkinson's disease.
KEEP IN MIND	• Amino acid supplements can temporarily reduce the effectiveness of levodopa. The amino acid tryptophan in the form of 5-HTP could cause tissue changes similar to the disease scleroderma if taken with carbidopa. Do not take amino acid supplements when taking these drugs. • Your body uses vitamin B_6 (pyridoxine) to break down levodopa. Discuss vitamin B_6 supplements with your medical practitioner, because taking them may lessen the effectiveness of the drug therapy. • High-protein foods can interfere with the body's absorption of levodopa. Discuss your diet with your medical practitioner. • Early studies suggest that levodopa depletes levels of S-adenosyl-l-methionine (SAMe). Taking SAMe supplements, however, could keep the levodopa from working as well. Discuss SAMe supplements with your medical practitioner before you try them. • Because iron interferes with the body's absorption of both carbidopa and levodopa, take iron or multivitamin supplements containing iron two hours apart from the drug.

Kava kava

CELECOXIB

BRAND NAME *Celebrex*

TYPE OF DRUG	Cyclooxygenase-2 (COX-2) inhibitor nonsteroidal anti-inflammatory drug (NSAID)
DESCRIPTION	COX-2 inhibitors are used to treat arthritis. They work by blocking the body's production of an enzyme that regulates pain and inflammation. COX-2 inhibitors are slightly less likely than are other NSAIDs to cause stomach irritation; they also don't thin the blood.
DON'T MIX WITH	**Salicylate–containing herbs.** The herbs meadowsweet *(Filipendula ulmaria)*, white willow bark *(Salix alba)*, and wintergreen *(Gaultheria procumbens)* contain salicylates. In combination with celecoxib, these herbs could cause severe stomach irritation.
DO TAKE WITH	**Milk thistle** *(Silybum marianum)*. Silymarin, an active compound in the herb milk thistle, may help protect your liver against irritation caused by celecoxib. Consider taking supplements (150 mg three to four times daily).
KEEP IN MIND	• Many NSAIDs reduce your absorption of folic acid (folate). Although there is no evidence that celecoxib does this, consider taking supplements (400 mcg daily).

Milk thistle

CEPHALOSPORIN

BRAND NAMES *Ceclor, Keflex, Duricef, Suprax, Vantin, others*

TYPE OF DRUG	Cephalosporin antibiotic
DESCRIPTION	Cephalosporin antibiotics are quite similar to penicillin antibiotics. In general, cephalosporin antibiotics kill the bacteria that cause infections and illness. They do not kill viruses, so they are not helpful for treating colds and flu.
DON'T MIX WITH	No known herbal interactions.
KEEP IN MIND	• Cephalosporin antibiotics kill not only the harmful bacteria that cause illness, but also the good bacteria that are normally found in your intestines; this can cause diarrhea. Consider taking probiotic supplements (at least 1.5 billion live organisms daily, including a mixture of *Lactobacillus acidophilus, Bifidobacterium bifidum,* and *Saccharomyces boulardii*).

CETIRIZINE, FEXOFENADINE

BRAND NAMES *Allegra, Zyrtec*

TYPE OF DRUG	Antihistamine
DESCRIPTION	Cetirizine (Zyrtec) and fexofenadine (Allegra) are very similar drugs prescribed to treat the symptoms of seasonal allergies, such as runny nose, sneezing, and itchy eyes. Cetirizine is also used to treat other allergy symptoms such as hives and rashes.
DON'T MIX WITH	**Ephedra** (*Ephedra* spp., also known as ma huang). This stimulant herb can worsen dry mouth, a side effect of both cetirizine and fexofenadine. Similarly avoid the related drugs ephedrine and pseudoephedrine, which are found in many nonprescription cold and allergy remedies. **Henbane** (*Hyascyamus niger*). This herb is toxic and should be used only when prescribed and closely monitored by a qualified practitioner. As cetirizine and fexofenadine have similar effects to henbane, such as dry mouth, dizziness, and drowsiness, they should never be used in combination with each other. **Sedative herbs.** Sedative herbs may cause excessive drowsiness when combined with cetirizine or fexofenadine. Avoid sedative herbs, including chamomile (*Matricaria recutita*), catnip (*Nepeta cataria*), kava kava (*Piper methysticum*), passionflower (*Passiflora incarnata*), St. John's wort (*Hypericum perforatum*), valerian (*Valeriana officinalis*), and others, as well as sedative dietary supplements such as 5-HTP, tryptophan, and SAMe.
KEEP IN MIND	• Although cetirizine and fexofenadine are less likely than other antihistamines to cause drowsiness and dizziness, these side effects can still occur and are made worse by alcohol. Do not consume alcohol while taking these drugs.

Passionflower

CHARCOAL, ACTIVATED CHARCOAL

BRAND NAMES *Actidose-Aqua, CharcoAid, Insta-Char, Liqui-Char*

TYPE OF DRUG	Antidote, adsorbent, laxative
DESCRIPTION	Activated charcoal is also used for the emergency treatment of some kinds of poisoning. When used alone, activated charcoal helps keep the poison from being absorbed from your stomach into your body. Activated charcoal combined with the sweetener sorbitol is a laxative that helps eliminate the poison from your body. Do not attempt to treat poisoning on your own with activated charcoal. Call for emergency help instead. Activated charcoal tablets are sometimes used to treat cases of mild diarrhea and intestinal gas.
DON'T MIX WITH	No known herbal interactions.
KEEP IN MIND	• Frequent use of activated charcoal tablets can block the body's absorption of prescription and nonprescription drugs, vitamins, minerals, and other nutrients. Discuss alternative nonprescription remedies with your physician.

CHLORPHENIRAMINE

TYPE OF DRUG Antihistamine

DESCRIPTION Chlorpheniramine is a nonprescription drug used to treat symptoms of seasonal allergies (sneezing, runny nose, and itchy, watering eyes) and colds and upper respiratory infections (including scratchy throat and nasal congestion). When used in nonprescription allergy and cold formulas, chlorpheniramine is sometimes combined with a decongestant drug such as pseudoephedrine *(p. 185).*

Acetaminophen *(p. 122)* and dextromethorphan *(p. 145)* are found in some cold and flu formulas. Decongestant drugs should be avoided by people with diabetes, heart disease, high blood pressure, and many other health problems. Acetaminophen should be avoided by people with liver disease. Read the label carefully.

DON'T MIX WITH **Ephedra** (*Ephedra* spp., also known as ma huang). This can worsen dry mouth, a side effect of chlorpheniramine. Avoid the related ephedrine and pseudoephedrine, found in cold and allergy remedies.
Henbane (*Hyoscyamus niger).* This is toxic and should be used only when prescribed and closely monitored by a qualified practitioner. Because chlorpheniramine and henbane have similar side effects (dry mouth, dizziness, and drowsiness), they should never be used together.

Sedative herbs. Sedative herbs may cause excessive drowsiness when combined with chlorpheniramine. Avoid chamomile (*Matricaria recutita*), catnip (*Nepeta cataria*), kava kava (*Piper methysticum*), passionflower (*Passiflora incarnata*), St. John's wort (*Hypericum perforatum*), valerian (*Valeriana officinalis*), and others, as well as sedative dietary supplements such as 5-HTP, tryptophan, and SAMe.

Valerian

KEEP IN MIND • Chlorpheniramine causes drowsiness. Avoid alcohol, which can make the drowsiness worse, and may interact

adversely with other ingredients in allergy and cold formulas.

CIMETIDINE

TYPE OF DRUG H2 blocker

DESCRIPTION Cimetidine sharply reduces the production of stomach acid. In prescription form (Tagamet), it is used to treat ulcers and

heartburn. In nonprescription form (Tagamet HB), it is used for mild heartburn.

DON'T MIX WITH **Caffeine-containing herbs.** Cimetidine can reduce the rate at which caffeine is eliminated from the body. Use caution if taking caffeine-containing herbs, including

guarana *(Paullinia cupana)*, kola nut *(Cola spp.)*, and maté *(Ilex paraguariensis)*, in conjunction with cimetidine as their stimulant effects may last longer.

DO TAKE WITH **Deglycyrrhizinated licorice** (DGL, derived from *Glycyrrhiza glabra*). DGL can speed ulcer healing as it stimulates the production of mucus that protects

the stomach lining and also has an anti-inflammatory effect. Consider taking licorice supplements (up to 250 mg 2 to 4 times daily).

KEEP IN MIND • Cimetidine and other H2 blockers reduce the absorption of some vitamins and minerals, including folic acid (folate), vitamin B_{12} (cobalamin), zinc, and iron. If you use these drugs on a regular basis, consider taking supplements (400 mcg daily of folic acid, 500 mcg daily for vitamin B_{12}, plus a daily multivitamin supplement with minerals). Take them at least two hours apart from cimetidine.

• Cimetidine may slow the elimination of caffeine. The stimulant effect of coffee, tea, colas, other caffeine-containing soft drinks, and medications containing caffeine *(p. 133)* may last longer.
• Magnesium supplements and calcium-, magnesium-, and magnesium/aluminum-based antacids may block the absorption of cimetidine. Take them at least two hours apart from cimetidine.

CIPROFLOXACIN

BRAND NAME *Cipro*

TYPE OF DRUG	Fluoroquinolone antibiotic
DESCRIPTION	Ciprofloxacin is a widely prescribed member of the fluoroquinolone family of antibacterial drugs. These drugs are used to treat infections against which antibiotics such as penicillin and tetracycline are less effective, such as urinary tract infections and sinus infections. Fluoroquinolones also treat infections in the bones and joints. The asthma drug theophylline can cause a potentially fatal heart arrhythmia if taken with ciprofloxacin. If you use theophylline, be certain to tell your physician.
DON'T MIX WITH	**Caffeine–containing herbs.** Ciprofloxacin can reduce the rate at which the body eliminates caffeine. Exercise caution when combining this drug with caffeine-containing herbs, including guarana *(Paullinia cupana)*, kola nut *(Cola* spp.*)*, and maté *(Ilex paraguariensis)*, as their stimulant effects may last longer.
KEEP IN MIND	• Dairy foods such as milk, yogurt, and cheese interfere with the absorption of ciprofloxacin. Discuss your intake of these foods with your medical practitioner. • The minerals calcium, iron, magnesium, and zinc can interfere with the absorption of ciprofloxacin. The reverse is also true: ciprofloxacin can interfere with the absorption of these minerals. Take mineral supplements, multivitamin supplements with minerals, and calcium- or magnesium-containing antacids two hours apart from ciprofloxacin. • Ciprofloxacin may slow down the elimination of caffeine. The stimulant effect of coffee, tea, colas, other caffeine-containing soft drinks, and drugs containing caffeine may last longer; use caution if consuming caffeine-containing substances when taking ciprofloxacin.

CISPLATIN

BRAND NAMES *Platinol, Platinol-AQ*

TYPE OF DRUG	Anticancer (antineoplastic)
DESCRIPTION	Cisplatin is an anticancer drug used primarily to treat cancer of the bladder, ovaries, and testes, but is also used to treat many other kinds of cancer. Cisplatin is a powerful drug that can interact adversely with other drugs. Be sure to discuss any other prescription and nonprescription drugs and dietary supplements you are taking, including those suggested here, with your medical practitioner.
DON'T MIX WITH	No known herbal interactions.
DO TAKE WITH	**Milk thistle** *(Silybum marianum)*. In animal studies, milk thistle, which contains an active compound silymarin, helps protect against liver damage from cisplatin. Although there are no human studies yet, many scientists believe milk thistle can be helpful. Discuss taking supplements with your medical practitioner (150 mg 3 to 4 times daily). **Natural nausea remedies.** Ginger *(Zingiber officinale)* capsules and the homeopathic remedy nux vomica 30C (once a day or as directed by your medical practitioner) may help relieve nausea and vomiting, which are common side effects of cisplatin. *Ginger*
KEEP IN MIND	• Cisplatin can deplete the body's stores of calcium, magnesium, phosphate, potassium, and sodium. Discuss taking iron-free multivitamin and mineral supplements with your medical practitioner. • Preliminary studies suggest that injections of glutathione, the body's most abundant natural antioxidant, can help relieve some of the side effects of cisplatin. N-acetyl cysteine (also called NAC) and selenium supplements can also help increase the glutathione level. Discuss this with your medical practitioner and consider taking supplements (NAC, 600 mg 3 times daily; selenium, 200 mcg daily).

CLARITHROMYCIN

BRAND NAME *Biaxin*

TYPE OF DRUG	Macrolide antibiotic
DESCRIPTION	Clarithromycin is used to treat bacterial infections. It is often prescribed for respiratory tract infections, ulcers, and skin infections. This drug has numerous interactions with other prescription drugs. Be certain to tell your physician about any other prescription and nonprescription drugs and dietary supplements you may already be taking. If you take any statin drug such as lovastatin *(p. 168)* or atorvastatin *(p. 129)*, do not take clarithromycin. The combination could cause a potentially fatal muscle disease.
DON'T MIX WITH	**Digitalis** (*Digitalis* spp., also known as foxglove). Clarithromycin can raise the level of both the dangerous herb digitalis and digoxin, a drug with similar effects. Do not mix the two.
KEEP IN MIND	• Clarithromycin kills not only the harmful bacteria that cause illness but also the good bacteria normally found in your intestines. This can cause diarrhea. Consider taking probiotic supplements (at least 1.5 billion live organisms daily, including a mixture of *Lactobacillus acidophilus, Bifidobacterium bifidum,* and *Saccharomyces boulardii*).

Foxglove

CLEMASTINE

BRAND NAMES *Antihist-I, Tavist, Tavist-D*

TYPE OF DRUG	Antihistamine
DESCRIPTION	Clemastine is a nonprescription drug used to treat symptoms of seasonal allergies, including sneezing, runny nose, and itchy and watering eyes. Clemastine (Tavist-D) is used to treat the symptoms of colds and upper respiratory infections, including scratchy throat and nasal congestion.
DON'T MIX WITH	**Ephedra** (*Ephedra* spp., also known as ma huang). This stimulant herb can worsen dry mouth, a side effect of clemastine. Similarly, avoid the related drugs ephedrine and pseudoephedrine, which are found in many nonprescription cold and allergy remedies. **Henbane** (*Hyoscyamus niger*). This herb is toxic and should be used only when prescribed and closely monitored by a licensed practitioner. Because both clemastine and henbane have similar side effects, such as dry mouth, dizziness, and drowsiness, they should never be used in combination with each other. **Sedative herbs.** When combined with clemastine, sedative herbs may cause excessive drowsiness. Avoid sedative herbs such as chamomile (*Matricaria recutita*), catnip (*Nepeta cataria*), kava kava (*Piper methysticum*), passionflower (*Passiflora incarnata*), St. John's wort (*Hypericum perforatum*), valerian (*Valeriana officinalis*), and others, as well as sedative dietary supplements such as tryptophan, 5-HTP, and SAMe.
KEEP IN MIND	• Clemastine causes drowsiness and difficulty concentrating. Because alcohol can make these side effects worse, do not consume alcohol if taking this drug.

St. John's wort

CLINDAMYCIN

BRAND NAME *Cleocin*

TYPE OF DRUG	Antibiotic
DESCRIPTION	Clindamycin is prescribed to treat bacterial infections, including vaginal infections, lung abscesses, infected wounds, and abdominal infections. It is also used topically to treat acne and rosacea. When taken orally, clindamycin is a very powerful drug that can cause colitis, a severe intestinal irritation.
DON'T MIX WITH	No known herbal interactions.
KEEP IN MIND	• Clindamycin kills not only the harmful bacteria that cause illness, but also the good bacteria normally found in your intestines; this can cause diarrhea. Consider taking probiotic supplements (at least 1.5 billion live organisms daily, including a mixture of *Lactobacillus acidophilus, Bifidobacterium bifidum*, and *Saccharomyces boulardii*).

CLOFIBRATE

BRAND NAME *Atromid-S*

TYPE OF DRUG	Antihyperlipidemic
DESCRIPTION	Clofibrate is prescribed primarily for people who have high triglyceride (a type of fat present in the blood) levels. It is also sometimes prescribed to reduce high cholesterol levels. Clofibrate can interact adversely with a number of drugs, especially blood thinners, statin drugs, and drugs used to treat diabetes. It can also cause liver damage and gallstones. Be certain to tell your physician about any other prescription and nonprescription drugs and dietary supplements you take. Because of the risk of side effects and interactions, clofibrate is used only when other, safer drugs haven't helped.
DON'T MIX WITH	No known herbal interactions.
DO TAKE WITH	**Milk thistle** *(Silybum marianum).* Silymarin, an active compound in the herb milk thistle, may help protect your liver against damage from clofibrate. Consider taking supplements (150 mg 3 to 4 times daily).
KEEP IN MIND	• Clofibrate may reduce your absorption of Vitamin B_{12}. Consider taking supplements (500 mcg daily, taken at least two hours apart from the drug). • To avoid stomach upset, take clofibrate with food or milk.

Milk thistle

CLOMIPRAMINE
BRAND NAME *Anafranil*

TYPE OF DRUG	Tricyclic antidepressant

DESCRIPTION

Clomipramine is used to treat depression. Like other tricyclic antidepressants, it works by affecting the way chemicals called neurotransmitters, including serotonin and norepinephrine, move in and out of the body's nerve endings.

DON'T MIX WITH

Ephedra (*Ephedra* spp., also known as ma huang). Taking ephedra with any tricyclic antidepressant raises your risk of serious high blood pressure and heart arrhythmias. Similarly, avoid the related drugs ephedrine and pseudoephedrine, found in many nonprescription cold and allergy remedies.
Sedative herbs. Sedative herbs may cause excessive drowsiness when combined with clomipramine. Avoid sedative herbs such as chamomile *(Matricaria recutita)*, catnip *(Nepeta cataria)*, kava kava *(Piper methysticum)*, passionflower *(Passiflora incarnata)*, St. John's wort *(Hypericum perforatum)*, valerian *(Valeriana officinalis)*, and others, as well as sedative dietary supplements such as 5-HTP, tryptophan, and SAMe.
St. John's wort *(Hypericum perforatum)*. Research suggests that this herb and clomipramine work in similar ways. Until more is known, do not take clomipramine in conjunction with St. John's wort.
Yohimbe *(Pausinystalia yohimbe)*. This dangerous herb is said to improve male sexual function. Do not use this herb when taking clomipramine; the combination may cause a dangerous rise in blood pressure.

Chamomile

KEEP IN MIND

• Heart problems can be a side effect of tricyclic antidepressants, possibly because these drugs lower your production of coenzyme Q_{10} (CoQ_{10} or ubiquinone). CoQ_{10} is needed to produce energy in your cells, including the cells of your heart. Consider taking supplements (20–50 mg daily).

CLONIDINE
BRAND NAME *Catapres*

TYPE OF DRUG	Antihypertensive

DESCRIPTION

Clonidine is prescribed for lowering high blood pressure. It is also sometimes prescribed to help people withdraw from their addiction to alcohol and other substances, including tobacco.

DON'T MIX WITH

Blood vessel relaxing herbs. Coleus *(Coleus forskohlii)*, garlic *(Allium sativum)*, ginkgo *(Ginkgo biloba)*, and hawthorn *(Crataegus oxyacantha)* relax your blood vessels and are sometimes used to treat high blood pressure. Although there have been no studies, it is possible that combining these herbs with clonidine could make your blood pressure drop too low.
Licorice *(Glycyrrhiza glabra)*. Glycyrrhizin, a compound naturally occurring in licorice, can cause an increase in blood pressure. If you are taking clonidine to lower blood pressure, avoid this herb unless it is deglycyrrhizinated licorice (DGL).
Yohimbe *(Pausinystalia yohimbe)*. This dangerous herb is sometimes used for erectile dysfunction; one of its side effects is a sharp rise in blood pressure. Never mix it with clonidine – dangerous changes in your blood pressure could occur.

Licorice

KEEP IN MIND

• Clonidine has a depressive effect, as does alcohol. Do not consume alcohol when taking this drug.
• Clonidine may reduce the bioavailability of coenzyme Q_{10} (CoQ_{10} or ubiquinone), which is needed for energy production within your body's cells. Consider taking CoQ_{10} supplements (20–50 mg daily).
• Vitamin E can increase blood pressure in certain susceptible people according to some studies. Consult your physician before taking vitamin E supplements if you have high blood pressure.

CODEINE	BRAND NAMES *Empirin, Phenergan, Robitussin AC, others*

TYPE OF DRUG	Narcotic analgesic
DESCRIPTION	Codeine is a powerful narcotic pain reliever used by itself or combined with a nonsteroidal anti-inflammatory drug such as aspirin *(p. 128)* or acetaminophen *(p. 122)*. Codeine is also used as a prescription cough suppressant by itself or in combination with other drugs (Phenergan, Robitussin AC).
DON'T MIX WITH	**Tannin-containing herbs.** Herbs that are high in tannin, including black walnut *(Juglans nigra)*, red raspberry *(Rubus idaeus)*, oak *(Quercus* spp.*)*, uva ursi *(Arctostaphylos uva-ursi)*, and witch hazel *(Hamamelis virginiana)*, can interfere with the body's absorption of codeine, as can the tannins in tea. Do not consume any of these substances within two hours of taking this drug.
KEEP IN MIND	• Codeine causes drowsiness, impaired judgment, and loss of coordination. Alcohol makes these side effects worse. Do not consume alcohol while taking this drug. • Constipation is a common side effect of codeine. To lessen this problem, eat plenty of high-fiber foods, such as fresh fruits and vegetables and whole grains, and drink 64 ounces of water daily.

COLCHICINE	BRAND NAMES *This drug is sold only in generic form.*

TYPE OF DRUG	Antigout
DESCRIPTION	Colchicine relieves pain and inflammation in people with gout. It is also used long-term to prevent gout attacks. Colchicine is a good example of a traditional herbal remedy that has become a standard drug. The original source of this drug is a type of crocus called *Colchicum autumnale.*
DON'T MIX WITH	**Tannin-containing herbs.** Herbs that are high in tannin, including black walnut *(Juglans nigra)*, red raspberry *(Rubus idaeus)*, oak *(Quercus* spp.*)*, uva ursi *(Arctostaphylos uva-ursi)*, and witch hazel *(Hamamelis virginiana)*, can interfere with your absorption of colchicine, as can the tannins in tea. Do not consume any of these substances within two hours of taking this drug.
KEEP IN MIND	• Colchicine may make you much more sensitive to alcohol. As alcohol is also not recommended for people suffering from gout, do not consume alcohol while taking this drug. • Colchicine may block your absorption of vitamin B_{12} (cobalamin). If you use this drug on a regular basis, consider taking supplements (500 mcg daily). Colchicine may also block your absorption of beta carotene, which your body uses to produce vitamin A. Consider taking supplements of mixed carotenes (25,000 IU daily).

CONJUGATED ESTROGEN

BRAND NAMES *Cenestin, Premarin, Premphase, Prempro*

TYPE OF DRUG	Estrogen/progesterone hormone replacement

Conjugated estrogens combine several different estrogen-like hormones into one medication (Premarin, Cenestin). Conjugated estrogens are often combined with a semisynthetic compound called medroxyprogesterone (Prempro, Premphase). These drugs are prescribed to treat the symptoms of menopause, including hot flashes and vaginal dryness, and to help prevent osteoporosis in women.

DON'T MIX WITH

Red clover

Black cohosh (*Cimicifuga racemosa*). Black cohosh contains phytoestrogens, plant hormones similar to human estrogen. Combining it with prescription estrogen drugs could raise your estrogen level too high.

Chaste tree (*Vitex agnus-castus*). Chaste tree affects your levels of the hormone prolactin, which in turn can affect your natural production of estrogen and how your body uses supplemental estrogen.

Other estrogenic herbs. The herbs dong quai (*Angelica sinensis*) and red clover (*Trifolium pratense*) may have estrogen-like effects. Laboratory studies have shown that the herbs licorice (*Glycyrrhiza glabra*), thyme (*Thymus* spp.), turmeric (*Curcuma longa*), hops (*Humulus lupulus*), and vervain (*Verbena* spp. and *V. hastata*) may also modulate estrogen activity. Discuss the use of these herbs with your medical practitioner before using them.

KEEP IN MIND

• Studies have shown that soy isoflavones (estrogen-like substances) can help to relieve menopause symptoms. Ipriflavone, a type of soy isoflavone, can help prevent osteoporosis. Combining soy isoflavones with prescription estrogen drugs could raise your estrogen levels too high. If you want to use soy isoflavones in combination with or instead of supplemental estrogen, discuss it with your physician first.

CYCLOPHOSPHAMIDE

BRAND NAMES *Cytoxan, Neosar*

TYPE OF DRUG	Anticancer

DESCRIPTION

Cyclophosphamide is a drug used in chemotherapy for various types of cancer. It is a powerful drug that can have severe side effects and interact adversely with a number of other drugs. Be certain to tell your physician about any other prescription and nonprescription drugs and dietary supplements you take.

DON'T MIX WITH

Rosemary

Antioxidant herbs. In theory, herbs with high antioxidant activity could reduce the effectiveness of cyclophosphamide. Until more is known, avoid herbs such as ginkgo (*Ginkgo biloba*), lemon balm (*Melissa officinalis*), mint (*Mentha* spp.), oregano (*Origanum vulgare*), rosemary (*Rosmarinus officinalis*), thyme (*Thymus* spp.), and turmeric (*Curcuma longa*). Also avoid grapeseed and pine bark extract, including Pycnogenol, because of their antioxidant properties.

DO TAKE WITH

Natural nausea remedies. Ginger (*Zingiber officinale*) capsules or tea and the homeopathic remedy nux vomica 30C may help relieve nausea and vomiting, common side effects of cyclophosphamide. Discuss these remedies and dosage recommendations with your medical practitioner before trying them.

Turkey tail (*Coriolus versicolor*). Called yun zhi in Chinese and kawaratake in Japanese, turkey tail is a type of mushroom. A substance in turkey tail called PSK may help protect the immune system from the damaging effects of chemotherapy drugs such as cyclophosphamide. Discuss turkey tail with a physician and consider taking supplements (625 mg 1 to 2 times daily).

KEEP IN MIND

• Although there are no studies, it is possible that the antioxidant vitamins A, C, and E and beta carotene could reduce the effectiveness of cyclophosamide. Other studies suggest that these vitamins might be helpful. Discuss vitamin supplements with your physician.

CYCLOSPORINE	BRAND NAMES *Neoral, Sandimmune*
TYPE OF DRUG	Immunosuppressant
DESCRIPTION	Cyclosporine suppresses the body's immune system and prevents the rejection of transplanted organs. This very powerful drug is also sometimes used to treat other serious conditions, including aplastic anemia, ulcerative colitis, multiple sclerosis, and severe psoriasis. Cyclosporine has several serious side effects and interacts adversely with a number of drugs. Be certain to tell your physician about any other prescription and nonprescription drugs and dietary supplements you take. Cyclosporine is usually used along with corticosteroid drugs such as prednisone *(p. 182)*.
DON'T MIX WITH	**St. John's wort** *(Hypericum perforatum)*. This herb significantly lowers the amount of cyclosporine you absorb, to the point where organ rejection might occur. Do not use this herb if you are taking cyclosporine.
KEEP IN MIND	• A substance in grapefruit or grapefruit juice may reduce the rate of elimination of cyclosporine. This can increase the amount of cyclosporine in your body to dangerous levels. Avoid grapefruit and grapefruit juice when taking this drug. • Cyclosporine increases the amount of potassium in your blood. Do not use potassium supplements or salt substitutes when taking this drug. • One study in 1996 showed that water-soluble vitamin E may be helpful for improving your absorption of cyclosporine. Discuss taking vitamin E supplements with your physician – do not start taking them on your own.

DESIPRAMINE	BRAND NAME *Norpramin*
TYPE OF DRUG	Tricyclic antidepressant
DESCRIPTION	Desipramine is used to treat depression. Like the other tricyclic antidepressants, it works by affecting the way chemicals called neurotransmitters, including serotonin and norepinephrine, move in and out of the body's nerve endings.
DON'T MIX WITH	**Ephedra** *(Ephedra* spp., also known as ma huang). Taking ephedra with any tricyclic antidepressant raises your risk of serious high blood pressure and heart arrhythmias. Similarly, avoid the related drugs ephedrine and pseudoephedrine, which are found in many nonprescription cold and allergy remedies. **Sedative herbs.** Sedative herbs may cause excessive drowsiness when combined with desipramine. Avoid sedative herbs such as chamomile *(Matricaria recutita)*, catnip *(Nepeta cataria)*, kava kava *(Piper methysticum)*, passionflower *(Passiflora incarnata)*, St. John's wort *(Hypericum perforatum)*, valerian *(Valeriana officinalis)*, and others, as well as sedative dietary supplements such as 5-HTP, tryptophan, and SAMe. **St. John's wort** *(Hypericum perforatum)*. Research suggests that this herb and desipramine work in similar ways. Until more is known, do not take desipramine in conjunction with St. John's wort. **Yohimbe** *(Pausinystalia yohimbe)*. This dangerous herb is said to improve male sexual function. Do not use this herb when taking desipramine; the combination may cause a dangerous rise in blood pressure. *Ephedra*
KEEP IN MIND	• Heart problems can be a side effect of tricyclic antidepressants, possibly because these drugs lower your production of coenzyme Q_{10} (CoQ_{10} or ubiquinone). CoQ_{10} is needed to produce energy in the body's cells, including the cells of the heart. Consider taking CoQ_{10} supplements (20–50 mg daily).

DEXAMETHASONE

BRAND NAMES *Decadron, Dexone, Hexadrol*

TYPE OF DRUG	Corticosteroid
DESCRIPTION	These hormones are used to treat a wide variety of severe disorders, particularly those that involve inflammation, including arthritis, psoriasis, allergies, asthma, and inflammatory bowel disease. They are also used to treat autoimmune diseases such as lupus erythematosus and transplant rejection. Corticosteroids are powerful drugs that can cause serious side effects and interact adversely with a wide range of drugs. Tell your physician about any other prescription and nonprescription drugs and dietary supplements you take.
DON'T MIX WITH	**Digitalis** (*Digitalis* spp., also known as foxglove). This dangerous herb is very similar to the heart drug digoxin *(p. 147)*, which may worsen the side effects of dexamethasone. Do not use either digitalis or digoxin if taking this drug. **Ephedra** (*Ephedra* spp., also known as ma huang). The herb ephedra naturally contains ephedrine, which can reduce the effectiveness of corticosteroids. Do not use it when taking dexamethasone. Similarly, avoid ephedrine *(p. 152)* and pseudoephedrine *(p. 185)*, which can be found in many nonprescription cold and allergy remedies.
KEEP IN MIND	• Corticosteroids can make you retain sodium, found in salt. Discuss reducing your salt intake with your physician. • Long-term use of corticosteroids can interfere with your body's absorption of calcium, which may lead to osteoporosis. Consider taking supplements (1,000 mg calcium daily, 400 IU vitamin D daily). Corticosteroids may also reduce your level of vitamin B_6 (pyridoxine). Consider taking supplements (50 mg daily). • Long-term use of corticosteroids may deplete your levels of magnesium. Consider taking supplements (300–400 mg daily). • Long-term use of corticosteroids can contribute to the development of diabetes. Consider taking a chromium picolinate supplement (200 mcg daily).

Foxglove

DEXTROMETHORPHAN

BRAND NAMES *Benylin DM, Robitussin, others*

TYPE OF DRUG	Cough suppressant
DESCRIPTION	Dextromethorphan helps stop coughing from colds, flu, upper respiratory infections, and allergies. It can be found in many nonprescription cough formulas, either by itself (Benylin DM), or in combination with other cough medicines and decongestants (Robitussin).
DON'T MIX WITH	**Sedative herbs.** When combined with dextromethorphan, these herbs may cause excessive drowsiness. Avoid sedative herbs such as chamomile *(Matricaria recutita)*, catnip *(Nepeta cataria)*, kava kava *(Piper methysticum)*, passionflower *(Passiflora incarnata)*, St. John's wort *(Hypericum perforatum)*, valerian *(Valeriana officinalis)*, and others, as well as sedative dietary supplements such as 5-HTP, tryptophan, and SAMe.
KEEP IN MIND	• Dextromethorphan can cause drowsiness. Alcohol makes this side effect worse; avoid consuming alcohol while taking this drug.

Kava kava

DIAZEPAM	BRAND NAME *Valium*

TYPE OF DRUG	Antianxiety
DESCRIPTION	Diazepam, along with other members of the benzodiazepine family such as alprazolam (Xanax) and chlordiazepoxide (Librium), is prescribed to relieve anxiety and tension; it is also used as a muscle relaxant. Benzodiazepine drugs are safe and effective and have few side effects, but they are potentially addictive.
DON'T MIX WITH	**Digitalis** (*Digitalis* spp., also known as foxglove). This dangerous herb is very similar to the heart drug digoxin (p. 147). Diazepam raises the level of digoxin in your blood. Do not take digitalis if you are taking diazepam. **Sedative herbs.** When combined with diazepam, these herbs may cause excessive drowsiness. Avoid sedative herbs such as chamomile *(Matricaria recutita)*, catnip *(Nepeta cataria)*, kava kava *(Piper methysticum)*, passionflower *(Passiflora incarnata)*, St. John's wort *(Hypericum perforatum)*, valerian *(Valeriana officinalis)*, and others, as well as sedative dietary supplements such as 5-HTP, tryptophan, and SAMe.
KEEP IN MIND	• Diazepam depresses your central nervous system, as does alcohol. Mixing the two may cause excessive drowsiness and potentially fatal breathing difficulties. • Do not take macrolide antibiotics, such as azithromycin *(p. 130)*, clarithromycin *(p. 139)*, erythromycin *(p. 153)*, and others, with any benzodiazepine drug. These drugs can raise your level of the benzodiazepine drug dangerously high.

Passionflower

DICYCLOMINE	BRAND NAMES *Bemote, Byclomine, Di Spaz, others*

TYPE OF DRUG	Antispasmodic
DESCRIPTION	Dicyclomine is prescribed for irritable bowel syndrome and related digestive problems.
DON'T MIX WITH	No known herbal interactions.
KEEP IN MIND	• A side effect of dicyclomine is a reduction in your ability to sweat. Avoid overheating. Another side effect of dicyclomine is constipation. To lessen this problem, eat plenty of high-fiber foods, such as fresh fruits and vegetables and whole grains, and drink 64 ounces of water daily. You may also want to discuss constipation remedies with your physician.

DIDANOSINE
BRAND NAME *Videx*

TYPE OF DRUG	Antiviral

DESCRIPTION

Didanosine is used in combination with AZT *(p. 130)* and the protease inhibitor indinavir *(p. 162)* as part of a "cocktail" of drugs to treat HIV infection and AIDS.

Didanosine is a very powerful drug that can have a number of extremely serious side effects. It can also interact badly with a number of other drugs. Be certain to tell your physician about any other prescription and nonprescription drugs and dietary supplements you take.

DON'T MIX WITH

No known herbal interactions.

DO TAKE WITH

Lentinan, a complex sugar found in shiitake mushrooms, may help didanosine work better. Lentinan must be given by injection; eating a lot of shiitake mushrooms will not have any effect. Discuss this supplement with your medical practitioner. **Milk thistle** (*Silybum marianum*). Silymarin, an active compound in the herb milk thistle, may help protect your liver against damage from didanosine. Consider taking supplements (150 mg 3 to 4 times daily).

Milk thistle

DIGOXIN
BRAND NAME *Lanoxin*

TYPE OF DRUG	Digitalis glycoside

DESCRIPTION

Digoxin (Lanoxin) and the related drug digitoxin (Crystodigin) are prescribed to treat congestive heart failure and other heart conditions that make your heart beat very rapidly, such as tachycardia.

DON'T MIX WITH

Digitalis (*Digitalis* spp., also known as foxglove). This dangerous herb acts in ways very similar to digoxin. Never combine the two – a potentially fatal increase in your digoxin level will occur. **Herbal diuretics.** If you are taking a prescription diuretic, do not take nonprescription or herbal diuretics including bilberry leaf (*Vaccinium myrtillus*), burdock (*Arctium lappa*), damiana (*Turnera diffusa*), dandelion (*Taraxacum officinale*), fennel seed (*Foeniculum vulgare*), goldenrod (*Solidago virgaurea*), horsetail (*Equisetum arvense*), kava kava (*Piper methysticum*), kola nut (*Cola* spp.), marshmallow (*Althaea officinalis*), maté (*Ilex paraguariensis*), parsley (*Petroselinum* spp.), sarsaparilla (*Smilax* spp.), saw palmetto (*Serenoa repens*), uva ursi (*Arctostaphylos uva-ursi*), vervain (*Verbena* spp), and yarrow (*Achillea millefolium*).

Hawthorn (*Crataegus* spp.). The herb hawthorn is often used to treat mild congestive heart failure. Combining the two may cause problems as they both are used to treat the same condition and may have additive effects. **Herbal laxatives.** Using herbal laxatives such as cascara sagrada (*Rhamnus purshiana*) and senna (*Senna alexandrina*) can decrease the level of digoxin in your blood and can also deplete your potassium level. Do not use them if taking this drug. **Licorice** (*Glycyrrhiza glabra*). Large amounts of licorice can reduce the body's levels of potassium. Since digoxin also reduces potassium levels, do not combine the two as it may cause your potassium level to become dangerously low. This effect does not occur as readily with deglycyrrhizinated licorice (DGL) or with artificial licorice flavoring.

Dandelion

DILTIAZEM

BRAND NAMES *Cardizem, Dilacor, Tiamate, Tiazac, others*

TYPE OF DRUG	Calcium channel blocker
DESCRIPTION	Diltiazem is prescribed for high blood pressure, angina, and to help prevent a second heart attack. Diltiazem is a calcium channel blocker, a drug that causes blood vessels to relax and widen.
DON'T MIX WITH	No known herbal interactions.
DO TAKE WITH	**Milk thistle** (*Silybum marianum*). Silymarin, an active substance in the herb milk thistle, may protect against liver damage from diltiazem. Consider taking supplements (150 mg 3 to 4 times daily).
KEEP IN MIND	• A substance in grapefruit or grapefruit juice may reduce the rate of excretion of other calcium channel blocker drugs such as felodipine and nifedipine (*p. 173*). This can cause a dangerous increase in the amount of these drugs in your blood. Although there have been no reports of a similar effect with diltiazem, until more is known, do not eat grapefruit or drink grapefruit juice if you take any calcium channel blocker.

Milk thistle

DIMENHYDRINATE

BRAND NAMES *Dimetabs, Dramamine, Marmine, Nico-Vert, Triptone, others*

TYPE OF DRUG	Antihistamine and antiemetic
DESCRIPTION	Dimenhydrinate is used to treat and prevent nausea, vomiting, and dizziness from motion sickness. This drug is a combination of two drugs, diphenhydramine (*see right*) and chlorotheophylline.
DON'T MIX WITH	**Henbane** (*Hyoscyamus niger*). This herb is toxic and should be used only when prescribed and closely monitored by a qualified practitioner. Because both dimenhydrinate and henbane have similar side effects, such as dry mouth, dizziness and drowsiness, they should never be used in combination with each other. **Sedative herbs.** When combined with dimenhydrinate, these herbs may cause excessive drowsiness. Avoid sedative herbs such as chamomile (*Matricaria recutita*), catnip (*Nepeta cataria*), kava kava (*Piper methysticum*), passionflower (*Passiflora incarnata*), St. John's wort (*Hypericum perforatum*), valerian (*Valeriana officinalis*), and others, as well as sedative dietary supplements such as 5-HTP, tryptophan, and SAMe.
KEEP IN MIND	• Dimenhydrinate causes drowsiness. Alcohol makes this effect worse; do not consume alcohol if taking this drug.

St. John's wort

DIPHENHYDRAMINE

BRAND NAMES *Anacin PM, Benadryl, Benylin, Excedrin PM, Nytol, Sleep-Eze, Sominex, Tylenol PM*

TYPE OF DRUG	Antihistamine

DESCRIPTION

Diphenhydramine is an antihistamine used to treat the symptoms of seasonal allergies, such as runny nose, itchy eyes, and scratchy throat, and to relieve other allergy symptoms such as rashes and hives (Benadryl, Benylin). Diphenhydramine is used in nonprescription sleep aids either by itself (Nytol, Sleep-Eze, Sominex) or in combination with other ingredients (Anacin PM, Excedrin PM, Tylenol PM).

Henbane *(Hyoscyamus niger)*. This herb is toxic and should be used only when prescribed and closely monitored by a qualified practitioner. Because diphenhydramine and henbane have similar side effects, such as dry mouth, dizziness, and drowsiness, they should never be used in combination with each other.
Sedative herbs. When combined with diphenhydramine, these herbs may cause excessive drowsiness. Avoid sedative herbs such as chamomile *(Matricaria recutita)*, catnip *(Nepeta cataria)*, kava kava *(Piper methysticum)*, passionflower *(Passiflora incarnata)*, St. John's wort *(Hypericum perforatum)*, valerian *(Valeriana officinalis)*, and others, as well as sedative dietary supplements such as 5-HTP, tryptophan, and SAMe.

Chamomile

KEEP IN MIND

• Diphenhydramine causes drowsiness. Alcohol makes this effect worse; do not consume alcohol if taking this drug.
• The hormone melatonin is used as a natural sleep aid. Because little is known about possible drug interactions, do not combine it with diphenhydramine or any other prescription or nonprescription sleep aids. To do so may make you dangerously drowsy.

DISULFIRAM

BRAND NAME *Antabuse*

TYPE OF DRUG	Alcohol abuse deterrent

DESCRIPTION

Disulfiram is prescribed to help people avoid drinking alcohol. The drug causes a very unpleasant reaction, including headache, nausea, vomiting, sweating, and dizziness, when the patient drinks or comes into physical contact with even a very small amount of alcohol.

DON'T MIX WITH

Sedative herbs. When combined with disulfiram, these herbs may cause excessive drowsiness. Avoid sedative herbs such as chamomile *(Matricaria recutita)*, catnip *(Nepeta cataria)*, kava kava *(Piper methysticum)*, passionflower *(Passiflora incarnata)*, St. John's wort *(Hypericum perforatum)*, valerian *(Valeriana officinalis)*, and others, as well as sedative dietary supplements such as 5-HTP, tryptophan, and SAMe.
Caffeine-containing herbs. Disulfiram, in combination with caffeine, may cause excessive stimulation. Avoid the herbs guarana *(Paullinia cupana)*, kola nut *(Cola spp.)*, and maté *(Ilex paraguariensis)* as they all contain caffeine.

Valerian

KEEP IN MIND

• Avoid alcohol in any form, even aftershaves and perfumes and the fumes from alcohol-containing chemicals such as paint thinner. Read the ingredients label on all products carefully. Avoid elixir or liquid cough, cold, flu, and diarrhea remedies that contain alcohol. Avoid mouthwashes and gargles. Avoid vinegar and any food or sauce that may contain traces of alcohol.
• Coffee, tea, chocolate, and cola drinks naturally contain caffeine; it is also added to many soft drinks and "energy-boosting" products. Avoid all of these products if you take disulfiram.

DOXEPIN

BRAND NAME *Sinequan*

TYPE OF DRUG	Tricyclic antidepressant
DESCRIPTION	Doxepin is used to treat depression. Like other tricyclic antidepressants, it works by affecting the way chemicals called neurotransmitters, including serotonin and norepinephrine, move in and out of the body's nerve endings.
DON'T MIX WITH	**Ephedra** (*Ephedra* spp., also known as ma huang). Taking ephedra with any tricyclic antidepressant raises your risk of serious high blood pressure and heart arrhythmias. Similarly, avoid the related drugs ephedrine and pseudoephedrine, which are found in many non-prescription cold and allergy remedies. **Sedative herbs.** Sedative drugs may cause excessive drowsiness when combined with doxepin. Avoid sedative herbs such as chamomile (*Matricaria recutita*), catnip (*Nepeta cataria*), kava kava (*Piper methysticum*), passionflower (*Passiflora incarnata*), St. John's wort (*Hypericum perforatum*), valerian (*Valeriana officinalis*), and others, as well as sedative dietary supplements such as 5-HTP, tryptophan, and SAMe. **St. John's wort** (*Hypericum perforatum*). Research suggests that this herb and doxepin work in similar ways. Until more information is known, do not take it in conjunction with St. John's wort. **Yohimbe** (*Pausinystalia yohimbe*). This dangerous herb is said to improve male sexual function. Do not use this herb when taking doxepin; the combination may cause a dangerous rise in blood pressure.
KEEP IN MIND	• Heart problems can be a side effect of tricyclic antidepressants, possibly because these drugs lower your production of coenzyme Q_{10} (CoQ_{10} or ubiquinone). CoQ_{10} is needed to produce energy in your cells, including the cells of the heart. Consider taking CoQ_{10} supplements (20–50 mg daily).

Ephedra

DOXORUBICIN

BRAND NAMES *Adriamycin, Rubex*

TYPE OF DRUG	Anticancer
DESCRIPTION	Doxorubicin is a very toxic drug used to treat many types of cancer. Because doxorubicin works by interfering with the growth not only of cancer cells but also of normal cells, this drug has many serious side effects, including heart problems. Be sure to discuss any prescription or nonprescription drugs and dietary supplements you are taking with your medical practitioner.
DON'T MIX WITH	No known herbal interactions.
KEEP IN MIND	• The risk of heart damage from doxorubicin may be lowered if you take coenzyme Q_{10} (CoQ_{10} or ubiquinone) before treatments. Animal studies have shown that vitamins C and E may also have a protective effect. Discuss this with your physician and consider taking supplements (30–100 mg coenzyme Q_{10} daily, 1000 mg vitamin C daily, 400 IU vitamin E daily). • Doxorubicin can increase your risk of kidney stones. Drinking at least 64 ounces of fluids daily can help prevent this.

DOXYCYCLINE

BRAND NAMES *Doryx, Monodox, Vibramycin, others*

TYPE OF DRUG	Tetracycline antibiotic
DESCRIPTION	Doxycycline is prescribed for bacterial infections. It is often prescribed to prevent or treat traveler's diarrhea.
DON'T MIX WITH	**Berberine-containing herbs.** Goldenseal *(Hydrastis canadensis)*, barberry *(Berberis vulgaris)*, and Oregon grape *(Berberis acquifolium)* contain berberine, an antibacterial chemical. It is possible that berberine interferes with the body's absorption of tetracycline, a drug very similar to doxycycline. Until more information is known, do not use these herbs when taking doxycycline.
KEEP IN MIND	• The calcium in milk and dairy products can interfere with the absorption of doxycycline. Discuss your intake of these foods with your medical practitioner. • The aluminum, calcium, and magnesium in antacids can interfere with your absorption of doxycycline, as can the calcium, iron, magnesium, zinc, and other minerals in supplements and multivitamins with minerals. Take these antacids and supplements two hours apart from this drug. • Doxycycline kills not only the harmful bacteria that cause illness but also the good bacteria normally found in your intestines; this can cause diarrhea. Consider taking probiotic supplements (at least 1.5 billion live organisms daily, including a mixture of *Lactobacillus acidophilus, Bifidobacterium bifidum*, and *Saccharomyces boulardii*).

DOXYLAMINE

BRAND NAMES *Unisom*

TYPE OF DRUG	Antihistamine
DESCRIPTION	Doxylamine is an antihistamine, a type of drug usually used to treat allergies, but it is used primarily as a nonprescription sleep aid, either by itself (Unisom) or as an ingredient in nighttime cold formulas.
DON'T MIX WITH	**Henbane** *(Hyoscyamus niger)*. This herb is toxic and should be used only when prescribed and closely monitored by a qualified practitioner. Because both doxylamine and henbane have similar side effects, such as dry mouth, dizziness, and drowsiness, they should never be used in combination with each other. **Sedative herbs.** When combined with doxylamine, these herbs may cause excessive drowsiness. Avoid sedative herbs such as chamomile *(Matricaria recutita)*, catnip *(Nepeta cataria)*, kava kava *(Piper methysticum)*, passionflower *(Passiflora incarnata)*, St. John's wort *(Hypericum perforatum)*, valerian *(Valeriana officinalis)*, and others, as well as sedative dietary supplements such as 5-HTP, tryptophan, and SAMe. *Passionflower*
KEEP IN MIND	• Doxylamine causes drowsiness. Alcohol makes this effect worse. Do not consume alcohol if taking this drug. • The hormone melatonin is used as a natural sleep aid. Do not combine it with doxylamine or any other prescription or nonprescription sleep aid. To do so may cause dangerous drowsiness.

ECONAZOLE

TYPE OF DRUG	Antifungal
DESCRIPTION	Spectazole is an antifungal cream prescribed for fungal infections of the skin, including athlete's foot, jock itch, and ringworm.
DON'T MIX WITH	No known herbal interactions.
DO TAKE WITH	**Echinacea** (*Echinacea* spp). According to one study, women who took the herb echinacea while using econazole cream had fewer recurrences of vaginal yeast infections compared to women who used the cream alone. Consider taking supplements (500 mg 3 times daily) until infection clears.

EPHEDRINE

TYPE OF DRUG	Bronchodilator and decongestant
DESCRIPTION	In prescription and nonprescription forms, ephedrine is used to relieve asthma (Bronkaid, Primatene, others). As a nasal spray (Pretz-D) or in drops (Vicks Vatronol), it is used to treat nasal congestion. If you have asthma, discuss ephedrine products with your physician first before you try them.
DON'T MIX WITH	**Caffeine-containing herbs.** The stimulant effect of caffeine can make the side effects of ephedrine, such as nervousness, restlessness, insomnia, and dizziness, worse. Avoid caffeine-containing herbs, including guarana *(Paullinia cupana)*, kola nut *(Cola* spp.), and maté *(Ilex paraguariensis)*. **Ephedra** (*Ephedra* spp., also known as ma huang). Ephedrine was originally isolated from ephedra. Taking ephedra with any product containing ephedrine could increase the side effects of the drug, including nervousness, insomnia, dizziness, high blood pressure, and heart arrhythmias. **Tannin-containing herbs.** Herbs that are high in tannin, including black walnut *(Juglans nigra)*, red raspberry *(Rubus idaeus)*, oak *(Quercus* spp.), uva ursi *(Arctostaphylos uva-ursi)*, and witch hazel *(Hamamelis virginiana)*, can interfere with your absorption of ephedrine, as can the tannins in tea. Take them two hours apart from this drug.
KEEP IN MIND	• The side effects of ephedrine, such as nervousness, restlessness, insomnia, and dizziness, may be worsened by caffeine's stimulant effect. Coffee, tea, and cola drinks naturally contain caffeine; it is also added to many soft drinks and "energy-boosting" products. Avoid these if taking ephedrine.

Witch hazel

EPINEPHRINE

BRAND NAMES *EpiPen, Primatene Mist, others*

TYPE OF DRUG	Bronchodilator
DESCRIPTION	Epinephrine is the synthetic form of adrenaline. As a nonprescription drug, epinephrine is sold as a mist to be inhaled into the lungs to treat asthma symptoms. If you have asthma, discuss epinephrine with your physician before you try it. As a prescription drug, epinephrine is sold as EpiPen, an auto injector used for treating anaphylactic shock caused by severe allergic reactions, such as those caused by bee stings.
DON'T MIX WITH	**Caffeine-containing herbs.** The stimulant effect of caffeine can make the side effects of epinephrine, such as nervousness, restlessness, insomnia, and dizziness, worse. Avoid all caffeine-containing herbs, including guarana (*Paullinia cupana*), kola nut (*Cola* spp.), and maté (*Ilex paraguariensis*). **Ephedra** (*Ephedra* spp., also known as ma huang). The drug ephedrine, which is very similar to epinephrine, was originally isolated from ephedra. Taking ephedra with any product containing epinephrine could increase the side effects of the drug, including nervousness, insomnia, dizziness, high blood pressure, and heart arrhythmias.
KEEP IN MIND	• Frequent use of epinephrine mist may lower your levels of vitamin C, potassium, and magnesium. Consider taking supplements (daily multivitamin with minerals). • The side effects of epinephrine, such as nervousness, restlessness, insomnia, and dizziness, may be worsened by caffeine's stimulant effect. Coffee, tea, and cola drinks naturally contain caffeine; it is also added to many soft drinks and "energy-boosting" products. Avoid these if taking epinephrine.

Ephedra

ERYTHROMYCIN

BRAND NAMES *Benzamycin, E-Mycin, Eryc, Ery-Tab, Ilotycin, others*

TYPE OF DRUG	Macrolide antibiotic
DESCRIPTION	Erythromycin is used to treat a wide range of bacterial infections and is often prescribed for acne and skin infections. This drug has numerous interactions with other prescription drugs. Be certain to tell your physician about any other prescription and nonprescription drugs and dietary supplements you may already be taking before you try this. If you take any statin drug such as lovastatin *(p. 168)* or atorvastatin *(p. 129)*, do not take erythromycin. The combination could cause a potentially fatal muscle disease.
DON'T MIX WITH	**Digitalis** (*Digitalis* spp., also known as foxglove). Erythromycin can raise your blood level of the dangerous herb digitalis and also digoxin, a drug with similar effects. Do not mix digitalis and erythromycin.
KEEP IN MIND	• Erythromycin interferes with your absorption of folic acid, vitamin B_6, and vitamin B_{12}, as well as calcium and magnesium. To prevent deficiencies, take a daily multivitamin/mineral supplement at least two hours apart from when you take erythromycin. • Erythromycin kills not only the harmful bacteria that cause illness but also the good bacteria that are normally found in your intestines; this can cause diarrhea. Consider taking probiotic supplements (at least 1.5 billion live organisms daily, including a mixture of *Lactobacillus acidophilus, Bifidobacterium bifidum,* and *Saccharomyces boulardii*). • Bromelain, an enzyme found in pineapples, increases the body's absorption of erythromycin. This may help people with severe infections or infections that don't respond to erythromycin. Discuss bromelain with your physician before you try it.

Pineapple

153

ESTRADIOL

BRAND NAMES *Alora, CombiPatch, Estrace, Estraderm, FemPatch, Vivelle, others*

TYPE OF DRUG	Estrogen hormone replacement

DESCRIPTION Estradiol is prescribed to replace estrogen in menopausal women. It is used to treat menopause symptoms, such as hot flashes and vaginal dryness, and to help prevent osteoporosis. It is also used to treat some forms of breast cancer and prostate cancer.

DON'T MIX WITH

Black cohosh (*Cimicifuga racemosa*). Black cohosh contains phytoestrogens, plant hormones similar to human estrogen. Combining it with estradiol could raise the body's estrogen level too high. **Chaste tree** (*Vitex agnus-castus*). Chaste tree affects your levels of the hormone prolactin, which in turn can affect estrogen and how your body uses estradiol.

Black cohosh

Other estrogenic herbs. The herbs dong quai (*Angelica sinensis*) and red clover (*Trifolium pratense*) may have estrogen-like effects. Laboratory studies have shown that the herbs licorice (*Glycyrrhiza glabra*), thyme *(Thymus spp.)*, turmeric (*Curcuma longa*), hops *(Humulus lupulus)*, and vervain (*Verbena* spp. and *V. hastata*) may modulate estrogen activity. Discuss the use of these herbs with your medical practitioner before using them if you already take estradiol.

KEEP IN MIND

• Estradiol may block the body's absorption of folic acid (folate). Consider taking supplements (400 mcg daily).
• Estradiol may decrease the body's levels of vitamin C, magnesium, and zinc. Consider taking a daily multivitamin with minerals.

• Studies have shown that soy isoflavones (estrogenlike substances) can help to relieve menopausal symptoms. Ipriflavone, a type of soy isoflavone, can help prevent osteoporosis. Combining soy isoflavones with estradiol could raise your estrogen level too high. If you want to use soy isoflavones in combination with or instead of estradiol, discuss the decision with your physician.

ETODOLAC

BRAND NAMES *Lodine, Lodine XL*

TYPE OF DRUG	Nonsteroidal anti-inflammatory drug (NSAID)

DESCRIPTION Etodolac is an NSAID used to treat arthritis, bursitis, tendinitis, and mild to moderate pain.

DON'T MIX WITH No known herbal interactions.

DO TAKE WITH **Deglycyrrhizinated licorice** (DGL derived from *Glycyrrhiza glabra*). The soothing and anti-inflammatory properties of DGL can help prevent stomach irritation often caused by etodolac. Consider taking supplements (400 mg 2 to 4 times daily).

KEEP IN MIND

• Etodolac may cause sodium and water retention. Discuss salt restrictions with your physician.

• Etodolac may cause drowsiness, dizziness, or blurred vision. Alcohol can make these side effects worse; do not consume alcohol if you take this drug.

FAMOTIDINE

BRAND NAMES *Pepcid, Pepcid AC*

TYPE OF DRUG	H2 blocker
DESCRIPTION	Famotidine sharply reduces the body's production of stomach acid. In prescription form (Pepcid), it is used to treat ulcers, heartburn, and gastroesophageal reflux disease (GERD). In nonprescription form (Pepcid AC), it is used for mild heartburn.
DON'T MIX WITH	No known herbal interactions.

DO TAKE WITH

Licorice

Deglycyrrhizinated licorice (DGL, derived from *Glycyrrhiza glabra*). DGL can speed ulcer healing as it stimulates the production of mucus that protects the stomach lining and also has an anti-inflammatory effect. Consider taking supplements (250 mg 2 to 4 times daily).

KEEP IN MIND

• Famotidine and other H2 blockers reduce the body's absorption of some vitamins and minerals, including folic acid (folate), vitamin B_{12} (cobalamin), zinc, and iron. If you use these drugs on a regular basis, consider taking supplements (400 mcg daily of folic acid, 500 mcg daily of vitamin B_{12}, plus a daily multivitamin supplement with minerals). Take them at least two hours apart from famotidine.
• Magnesium supplements and calcium-, magnesium-, and magnesium/aluminum-based antacids may block the body's absorption of famotidine. Take them at least two hours apart from famotidine.

FLUOXETINE HYDROCHLORIDE

BRAND NAMES *Prozac, Sarafem*

TYPE OF DRUG	Selective serotonin reuptake inhibitor (SSRI)
DESCRIPTION	Fluoxetine is used to treat depression, obsessive-compulsive disorder, bulimia, anorexia, social phobias, and a number of other disorders. SSRI drugs affect the way the body uses the neurotransmitter serotonin.

DON'T MIX WITH

Valerian

Sedative herbs. When combined with fluoxetine, these herbs may cause excessive drowsiness. Avoid sedative herbs such as chamomile (*Matricaria recutita*), catnip (*Nepeta cataria*), kava kava (*Piper methysticum*), passionflower (*Passiflora incarnata*), St. John's wort (*Hypericum perforatum*), and valerian (*Valeriana officinalis*).

St. John's wort (*Hypericum perforatum*). Although there have been no reports of dangerous interactions, it is possible that combining this herb with fluoxetine could raise your serotonin levels too high. This may cause a serious condition called serotonin syndrome. If you wish to take St. John's wort instead of fluoxetine, discuss it with your physician.

DO TAKE WITH

Ginkgo (*Ginkgo biloba*). Sexual dysfunction in both men and women is a fairly common side effect of fluoxetine. Ginkgo may be helpful in lessening this problem. Consider taking supplements (60 mg *Ginkgo biloba* extract standardized to 24 percent ginkgo flavone glycosides three times daily).

KEEP IN MIND

• Don't use the dietary supplements 5-HTP, tryptophan, or SAMe if you take fluoxetine. Both the supplements and the drug increase serotonin levels, which may rise too high.

• A study in 1995 showed fluoxetine lowers levels of the hormone melatonin. Discuss this with your physician and consider taking supplements (1–3 mg daily).
• Fluoxetine doesn't work well if your folic acid level is low. Consider taking supplements (400 mcg daily).

FLUVASTATIN

TYPE OF DRUG	Statin cholesterol-lowering agent
DESCRIPTION	Fluvastatin is prescribed to lower high cholesterol, slow or prevent hardening of the arteries, and reduce the risk of heart attack and stroke.
DON'T MIX WITH	No known herbal interactions.
DO TAKE WITH	**Milk thistle** *(Silybum marianum)*. Although there are no studies of statin drugs to date, silymarin, an active compound in the herb milk thistle, may protect against the liver damage that can occur as a side effect of this type of drug. Consider taking supplements (150 mg 3 to 4 times daily).
KEEP IN MIND	• Lovastatin, a drug similar to fluvastatin, interacts adversely with grapefruit juice. Don't take fluvastatin with grapefruit juice. • High doses of niacin (2–3 grams daily) can also lower cholesterol. Combining high-dose niacin with some statin drugs, however, can lead to a serious muscle disorder. There are no studies of niacin and fluvastatin, but until more information is known, avoid high-dose niacin. The amount of niacin in a daily multivitamin or B vitamin supplement is not enough to cause problems. • Red yeast rice, sold as Cholestin, works in a way similar to the statin drugs. Do not use red yeast rice with fluvastatin. • According to one study, statin drugs can gradually raise vitamin A levels. Until more is known, do not take vitamin A supplements. The vitamin A contained in a daily multivitamin is not enough to cause problems. • Studies show that taking statin drugs can lower your level of coenzyme Q_{10} (CoQ_{10} or ubiquinone), a substance needed for energy production in your cells. Consider taking supplements (100 mg daily).

FLUVOXAMINE

TYPE OF DRUG	Selective serotonin reuptake inhibitor (SSRI)
DESCRIPTION	Fluvoxamine is used to treat obsessive-compulsive disorder and depression. SSRI drugs such as fluvoxamine affect the way the body uses the neurotransmitter serotonin.
DON'T MIX WITH	**Sedative herbs.** When combined with fluvoxamine, these herbs may cause excessive drowsiness. Avoid sedative herbs such as chamomile *(Matricaria recutita)*, catnip *(Nepeta cataria)*, kava kava *(Piper methysticum)*, passionflower *(Passiflora incarnata)*, St. John's wort *(Hypericum perforatum)*, and valerian *(Valeriana officinalis)*. *St. John's wort* **St. John's wort** *(Hypericum perforatum)*. Although there have been no reports of dangerous interactions, it is possible that combining this herb with fluvoxamine could raise serotonin levels too high. This may cause a serious condition called serotonin syndrome. If you wish to take St. John's wort instead of fluvoxamine, discuss it with your physician.
DO TAKE WITH	**Ginkgo** *(Ginkgo biloba)*. Sexual dysfunction in both men and women is a fairly common side effect of fluvoxamine. Ginkgo may be helpful in lessening this problem. Consider supplements (60 mg ginkgo extract standardized to 24 percent ginkgo flavone glycosides three times daily).
KEEP IN MIND	• Fluvoxamine can cause drowsiness and dizziness. Alcohol can make these side effects worse. Do not combine the two. • Do not use the dietary supplements 5-HTP, tryptophan, or SAMe if you take fluvoxamine. Both the supplements and the drug increase your serotonin level; it may rise too high, causing a serious condition called serotonin syndrome.

FUROSEMIDE

BRAND NAME *Lasix*

TYPE OF DRUG	Loop diuretic
DESCRIPTION	Loop diuretics are used to treat congestive heart failure, high blood pressure, and other conditions such as edema. Furosemide is a powerful diuretic (a drug that removes water from the body) that also depletes the body's levels of potassium and magnesium. Discuss your diet and taking supplements with your physician.
DON'T MIX WITH	**Digitalis** (*Digitalis* spp., also known as foxglove). This dangerous herb is very similar to the heart drug digoxin *(p. 147)*, which can cause dangerous side effects when taken in combination with furosemide. Digitalis can cause the same sort of problems and should not be combined with furosemide. **Licorice** (*Glycyrrhiza glabra*). The potassium-depleting effect of furosemide is worsened by licorice. This effect does not occur with deglycyrrhizinated licorice (DGL) or with artificial licorice flavoring. **Herbal diuretics.** Avoid herbal diuretics as their effects, added to that of furosemide, may be dangerous. Herbal diuretics include bilberry leaf *(Vaccinium myrtillus)*, buchu *(Barosma betulina)*, burdock *(Arctium lappa)*, couch grass *(Agropyron repens)*, damiana *(Turnera diffusa)*, dandelion *(Taraxacum officinale)*, fennel seed *(Foeniculum vulgare)*, goldenrod *(Solidago virgaurea)*, horsetail *(Equisetum arvense)*, kava kava *(Piper methysticum)*, kola nut *(Cola* spp.), marshmallow *(Althaea officinalis)*, maté *(Ilex paraguariensis)*, parsley *(Petroselinum* spp.), sarsaparilla *(Smilax* spp.), saw palmetto *(Serenoa repens)*, uva ursi *(Arctostaphylos uva-ursi)*, vervain *(Verbena* spp. and *V. hastata)*, and yarrow *(Achillea millefolium)*. Any other non-prescription diuretics should also be avoided.

Bilberry

GEMFIBROZIL

BRAND NAMES *Lopid, Apo-Gemfibrozil Canada, Novo-Gemfibrozil Canada*

TYPE OF DRUG	Cholesterol-lowering agent
DESCRIPTION	Gemfibrozil is prescribed for people with very high triglycerides (a type of blood fat), high LDL cholesterol, and low HDL cholesterol. In general, it is used only when other treatments have failed.
DON'T MIX WITH	No known herbal interactions.
KEEP IN MIND	• Red yeast rice. This dietary supplement, sold as Cholestin, works in a similar way to statin drugs, such as lovastatin *(p. 168)*. Combining the statin drugs with gemfibrozil can lead to a potentially fatal muscle disease. Do not combine red yeast rice with gemfibrozil because the same interaction may occur. • Gemfibrozil may cause dizziness or blurred vision. Alcohol makes these side effects worse. Do not consume alcohol if taking this drug.

GENTAMICIN, GENTAMICIN SULFATE
BRAND NAMES *Garamycin, Genoptic, Ocu-Mycin, others*

TYPE OF DRUG	Aminoglycoside antibiotic
DESCRIPTION	Gentamicin is a powerful antibiotic that is given intravenously or by injection (Garamycin) to treat bacterial infections. It is also used in eyedrops to treat eye infections (Genoptic, Ocu-Mycin, others).
DON'T MIX WITH	No known herbal interactions.
KEEP IN MIND	• Intravenous or injected gentamicin (but not in eyedrops) kills not only the harmful bacteria that cause illness but also the good bacteria that are normally found in your intestines; this can cause diarrhea. Consider probiotic supplements (at least 1.5 billion live organisms daily, including a mixture of *Lactobacillus acidophilus, Bifidobacterium bifidum,* and *Saccharomyces boulardii*).

GLIPIZIDE
BRAND NAMES *Glucotrol, Glucotrol XL*

TYPE OF DRUG	Sulfonylurea antidiabetic drug
DESCRIPTION	Glipizide is prescribed to lower blood sugar in people with non-insulin-dependent (Type 2 or adult-onset) diabetes.
DON'T MIX WITH	No known herbal interactions.
DO TAKE WITH	**Note:** You may be able to reduce the amount of glipizide you need by taking one of the following herbs, or chromium picolinate *(see* Keep in Mind *section)*. In order to make sure that you are receiving the right amount of medication, it is extremely important for you to discuss your use and dosage of these herbs or this supplement with your physician before you try them. **Fenugreek** *(Trigonella foenum-graecum)*. In very large doses (25 or more grams daily) fenugreek seeds can help lower blood sugar levels in diabetics. Discuss fenugreek with your physician before you try it; your glipizide dose may have to be adjusted. **Gurmar** *(Gymnema sylvestre)*. This herb from India may help lower blood sugar levels in diabetics. Consider taking supplements (100 mg 3 times daily). Discuss gurmar with your physician before you try it; your glipizide dose may have to be adjusted. **Other herbs.** Bitter melon *(Momordica charantia)*, burdock *(Arctium lappa)*, dandelion *(Taraxacum officinale)*, garlic *(Allium sativum)*, and ginseng *(Panax ginseng)* are among the herbs that are traditionally recommended for lowering blood sugar in diabetics. Use these herbs with caution and discuss them with your physician first. Your glipizide dose may have to be adjusted.
Fenugreek	
KEEP IN MIND	• The mineral chromium can be helpful for lowering blood sugar in diabetics. Consider taking supplements in the form of chromium picolinate (500–1,000 mcg daily). Discuss chromium picolinate with your physician before you try it; your glipizide dose may have to be adjusted.

GLYBURIDE

BRAND NAMES *DiaBeta, Glynase PresTab, Micronase*

TYPE OF DRUG	Sulfonylurea antidiabetic drug
DESCRIPTION	Glyburide is prescribed to lower blood sugar in people with non-insulin-dependent (Type 2 or adult-onset) diabetes.
DON'T MIX WITH	No known herbal interactions.
DO TAKE WITH	**Note:** You may be able to reduce the amount of glyburide you need by taking one of the following herbs, or chromium picolinate *(see* Keep in Mind *section).* In order to make sure that you are receiving the right amount of medication, it is extremely important for you to discuss your use and dosage of these herbs or this supplement with your physician before you try them. **Fenugreek** *(Trigonella foenum-graecum).* In very large doses (25 or more grams daily) fenugreek seeds can help lower blood sugar levels in diabetics. Discuss fenugreek with your physician before you try it; your glyburide dose may have to be adjusted. **Gurmar** *(Gymnema sylvestre).* This herb from India may help lower blood sugar levels in diabetics. Discuss gurmar with your physician before you try it; your glyburide dose may have to be adjusted. Consider taking supplements (100 mg 3 times daily). **Other herbs.** Bitter melon *(Momordica charantia),* burdock *(Arctium lappa),* dandelion *(Taraxacum officinale),* garlic *(Allium sativum),* and ginseng *(Panax ginseng)* are among the herbs that are traditionally recommended for lowering blood sugar in diabetics. Use these herbs with caution and discuss them with your physician first. Your glyburide dose may have to be adjusted.
KEEP IN MIND	• The mineral chromium can be helpful for lowering blood sugar in diabetics. Consider taking supplements in the form of chromium picolinate (500–1,000 mcg daily). Discuss this with your physician first; the glyburide dose may have to be adjusted.

Dandelion

HALOPERIDOL

BRAND NAME *Haldol*

TYPE OF DRUG	Antipsychotic
DESCRIPTION	Haloperidol is prescribed to treat psychotic disorders, schizophrenia, Tourette's syndrome, and acute psychiatric conditions.
DON'T MIX WITH	**Caffeine-containing herbs.** Research suggests caffeine can reduce the absorption of haloperidol. Do not use the herbs guarana *(Paullinia cupana),* kola nut *(Cola spp.),* and maté *(Ilex paraguariensis)* within two hours of taking this drug. **Sedative herbs.** When combined with haloperidol, sedative herbs may cause excessive drowsiness. Avoid sedative herbs such as chamomile *(Matricaria recutita),* catnip *(Nepeta cataria),* kava kava *(Piper methysticum),* passionflower *(Passiflora incarnata),* St. John's wort *(Hypericum perforatum),* valerian *(Valeriana officinalis),* and others, as well as sedative dietary supplements such as 5-HTP, tryptophan, and SAMe.
KEEP IN MIND	• Haloperidol can cause drowsiness. Alcohol can make this side effect worse. Do not consume alcohol if taking this drug. • Caffeine may reduce the absorption of haloperidol. Coffee, tea, chocolate, and cola drinks naturally contain caffeine; it is also added to many soft drinks and "energy-boosting" products. Avoid all these drinks and products for two hours before and after taking haloperidol.

Kava kava

HEPARIN	BRAND NAMES *This drug is sold only in generic form*

TYPE OF DRUG	Anticoagulant
DESCRIPTION	Heparin is a very powerful blood-thinning drug that is given by injection to prevent and treat blood clots. Be sure to tell your medical practitioner about any prescription or nonprescription drugs and herbs or supplements you are taking.
DON'T MIX WITH	**Blood-thinning herbs.** A number of herbs have known or possible anticoagulant action and may cause an increased risk of bleeding when used with heparin. Avoid dan shen *(Salvia miltiorrhiza)*, devil's claw *(Harpagophytum procumbens)*, garlic *(Allium sativum)*, ginger *(Zingiber officinale)*, ginkgo *(Ginkgo biloba)*, ginseng *(Panax ginseng)*, and sweet woodruff *(Galium odoratum)*. Foods containing garlic and ginger in moderate amounts are unlikely to cause any problems. In addition, the herbs dong quai *(Angelica sinensis)*, fenugreek *(Trigonella foenum-graecum)*, horse chestnut *(Aesculus hippocastanum)*, and red clover *(Trifolium pratense)* contain small amounts of chemicals similar to warfarin, another powerful blood-thinning drug *(p. 195)*, and should be avoided when taking heparin.
KEEP IN MIND	• High doses of vitamin C (more than 3,000 mg daily) might reduce the blood-thinning effect of heparin. High doses of vitamin E may cause an increased risk of bleeding when used with heparin. In addition, dietary supplements such as phosphatidyl serine and fish oil may interact adversely with heparin. In general, avoid any dietary supplements when taking heparin unless you have discussed them with your medical practitioner.

Devil's claw

HYDRALAZINE	BRAND NAME *Apresoline*

TYPE OF DRUG	Antihypertensive
DESCRIPTION	Hydralazine is usually prescribed to lower high blood pressure. It is sometimes prescribed to treat congestive heart failure. This drug can make some heart problems worse and could cause angina or a heart attack. Be certain to tell your physician if you have ever had any heart trouble.
DON'T MIX WITH	**Blood vessel relaxing herbs.** Coleus *(Coleus forskohlii)*, garlic *(Allium sativum)*, ginkgo *(Ginkgo biloba)*, and hawthorn *(Crataegus oxyacantha)* relax your blood vessels and are sometimes used to treat high blood pressure. Although there have been no studies, it is possible that combining these herbs with hydralazine could make your blood pressure drop too low.
KEEP IN MIND	• Hydralazine works by opening up your blood vessels. Alcohol has a similar effect. Do not consume alcohol while taking this drug because your blood pressure may drop too low. • Hydralazine can make you eliminate extra vitamin B_6 (pyridoxine), which could cause a deficiency. Discuss this with your physician and consider taking supplements (50 mg daily).

Ginkgo

HYDROCORTISONE

BRAND NAMES *Cortef, Hydrocortone*

TYPE OF DRUG	Corticosteroid

DESCRIPTION

Corticosteroids such as hydrocortisone are synthetic hormones used to treat a wide variety of severe disorders, particularly those that involve inflammation, including arthritis, psoriasis, allergies, asthma, and inflammatory bowel disease. They also treat autoimmune diseases such as lupus erythematosus and transplant rejection.

Hydrocortisone in small amounts is used in many nonprescription creams to relieve itching from poison ivy, insect bites, mild psoriasis, and other minor skin irritations. The amount of hydrocortisone in these creams is not enough to cause interactions in most people.

DON'T MIX WITH

Foglove

Digitalis (*Digitalis* spp., also known as foxglove). This dangerous herb is very similar to the heart drug digoxin *(p. 147)*, which may worsen the side effects of hydrocortisone. Digitalis may cause the same problem as digoxin.

Ephedra (*Ephedra* spp., also known as ma huang). The herb ephedra naturally contains ephedrine, which reduces the effectiveness of corticosteroids. Do not use it when taking hydrocortisone. Similarly, avoid the drugs ephedrine *(p. 152)* and pseudoephedrine *(p. 185)*, which are found in many nonprescription cold and allergy remedies.

KEEP IN MIND

• Corticosteroids can cause the retention of sodium, which is found in salt. Discuss salt restrictions with your physician.
• Long-term use of corticosteroids may cause osteoporosis. Consider taking supplements (1,000 mg calcium daily, 400 IU vitamin D daily). Corticosteroids may also reduce your levels of vitamin B_6 (pyridoxine) and

magnesium. Consider taking supplements (50 mg pyridoxine daily and 300–400 mg magnesium daily).
• Because this drug reduces the body's levels of chromium, long-term use of corticosteroids may contribute to the development of diabetes. Consider taking supplements (200 mcg chromium picolinate daily).

IBUPROFEN

BRAND NAMES *Advil, Arthritis Foundation, Midol, Motrin, Nuprin, others*

TYPE OF DRUG	Nonsteroidal anti-inflammatory drug (NSAID)

DESCRIPTION

Ibuprofen is an NSAID used to treat arthritis, headaches, menstrual discomfort, and mild to moderate pain. It is also used to treat fever and swelling. Ibuprofen is sold as both a prescription drug (Motrin) and nonprescription drug (Advil, Arthritis Foundation, Midol, Nuprin, others).

DON'T MIX WITH No known herbal interactions.

DO TAKE WITH

Deglycyrrhizinated licorice (DGL, derived from *Glycyrrhiza glabra*). DGL stimulates the production of mucus that protects the stomach lining and also has an anti-inflammatory effect. It may help prevent the stomach irritation often caused by ibuprofen. Consider taking supplements (250 mg 2 to 4 times daily).

KEEP IN MIND

• Ibuprofen can irritate your stomach. Alcohol can make this effect worse. Do not combine alcohol and this drug.
• Take ibuprofen with food to reduce the risk of stomach irritation.

IMIPRAMINE	BRAND NAMES *Tofranil, Tofranil-PM*

TYPE OF DRUG	Tricyclic antidepressant
DESCRIPTION	Imipramine is used to treat depression. Like other tricyclic antidepressants, it works by affecting the way chemicals called neurotransmitters, including serotonin and norepinephrine, move in and out of the body's nerve endings.
DON'T MIX WITH *Passionflower*	**Ephedra** (*Ephedra* spp., also known as ma huang). Taking ephedra with any tricyclic antidepressant increases your risk of serious high blood pressure and heart arrhythmias. Similarly, avoid the related drugs ephedrine and pseudoephedrine, which can usually be found in many nonprescription cold and allergy remedies. **Sedative herbs.** Sedative herbs may cause excessive drowsiness when combined with imipramine. Avoid sedative herbs such as chamomile *(Matricaria recutita)*, catnip *(Nepeta cataria)*, kava kava *(Piper methysticum)*, passionflower *(Passiflora incarnata)*, St. John's wort *(Hypericum perforatum)*, valerian *(Valeriana officinalis)*, and others, as well as sedative dietary supplements such as 5-HTP, tryptophan, and SAMe. **St. John's wort** *(Hypericum perforatum)*. Research suggests that this herb and imipramine work in similar ways. Until more is known, do not take imipramine in conjunction with St. John's wort. **Yohimbe** *(Pausinystalia yohimbe)*. This dangerous herb is said to improve male sexual function. Do not use this herb when taking imipramine; the combination may cause a dangerous rise in blood pressure.
KEEP IN MIND	• Heart problems can be a side effect of tricyclic antidepressants, possibly because these drugs lower your production of coenzyme Q_{10} (CoQ_{10} or ubiquinone). CoQ_{10} is needed to produce energy in your cells, including the cells of your heart. Consider taking CoQ_{10} supplements (20–50 mg daily).

INDINAVIR	BRAND NAME *Crixivan*

TYPE OF DRUG	Antiviral
DESCRIPTION	Indinavir is used in combination with the antiviral drug AZT *(p. 130)* as part of a "cocktail" of drugs to treat HIV infection and AIDS. Indinavir has a number of serious side effects, including increased cholesterol and blood glucose levels. Indinavir can interact adversely with a number of drugs, including drugs to control cholesterol and triglycerides. Be certain to tell your physician about any other prescription and nonprescription drugs and dietary supplements you take.
DON'T MIX WITH	**St. John's wort** *(Hypericum perforatum)*. Your absorption of protease inhibitors is seriously reduced by this herb. Do not use it if you are taking indinavir.
DO TAKE WITH	**Milk thistle** *(Silybum marianum)*. Silymarin, an active compound in the herb milk thistle, may help protect your liver against damage from indinavir. Discuss this with your medical practitioner and consider taking supplements (150 mg 3 to 4 times daily).
KEEP IN MIND	• Indinavir works best if you take it on an empty stomach. Fatty foods block your absorption of the drug. • To avoid the risk of kidney stones, drink plenty of liquids (at least 64 ounces a day).

INDOMETHACIN

BRAND NAMES *Indochron E-R, Indocin, Indocin SR*

TYPE OF DRUG	Nonsteroidal anti-inflammatory drug (NSAID)
DESCRIPTION	Indomethacin is a prescription NSAID used to treat arthritis, tendinitis, bursitis, menstrual discomfort, and migraine. It can interact adversely with many drugs frequently prescribed for high blood pressure and heart problems. Be certain to tell your physician about all prescription and nonprescription drugs and dietary supplements you take.
DON'T MIX WITH	No known herbal interactions.
DO TAKE WITH	**Deglycyrrhizinated licorice** (DGL, derived from *Glycyrrhiza glabra*). DGL stimulates the production of mucus that protects the stomach lining and also has an anti-inflammatory effect. It may help prevent the stomach irritation often caused by indomethacin. Consider taking supplements (up to 250 mg 2 to 4 times daily).
KEEP IN MIND	• Indomethacin can irritate your stomach. Alcohol can make this effect worse. Do not combine alcohol with this drug. • Take indomethacin with food to reduce the risk of stomach irritation. • Indomethacin may reduce your absorption of vitamins and minerals such as vitamin C and calcium. Consider taking a daily multivitamin supplement with minerals at least two hours apart from the drug.

INFLUENZA VACCINE

BRAND NAMES *Fluogen, Flu-Shield, Fluvirin, Fluzone*

TYPE OF DRUG	Influenza vaccine
DESCRIPTION	Influenza vaccines are administered as a protective measure against catching the flu; they may also keep the flu from being as severe if you do catch it. The vaccines are modified annually to protect against the flu strains researchers believe are most likely to occur that season.
DON'T MIX WITH	No known herbal interactions.
DO TAKE WITH	**Ginseng** (*Panax ginseng*). A well-conducted study in 1996 showed that ginseng may help the flu vaccine work better by increasing antibody production and decreasing the frequency of colds and flus. The dose used in the study was 100 mg taken twice daily for four weeks before vaccination and eight weeks afterward.

Ginseng

INSULIN	BRAND NAMES *Humalog, Humulin, Iletin, Novolin, Velosulin, others*
TYPE OF DRUG	Antidiabetic
DESCRIPTION	Insulin drugs are very similar to the hormone insulin produced by your pancreas. They are used by people with insulin-dependent (juvenile or Type 1 diabetes) diabetes to replace the insulin their pancreas doesn't make. These drugs are also used by some people with non-insulin-dependent (adult-onset or Type 2) diabetes. Insulin must be injected. Because many drugs interact with insulin, be certain to tell your physician about any prescription and nonprescription and dietary supplements you take.
DON'T MIX WITH	No known herbal interactions.
DO TAKE WITH	**Note:** You may be able to reduce the amount of insulin you need by taking one of the following herbs. In order to make sure that you are receiving the right amount of medication, it is extremely important for you to discuss your use and dosage of this supplement or these herbs with your physician before you try them. **Fenugreek** *(Trigonella foenum-graecum)*. In very large doses (25 or more grams daily) fenugreek seeds can help lower blood sugar levels in people with diabetes. Discuss fenugreek with your physician before you actually try it; your insulin dose may have to be adjusted. **Gurmar** *(Gymnema sylvestre)*. This herb from India may help lower blood sugar levels in diabetics. Consider taking supplements (100 mg 3 times daily). Discuss gurmar with your physician before you try it; your insulin dose may have to be adjusted. **Other herbs:** Bitter melon *(Momordica charantia)*, burdock *(Arctium lappa)*, dandelion *(Taraxacum officinale)*, garlic *(Allium sativum)*, and ginseng *(Panax ginseng)* are among the herbs that are traditionally recommended for lowering blood sugar in people with diabetes. Use these herbs with caution and discuss them with your physician first. The insulin dose may have to be adjusted.

Fenugreek

INTERFERON	BRAND NAMES *Actimmune, Alferon N, Avonex, Betaseron, Rebif, others*
TYPE OF DRUG	Antiviral
DESCRIPTION	Interferon is an antiviral drug prescribed for hepatitis C and other viral infections. It is also used to treat multiple sclerosis, some kinds of cancer, and other diseases. Because interferon can cause liver damage and other problems, you will need to be carefully monitored by your medical practitioner.
DON'T MIX WITH	**Bupleurum** *(Bupleurum* spp.). Combining bupleurum in any form with interferon can lead to a dangerous form of lung disease. Never mix the two. This herb, also known as hare's ear (chai hu) or thorewax root, is sometimes recommended by herbalists for a wide variety of ailments. It is found in some Japanese herbal combination formulas for treating liver disease, including the products known as sho-saiko-to and xino-chai-hu-tang.
KEEP IN MIND	• Preliminary research indicates that it is possible that the dietary supplement n-acetyl-cysteine (NAC) may enhance the effectiveness of interferon. Discuss this with your medical practitioner and consider taking supplements (600 mg three times daily).

ISONIAZID

TYPE OF DRUG	Antitubercular
DESCRIPTION	Isoniazid, either by itself (INH, Laniazid) or in combination with rifampin (Rifamate, Rimactane) is an antibiotic prescribed to treat tuberculosis.
DON'T MIX WITH	**St. John's wort** (*Hypericum perforatum*). Isoniazid has some effects similar to monoamine oxidase inhibitor (MAOI) drugs. St. John's wort may work in a way similar to these drugs. Until more is known, do not mix St. John's wort with isoniazid. The combination could worsen isoniazid's side effects, including flulike symptoms, nausea, dizziness, drowsiness, and headache.

St. John's wort

KEEP IN MIND
• Combining alcohol with isoniazid can cause a number of unpleasant side effects, including headache and nausea.
• Isoniazid has some effects similar to monoamine oxidase inhibitor (MAOI) drugs such as phenelzine *(p. 180)*. Like MAOI drugs, isoniazid may interact adversely with foods containing the amino acid tyramine, such as alcohol, cheese and other dairy foods, fermented foods such as sauerkraut and pickles, bologna, salami, pepperoni, liver, pickled herring, caffeine, and chocolate. Symptoms include diarrhea, vasodilation (flushing), and dangerous changes in your blood pressure, among others. Discuss food restrictions with your physician and follow them carefully.
• Combining isoniazid with supplements of the amino acid tryptophan, sold as 5-HTP and often used as a natural sedative, may cause excessive drowsiness.
• Isoniazid can interfere with the action of vitamin B_6 (pyridoxine) and the absorption of other vitamins and minerals. Consider taking a daily multivitamin and mineral supplement containing 50 mg of vitamin B_6 at least two hours apart from the drug.

ISOSORBIDE DINITRATE

TYPE OF DRUG	Antianginal
DESCRIPTION	Isosorbide is prescribed to relieve the heart or chest pain of angina and to treat congestive heart failure and some other heart problems. This drug is sometimes used in sublingual (under the tongue) tablets to provide immediate relief from angina pain.
DON'T MIX WITH	No known herbal interactions.
KEEP IN MIND	• One study in 1989 suggested that the dietary supplement n-acetyl-cysteine (NAC) may help isosorbide work better. Discuss NAC supplements with your physician before you try them.

METRONIDAZOLE — BRAND NAMES *Flagyl, Helidac, MetroGel, Protostat, others*

TYPE OF DRUG	Antibiotic
DESCRIPTION	Metronidazole is an antibiotic used to treat bacterial, fungal, and parasitic infections, particularly infections of the vagina, bone, brain, and urinary tract. In combination with bismuth subsalicylate *(p. 131)* and tetracycline *(p. 190)*, metronidazole (Flagyl) is used to treat ulcers caused by *Helicobacter pylori* infection.
DON'T MIX WITH	No known herbal interactions.

DO TAKE WITH

Licorice

Deglycyrrhizinated licorice (DGL, derived from *Glycyrrhiza glabra*). DGL can speed ulcer healing as it stimulates the production of mucus that protects the stomach lining and also has an anti-inflammatory effect. Consider taking supplements (up to 250 mg 2 to 4 times daily).

Milk thistle *(Silybum marianum)*. Silymarin, an active compound in the herb milk thistle, may help protect your liver against damage from metronidazole. Consider taking supplements (150 mg 3 to 4 times daily).

KEEP IN MIND

• Metronidazole kills not only the harmful bacteria that cause illness but also the good bacteria normally found in your intestines; this can cause diarrhea. Consider taking probiotic supplements (at least 1.5 billion live organisms daily, including a mixture of *Lactobacillus acidophilus, Bifidobacterium bifidum,* and *Saccharomyces boulardii*).

• Do not drink alcohol while taking metronidazole. Severe side effects, including vasodilation (flushing), headache, and nausea may occur. Vinegar may have a similar effect. Avoid salad dressings, pickles, and other foods containing vinegar.

NAPROXEN — BRAND NAMES *Aleve, Anaprox, Naprelan, Naprosyn, others*

TYPE OF DRUG	Nonsteroidal anti-inflammatory drug (NSAID)
DESCRIPTION	Naproxen is used mostly to relieve pain, swelling, and stiffness from arthritis, tendinitis, and bursitis. It is also used to lower fevers, relieve menstrual discomfort, and to treat mild to moderate pain. Naproxen is available in prescription (Anaprox, Naprelan, Naprosyn, others) and nonprescription (Aleve, others) strengths.
DON'T MIX WITH	No known herbal interactions.
DO TAKE WITH	**Deglycyrrhizinated licorice** (DGL, derived from *Glycyrrhiza glabra*) stimulates the production of mucus that protects the stomach lining and also has an anti-inflammatory effect. It may help prevent the stomach irritation often caused by naproxen. Consider taking supplements (up to 250 mg 2 to 4 times daily).

KEEP IN MIND

• Naproxen can raise the amount of potassium in your body. Avoid potassium supplements or salt substitutes while taking this drug. Discuss your intake of foods high in potassium, such as bananas and orange juice, with your medical practitioner.
• Naproxen may make you retain sodium and water. Discuss restricting your salt intake with your physician.

• Naproxen may cause drowsiness, dizziness, or blurred vision. Alcohol can make these side effects worse – don't consume alcohol while taking this drug.
• Take naproxen with food to avoid stomach irritation.

NEFAZODONE
BRAND NAME *Serzone*

TYPE OF DRUG	Antidepressant
DESCRIPTION	Nefazodone is prescribed to treat depression.
DON'T MIX WITH	**Digitalis** (*Digitalis* spp., also known as foxglove). This dangerous herb is very similar to the heart drug digoxin (p. 147). Nefazodone increases the amount of digoxin in your blood, possibly to dangerous levels, and may have the same effect with digitalis. Do not use this herb if taking nefazodone. **Sedative herbs.** Although there have been no studies, it is possible that nefazodone in combination with natural sedatives could cause excessive drowsiness. Until more information is known, avoid sedative herbs such as chamomile (*Matricaria recutita*), catnip (*Nepeta cataria*), kava kava (*Piper methysticum*), passionflower (*Passiflora incarnata*), valerian (*Valeriana officinalis*), and others, as well as sedative dietary supplements such as 5-HTP, tryptophan, and SAMe, when taking nefazodone. **St. John's wort** (*Hypericum perforatum*). St. John's wort and nefazodone may work in similar ways. To avoid increasing the effect of the drug, do not take St. John's wort.
KEEP IN MIND	• Do not combine nefazodone with alcohol. The combination may cause dangerous drowsiness.

Valerian

NICOTINE
BRAND NAMES *Habitrol, Nicoderm, Nicorette, Nicotrol, ProStep*

TYPE OF DRUG	Smoking cessation product
DESCRIPTION	Nicotine replacement products are used to help people quit smoking by easing the symptoms of nicotine withdrawal. Nicotine is available as a prescription skin patch (Habitrol), as a nonprescription chewing gum (Nicorette), and as a nonprescription skin patch (Nicoderm, Nicotrol, ProStep). Nicotine overdose can be dangerous and even fatal. Follow the directions given by your physician or the package insert.
DON'T MIX WITH	**Lobelia** (*Lobelia inflata*). Because the effects of lobelia on your body are similar to those of nicotine, lobelia is sometimes recommended as an aid to quitting smoking. Although there have been no reported interactions between lobelia and nicotine, combining the two could increase the risks of nicotine side effects such as dizziness, fatigue, irritability, dry mouth, and headaches. Use lobelia cautiously and only under the supervision of a physician.
KEEP IN MIND	• Do not eat or drink anything just before, while, or just after you chew nicotine gum. Caffeine, soft drinks, fruit juice, and wine can block your absorption of nicotine.

NIFEDIPINE

BRAND NAMES *Adalat, Procardia*

TYPE OF DRUG	Calcium channel blocker
DESCRIPTION	Nifedipine, prescribed for high blood pressure and angina, is a calcium channel blocker, a drug that causes blood vessels to relax and widen.
DON'T MIX WITH	No known herbal interactions.
KEEP IN MIND	• A substance in grapefruit or grapefruit juice may cause the liver to reduce the rate of elimination of nifedipine. This can increase the amount of the drug in your body to dangerous levels. Avoid grapefruit and grapefruit juice when taking nifedipine.

NITROFURANTOIN

BRAND NAMES *Furadantin, Macrobid, Macrodantin*

TYPE OF DRUG	Urinary tract anti-infective
DESCRIPTION	Nitrofurantoin is prescribed to treat bacterial urinary tract infections, including cystitis. Nitrofurantoin can cause liver damage when taken with oral antidiabetes drugs such as glipizide *(p. 158)* or glyburide *(p. 159)*. It can also interact adversely with some antibiotics and other drugs. Be certain to tell your physician about all prescription and nonprescription drugs and dietary supplements you take.
DON'T MIX WITH	No known herbal interactions.
KEEP IN MIND	• The magnesium in many nonprescription antacids reduces the amount of nitrofurantoin you absorb. Ask your physician or pharmacist to recommend a different kind of antacid. • Long-term use of nitrofurantoin could block your absorption of folic acid (folate). Consider taking folic acid supplements (400 mcg daily) taken at least two hours apart from the drug. • Take nitrofurantoin with food to improve absorption and avoid stomach upset.

NITROGLYCERIN

BRAND NAMES *This drug is sold only in generic form*

TYPE OF DRUG	Antianginal drug
DESCRIPTION	Nitroglycerin is a very powerful drug used to treat angina and chest pain. It is also used to treat heart failure and high blood pressure.

DON'T MIX WITH

Ephedra

Caffeine-containing herbs. Because caffeine acts as a stimulant and can raise the body's blood pressure and increase the heart rate, do not use it if taking nitroglycerin. Avoid caffeine-containing herbs, including guarana *(Paullinia cupana)*, kola nut *(Cola* spp.*)*, and maté *(Ilex paraguariensis)*. **Ephedra** *(Ephedra* spp., also known as ma huang*)*. Taking the stimulant herb ephedra when taking nitroglycerin raises your risk of dangerous high blood pressure and heart arrhythmias. Similarly, avoid the drugs ephedrine and pseudoephedrine, which are found in many nonprescription cold and allergy remedies. **Yohimbe** *(Pausinystalia yohimbe)*. This dangerous herb is sometimes used for erectile dysfunction; one of its side effects is a sharp increase in blood pressure. Never use yohimbe if you are taking nitroglycerin.

KEEP IN MIND

• Do not combine nitroglycerin and alcohol. Serious and possibly fatal side effects, such as a rapid drop in blood pressure, may occur.

• The stimulant effect of caffeine may be dangerous if combined with nitroglycerin. If taking this drug, avoid caffeine-containing products and drinks including coffee, tea, cola drinks, many soft drinks, and certain "energy-boosting" products.

NITROUS OXIDE

BRAND NAME *This drug is sold only in generic form*

TYPE OF DRUG	Anesthetic gas
DESCRIPTION	Nitrous oxide, also known as laughing gas, is an anesthetic gas sometimes used during dental work and surgery. When used during dental work, nitrous oxide causes deep relaxation; when used for surgery, it causes deep relaxation or unconsciousness. In general, nitrous oxide is used as a surgical anesthetic only if the patient can't be given other anesthetic drugs. If you take prescription drugs or have a chronic health problem and plan to have nitrous oxide for dental work, discuss it with your physician and your dentist first.

DON'T MIX WITH

Sedative herbs. Do not use sedative herbs within 48 hours before or after using nitrous oxide; you may become overly sedated. Avoid sedative herbs such as chamomile *(Matricaria recutita)*, catnip *(Nepeta cataria)*, kava kava *(Piper methysticum)*, passionflower *(Passiflora incarnata)*, St. John's wort *(Hypericum perforatum)*, valerian *(Valeriana officinalis)*, and others, as well as sedative dietary supplements such as 5-HTP, tryptophan, and SAMe.

DO TAKE WITH

Ginger *(Zingiber officinale)*. Many patients are nauseated or vomit after awakening from nitrous oxide anesthesia. Ginger capsules can help prevent this effect. Discuss ginger with your dentist or physician and consider taking supplements (1 gram powdered ginger root in capsules 1 hour before anesthesia).

Ginger

NIZATIDINE

BRAND NAMES *Axid, Axid-AR*

TYPE OF DRUG	H2 blocker
DESCRIPTION	Nizatidine sharply reduces the body's production of stomach acid. In prescription form (Axid) it is used to treat ulcers and gastroesophageal reflux disease (GERD). In nonprescription form (Axid-AR) it is used for mild heartburn.
DON'T MIX WITH	No known herbal interactions.
DO TAKE WITH	**Deglycyrrhizinated licorice** (DGL, derived from *Glycyrrhiza glabra*). DGL can speed ulcer healing as it stimulates the production of mucus that protects the stomach lining and has an anti-inflammatory effect. Consider taking supplements (250 mg 2 to 4 times daily).
KEEP IN MIND	• Nizatidine and other H2 blockers reduce your absorption of a number of vitamins and minerals including folic acid (folate), vitamin B_{12} (cobalamin), zinc, and iron. If you use these drugs on a regular basis, consider taking a multivitamin and mineral supplement, along with additional folic acid (400 mcg daily) and vitamin B_{12} (500 mcg daily). Take these supplements at least two hours apart from nizatidine. • Magnesium supplements and calcium-, magnesium-, and magnesium/aluminum-based antacids may block your absorption of nizatidine. Take them at least two hours apart from this drug.

OMEPRAZOLE

BRAND NAME *Prilosec*

TYPE OF DRUG	Proton pump inhibitor
DESCRIPTION	Omeprazole "turns off" the body's production of stomach acid. It is used to treat ulcers, severe heartburn, and gastroesophageal reflux disease (GERD).
DON'T MIX WITH	No known herbal interactions.
DO TAKE WITH	**Deglycyrrhizinated licorice** (DGL, derived from *Glycyrrhiza glabra*). DGL can speed ulcer healing as it stimulates the production of mucus that protects the stomach lining and also has an anti-inflammatory effect. Consider supplements (up to 250 mg 2 to 4 times daily).
KEEP IN MIND	• Omeprazole may block your absorption of certain vitamins and minerals, particularly folic acid (folate), vitamin B_{12} (cobalamin) and iron. If you use omeprazole or another proton pump inhibitor regularly, take a multivitamin supplement with minerals at least two hours apart from taking the drug, and additional folic acid (400 mcg daily) and vitamin B_{12} (500 mcg daily).

Licorice

ORAL CONTRACEPTIVES   BRAND NAMES *Alesse, Brevicon, Genora, Loestrin, Necon, Ortho-Novum, others*

TYPE OF DRUG	Contraceptive
DESCRIPTION	Oral contraceptives are used to prevent pregnancy. They usually contain a mixture of the female hormones estrogen and progesterone *(p. 183)* in synthetic form; some types contain only progestin (progesterone). A number of prescription drugs can interact adversely with oral contraceptives or make them less effective. Be certain to tell your physician about all drugs and supplements you take.
DON'T MIX WITH	**Caffeine-containing herbs.** It is possible that consuming large amounts of caffeine may reduce the effectiveness. Discuss your intake of caffeine-containing herbs, such as guarana *(Paullinia cupana)*, kola nut *(Cola spp.)*, and maté *(Ilex paraguariensis)*, as well as other caffeine-containing herbs, with your medical practitioner. **Estrogenic herbs.** The herbs black cohosh *(Cimicifuga racemosa)*, chaste tree *(Vitex agnus-castus)*, dong quai *(Angelica sinensis)*, red clover *(Trifolium pratense)*, and the supplement soy isoflavones all have estrogenic or estrogen-like effects. Do not use them in combination with oral contraceptives, as contraceptive failure could occur. **Other estrogen- and progesterone-modulating herbs.** Laboratory studies have shown that the herbs damiana *(Turnera diffusa* 'Willdenow')*, hops *(Humulus lupulus)*, licorice *(Glycyrrhiza glabra)*, oregano *(Origanum vulgare)*, thyme *(Thymus spp.)*, turmeric *(Curcuma longa)*, and vervain *(Verbena spp.* and *V. hastata)* may modulate estrogen and/or progesterone activity. Discuss the use of these herbs with your physician before taking an oral contraceptive. **St. John's wort** *(Hypericum perforatum)*. Some women report irregular bleeding when combining this herb with oral contraceptives. Until more is known, do not take it with oral contraceptives without discussing with your physician.

Red clover

OXAPROZIN   BRAND NAME *Daypro*

TYPE OF DRUG	Nonsteroidal anti-inflammatory drug (NSAID)
DESCRIPTION	Oxaprozin is prescribed to treat pain and swelling from arthritis.
DON'T MIX WITH	**Photo-sensitizing herbs.** Oxaprozin may make your skin extremely sensitive to sunlight. Because St. John's wort *(Hypericum perforatum)* and dong quai *(Angelica sinensis)* also have this effect when taken for more than a few days, do not combine the drug with these herbs. Avoid direct sun and wear sunscreen. **Salicylate-containing herbs.** Taking these herbs with oxaprozin could cause severe side effects, including gastrointestinal bleeding. The herbs meadowsweet *(Filipendula ulmaria)*, white willow bark *(Salix alba)*, and wintergreen *(Gaultheria procumbens)* contain salicylates, a chemical similar to aspirin (another NSAID).
DO TAKE WITH	**Deglycyrrhizinated licorice** (DGL, derived from *Glycyrrhiza glabra*) stimulates the production of mucus that protects the stomach lining and also has an anti-inflammatory effect. It may help prevent the stomach irritation often caused by oxaprozin. Consider taking supplements (up to 250 mg 2 to 4 times daily).
KEEP IN MIND	• Oxaprozin can raise the amount of potassium in your body. Avoid potassium supplements or salt substitutes while taking this drug. Discuss your intake of valerian *(Valeriana officinalis)*, and others, as well as sedative dietary supplements such as 5-HTP, tryptophan, and SAMe, with your physician. • Oxycodone causes drowsiness, impaired judgment, and loss of coordination. Alcohol makes these side effects worse. Do not consume alcohol while taking this drug. • To prevent constipation, a common side effect of codeine, eat plenty of fresh fruits and vegetables and whole grains and drink plenty of water (at least 64 ounces a day).

OXYCODONE

BRAND NAMES *Percodan, Percocet, Roxicet, Roxiprin, others*

TYPE OF DRUG	Narcotic analgesic
DESCRIPTION	Oxycodone is a narcotic drug made from codeine. In combination with acetaminophen *(p. 122)* or aspirin *(p. 128)*, oxycodone is prescribed to relieve moderate to severe pain.
DON'T MIX WITH	**Sedative herbs.** When combined with oxycodone these herbs may cause excessive drowsiness. Avoid herbs such as chamomile *(Matricaria recutita)*, catnip *(Nepeta cataria)*, kava kava *(Piper methysticum)*, passionflower *(Passiflora incarnata)*, St. John's wort *(Hypericum perforatum)*, valerian *(Valeriana officinalis)*, and others, as well as sedative dietary supplements such as 5-HTP, tryptophan, and SAMe.

St. John's wort

KEEP IN MIND

• Oxycodone causes drowsiness, impaired judgment, and loss of coordination. Alcohol makes these side effects worse. Do not consume alcohol if taking this drug.

• To prevent constipation, a common side effect of codeine, eat plenty of fresh fruits and vegetables and whole grains and drink plenty of water (at least 64 ounces a day).

PACLITAXEL

BRAND NAME *Taxol*

TYPE OF DRUG	Anticancer
DESCRIPTION	Paclitaxel is a chemotherapy drug made from a type of yew tree. It is used to treat ovarian cancer, breast cancer, Kaposi's sarcoma, and a wide range of other cancers. Patients receiving paclitaxel are usually also given other drugs to help relieve or prevent side effects. Be sure to tell your medical practitioner about any prescription or nonprescription drugs and supplements you are taking.
DON'T MIX WITH	No known herbal interactions.

KEEP IN MIND

• Although studies are very preliminary, it is possible that the amino acid glutamine could help reduce the side effects of paclitaxel, especially muscle and joint pain. Discuss glutamine with your physician and consider taking supplements (10 grams 3 times daily, starting 24 hours after paclitaxel administration and continuing for 5 to 10 days).

• B vitamins can help prevent or relieve neuropathy (nerve pain and tingling) from paclitaxel. Discuss this with your medical practitioner and consider supplements (B-50 formula once daily). The dietary supplement lipoic acid may also help neuropathy. Discuss this with your physician and consider supplements (200 mg daily).

PANTOPROZOLE

BRAND NAME *Protonix*

TYPE OF DRUG	Proton pump inhibitor
DESCRIPTION	Pantoprazole "turns off" the body's production of stomach acid. It is used to treat ulcers, severe heartburn, and gastroesophageal reflux disease (GERD).
DON'T MIX WITH	No known herbal interactions.
DO TAKE WITH	**Deglycyrrhizinated licorice** (DGL, derived from *Glycyrrhiza glabra*). DGL can speed ulcer healing as it stimulates the production of mucus that protects the stomach lining and it also has an anti-inflammatory effect. Consider supplements (up to 250 mg 2 to 3 times daily).

Licorice

KEEP IN MIND	• Pantoprazole may block your absorption of certain vitamins and minerals, particularly folic acid (folate), vitamin B$_{12}$ (cobalamin), and iron. If you use pantoprazole or other proton pump inhibitors on a regular basis, take a multivitamin supplement with minerals at least two hours apart from taking the drug, and additional folic acid (400 mcg daily) and vitamin B$_{12}$ (500 mcg daily).

PAROXETINE

BRAND NAME *Paxil*

TYPE OF DRUG	Selective serotonin reuptake inhibitor (SSRI)
DESCRIPTION	Paroxetine is used to treat depression, obsessive-compulsive disorder, social phobias, panic disorder, and post-traumatic stress syndrome. Like all SSRI drugs, paroxetine affects the way the body uses the neurotransmitter serotonin.
DON'T MIX WITH	**Sedative herbs.** When combined with paroxetine these herbs may cause excessive drowsiness. Avoid sedative herbs such as chamomile *(Matricaria recutita)*, catnip *(Nepeta cataria)*, kava kava *(Piper methysticum)*, passionflower *(Passiflora incarnata)*, valerian *(Valeriana officinalis)*, and others. **St. John's wort** *(Hypericum perforatum)*. Although there have been no reports of dangerous interactions, it is possible that combining this herb with paroxetine could raise your serotonin levels too high. If you wish to take St. John's wort instead of paroxetine, discuss it with your physician.

Valerian

DO TAKE WITH	**Ginkgo** *(Ginkgo biloba)*. Sexual dysfunction in both men and women is a fairly common side effect of paroxetine. Ginkgo may be helpful for this problem. Consider taking supplements (60 mg ginkgo extract standardized to 24 percent ginkgo flavone glycosides 3 times daily).
KEEP IN MIND	• Paroxetine can cause drowsiness and dizziness. Alcohol can make these side effects worse. Do not consume alcohol when taking this drug. • Don't use the dietary supplements 5-HTP, tryptophan, or SAMe if you take paroxetine. They may cause your serotonin level to rise too high.

PENICILLAMINE
BRAND NAMES *Cuprimine, Depen*

TYPE OF DRUG	Chelating agent
DESCRIPTION	Penicillamine is used to treat severe rheumatoid arthritis, Wilson's disease, and cystinuria.
DON'T MIX WITH	No known herbal interactions.
KEEP IN MIND	• Penicillamine binds to the minerals copper, iron, magnesium, and zinc in your digestive tract; this prevents you from absorbing both the minerals and the drug. If you are taking penicillamine for rheumatoid arthritis, consider taking a daily multivitamin with minerals. Take the supplement two hours apart from the drug. If you are already taking penicillamine for Wilson's disease, do not take copper supplements in any form. • Penicillamine promotes excretion of vitamin B_6 (pyridoxine), consider taking supplements (50 mg daily).

PENICILLIN
BRAND NAMES *Betapen-VK, Pen-Vee K, Pfizerpen, V-Cillin K, Veetids, others*

TYPE OF DRUG	Antibiotic
DESCRIPTION	Penicillin is an antibiotic that kills bacteria that cause infections.
DON'T MIX WITH	No known herbal interactions.
KEEP IN MIND	• Bromelain, an enzyme found in pineapples, increases your absorption of penicillin. This may be helpful for people with severe infections or infections that don't respond to penicillin. Discuss bromelain supplements with your physician. • Penicillin kills not only the harmful bacteria that cause illness but also the good bacteria that are normally found in your intestines; this can cause diarrhea. Consider probiotic supplements (at least 1.5 billion live organisms daily, including a mixture of *Lactobacillus acidophilus, Bifidobacterium bifidum*, and *Saccharomyces boulardii*). • Drink fruit juices and carbonated beverages at least two hours apart from when you take penicillin. The acid in these drinks decreases activity of the drug before it can get into your bloodstream.

Pineapple

PHENELZINE SULFATE

BRAND NAME *Nardil*

TYPE OF DRUG	Monoamine oxidase inhibitor (MAOI)

DESCRIPTION

Phenelzine is an MAOI drug prescribed to treat depression, especially depression that does not respond to other drugs.

Foods that contain a substance called tyramine can cause a dangerous interaction with MAOI drugs *(see* Keep in mind *section)*, as can a number of other drugs.

DON'T MIX WITH

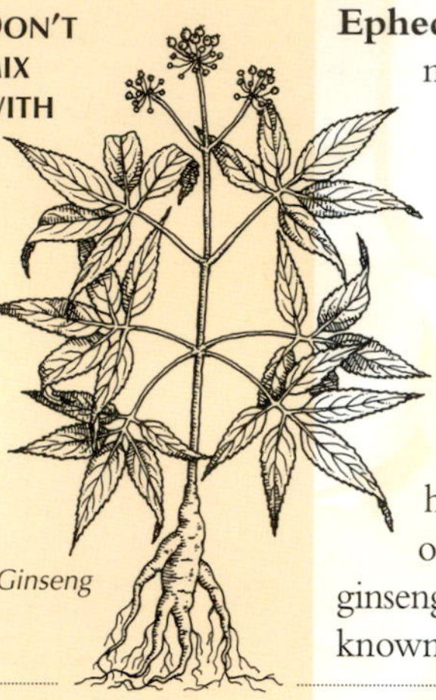

Ginseng

Ephedra (*Ephedra* spp., also known as ma huang). Taking ephedra with phenelzine raises your risk of serious high blood pressure and heart arrhythmias. Similarly, avoid the drugs ephedrine *(p. 152)* and pseudoephedrine *(p. 185)*, which are found in many nonprescription cold and allergy remedies.

Ginseng (*Panax ginseng*). There have been a few reports of a variety of adverse interactions between ginseng and phenelzine. Until more is known, avoid ginseng.

St. John's wort (*Hypericum perforatum*). Research suggests that this herb and phenelzine work in similar ways. To avoid increasing the effect of the drug, do not take St. John's wort.

Scotch broom (*Cytisus scoparius*). This herb, sometimes used to treat heart arrhythmias, contains a high amount of tyramine *(see* Keep in mind *section)*. Do not use this in conjunction with phenelzine.

KEEP IN MIND

• Combining phenelzine with tyramine, an amino acid found in many foods, can cause diarrhea, vasodilation (flushing), and dangerous changes in blood pressure, among other symptoms. Foods high in tyramine include alcohol, cheese, fava beans, fermented foods such as sauerkraut and miso soup, bologna, pepperoni, liver, pickled herring, yeast and protein supplements, and caffeine. Discuss food restrictions with your physician and then follow them carefully.

• Phenelzine may increase the effect of the amino acid tryptophan, sold as 5-HTP. This could cause excessive drowsiness.

PHENYLPROPANOLAMINE

BRAND NAMES *Dimetapp, DayQuil Allergy Relief, Tavist-D., Dexatrim, others*

TYPE OF DRUG	Antihistamine

DESCRIPTION

Phenylpropanolamine has been removed from the market by The US Food and Drug Administration because the drug may be associated with an increased risk of hemorrhagic stroke. Check the labels of any products you believe may contain phenylpropanolamine; if it is listed, discard the product.

PHENYTOIN

TYPE OF DRUG	Antiepileptic
DESCRIPTION	Phenytoin is prescribed to treat epilepsy as well as some heart rhythm problems.

DON'T MIX WITH

Caffeine–containing herbs. Phenytoin can cause nervousness, insomnia, confusion, and irritability. To avoid worsening these effects, avoid caffeine-containing herbs, including guarana *(Paullinia cupana)*, kola nut *(Cola* spp.*)*, and maté *(Ilex paraguariensis)*, as well as drinks and other products that contain caffeine.

Ephedra *(Ephedra* spp., also known as ma huang). Some side effects of phenytoin, including insomnia and nervousness, may be exacerbated by the stimulant herb ephedra. Do not use it if taking this drug. Similarly, avoid the drugs ephedrine *(p. 152)* and pseudoephedrine *(see p. 185)*, which are found in many nonprescription cold and allergy drugs.

KEEP IN MIND

• B vitamin supplements, especially vitamin B_6 (pyridoxine) decrease the effectiveness of phenytoin. However, phenytoin also blocks your absorption of B vitamins, especially folic acid (folate), to the point that supplements are usually prescribed to avoid deficiency. Discuss B vitamin supplements with your physician – you need to be monitored to make sure you have the correct levels of both the vitamins and phenytoin. Take B vitamin supplements at least two hours apart from this drug.

• Phenytoin can interfere with your body's absorption of calcium, which may lead to osteoporosis. Discuss calcium and vitamin D (needed for calcium absorption) supplements with your physician. When using calcium supplements, take them two hours apart from phenytoin; they may slow absorption of the drug.
• Pregnant women who take phenytoin may need supplements to prevent vitamin K deficiency in their babies. Discuss vitamin K and all other supplements with a physician.

POTASSIUM CHLORIDE

TYPE OF DRUG	Electrolyte replacement

DESCRIPTION

Potassium chloride is most commonly prescribed for people who are taking a diuretic, such as furosemide *(p. 157)*, which causes increased excretion of potassium. Note that potassium chloride is also an ingredient in many salt substitutes.

DON'T MIX WITH

Diuretic herbs. These could cause the elimination of more potassium than you get from supplements and food, especially if you also take a prescription diuretic. Avoid herbal diuretics, including bilberry leaf *(Vaccinium myrtillus)*, buchu *(Barosma betulina)*, burdock *(Arctium lappa)*, couch grass *(Agropyron repens)*, damiana *(Turnera diffusa)*, dandelion *(Taraxacum officinale)*, fennel seed *(Foeniculum vulgare)*, goldenrod *(Solidago virgaurea)*, horsetail *(Equisetum arvense)*, kava kava *(Piper methysticum)*, kola nut *(Cola* spp.*)*, marshmallow *(Althaea officinalis)*, maté *(Ilex paraguariensis)*, parsley *(Petroselinum* spp.*)*, sarsaparilla *(Smilax* spp.*)*, saw palmetto *(Serenoa repens)*, uva ursi *(Arctostaphylos uva-ursi)*, vervain *(Verbena* spp.*)*, and yarrow *(Achillea millefolium)*, and other herbal and nonprescription diuretics.

Licorice *(Glycyrrhiza glabra)*. This herb can raise your blood pressure to dangerous levels if combined with potassium supplements. Although deglycyrrhizinated licorice (DGL), used to prevent or treat ulcers and stomach irritation, does not contain the ingredient that raises blood pressure, it may still have an effect in combination with potassium supplements and should be avoided.

Dandelion

KEEP IN MIND

• If your physician has prescribed a potassium supplement, do not use salt substitutes – you could take in too much potassium. Many fruits and vegetables, and a number of other foods, are high in potassium. Discuss with your physician.

PRAVASTATIN	BRAND NAME *Pravachol*
TYPE OF DRUG	Statin cholesterol-lowering agent
DESCRIPTION	Pravastatin is prescribed to lower high cholesterol, slow or prevent hardening of the arteries, and reduce the risk of heart attack and stroke.
DON'T MIX WITH	No known herbal interactions.
DO TAKE WITH	**Milk thistle** *(Silybum marianum).* Pravastatin can cause liver damage. Silymarin, an active compound in milk thistle, may prevent or reduce the damage. Consider taking milk thistle supplements (150 mg 3 to 4 times daily).
KEEP IN MIND	• Lovastatin, a drug similar to pravastatin, interacts adversely with grapefruit juice. There are no studies of pravastatin and grapefruit juice, but similar problems are possible. Until more is known, do not take pravastatin with grapefruit juice. • The dietary supplement red yeast rice, sold as Cholestin, works in a way similar to the statin drugs. Do not use red yeast rice with pravastatin. • According to one study, statin drugs can gradually raise your vitamin A level. Until more is known, do not take vitamin A supplements with pravastatin. • Studies show that taking statin drugs can lower your level of coenzyme Q_{10} (CoQ_{10} or ubiquinone), a substance needed for energy production in your cells. Consider taking CoQ_{10} supplements (100 mg daily). • Two recent studies suggest that moderate doses of niacin (500 mg twice daily) along with pravastatin lowers cholesterol significantly more than taking the drug alone. Discuss niacin with your physician before you try it, however, because high doses of niacin interact adversely with some statin drugs.

PREDNISONE	BRAND NAMES *Deltasone, Liquid Pred, Meticorten, Orasone, Prednisone Intensol, Sterapred, others*
TYPE OF DRUG	Corticosteroid
DESCRIPTION	Corticosteroids such as prednisone are synthetic hormones used to treat a wide variety of severe disorders, particularly those that involve inflammation, including arthritis, psoriasis, allergies, asthma, and inflammatory bowel disease. Corticosteroids are also used to treat autoimmune diseases such as lupus erythematosus and transplant rejection.
DON'T MIX WITH	**Digitalis** (*Digitalis* spp., also known as foxglove). This dangerous herb is very similar to the heart drug digoxin *(p. 147),* which can worsen the side effects of prednisone. Digitalis may cause the same problem. *Foxglove* **Ephedra** (*Ephedra* spp., also known as ma huang). The herb ephedra naturally contains ephedrine, which can reduce the effectiveness of corticosteroids. Do not use it when taking prednisone. Similarly, avoid the drugs ephedrine *(p. 152)* and pseudoephedrine *(p. 185),* which can be found in many nonprescription cold and allergy remedies.
KEEP IN MIND	• Long-term use of corticosteroids may cause osteoporosis, probably because the drug interferes with your use of calcium and vitamin D. Studies show that taking supplements helps prevent corticosteroid-induced osteoporosis. Consider taking supplements (1,000 mg calcium daily, 400 IU vitamin D daily). Corticosteroids may also reduce your level of vitamin B_6 (pyridoxine) and magnesium. Consider taking supplements (50 mg pyroxidine and 300–400 mg magnesium daily). • Long-term use of corticosteroids reduces your level of chromium, which may contribute to the development of diabetes. Consider taking supplements (200 mcg chromium picolinate daily).

PROGESTERONE
BRAND NAMES *Amen, Crinone, Cycrin, Curretab, Depo-Provera, Prometrium, Provera*

TYPE OF DRUG	Progestin
DESCRIPTION	Progesterone (often in the semisynthetic form medroxyprogesterone) is prescribed to treat irregular menstrual bleeding, endometriosis, premenstrual syndrome (PMS), and some other problems. Combined with estrogen or in conjugated estrogens *(p. 143)*, it is used to treat menopause symptoms such as hot flashes. It is also used to treat sleep apnea and in formulations that prevent pregnancy.
DON'T MIX WITH	**Progesterone-modulating herbs.** Laboratory studies have shown that the herbs damiana *(Turnera diffusa)*, oregano *(Origanum vulgare)*, red clover *(Trifolium pratense)*, thyme *(Thyme spp.)*, turmeric *(Curcuma longa)*, and vervain *(Verbena spp.)* may modulate progesterone activity. Discuss the use of these herbs with your medical practitioner before using them if you take progesterone.

PROMETHAZINE
BRAND NAMES *Phenergan, others*

TYPE OF DRUG	Antihistamine
DESCRIPTION	Promethazine is an antihistamine used to treat seasonal allergies, motion sickness, and nausea and vomiting. In combination with codeine *(p. 142)* or extromethorphan, promethazine is used in prescription and nonprescription syrup cough remedies.
DON'T MIX WITH	**Henbane** *(Hyoscyamus niger)*. This herb is toxic and should be used only when prescribed and closely monitored by a qualified practitioner. As it has side effects similar to promethazine, such as heart palpitations, do not use the two together. **Sedative herbs.** Promethazine has a tranquilizing effect that can be heightened when taken in combination with sedative herbs such as such as German chamomile *(Matricaria recutita)*, catnip *(Nepeta cataria)*, kava kava *(Piper methysticum)*, passionflower *(Passiflora incarnata)*, St. John's wort *(Hypericum perforatum)*, valerian *(Valeriana officinalis)*, and others, as well as sedative dietary supplements such as 5-HTP, tryptophan, and SAMe.
KEEP IN MIND	• Promethazine often causes drowsiness and dizziness. Alcohol can make these side effects worse. Do not consume alcohol if taking this drug. • Long-term use of promethazine may increase your need for riboflavin (vitamin B$_2$). Consider taking supplements (a B-50 formula daily).

Kava kava

PROPOXYPHENE

BRAND NAMES *Darvon, Darvocet*

TYPE OF DRUG	Narcotic analgesic
DESCRIPTION	Propoxyphene is a prescription drug used to relieve mild to moderate pain. It is used by itself or combined with a nonsteroidal anti-inflammatory drug such as aspirin *(p. 128)* or acetaminophen *(p. 122)*; caffeine is also found in some formulas. Propoxyphene is potentially addictive and must be used with caution. The antacid cimetidine *(p. 137)* may cause serious side effects when taken with propoxyphene. Discuss alternative antacids with your medical practitioner or pharmacist.
DON'T MIX WITH	**Sedative herbs.** When combined with propoxyphene, these herbs may cause excessive drowsiness. Avoid sedative herbs such as chamomile *(Matricaria recutita)*, catnip *(Nepeta cataria)*, kava kava *(Piper methysticum)*, passionflower *(Passiflora incarnata)*, St. John's wort *(Hypericum perforatum)*, valerian *(Valeriana officinalis)*, and others, as well as sedative dietary supplements such as 5-HTP, tryptophan, and SAMe.
KEEP IN MIND	• Propoxyphene causes drowsiness. Alcohol makes this side effect worse. Do not consume alcohol if taking this drug. • To avoid constipation, a common side effect of propoxyphene, eat plenty of high-fiber foods, such as fresh fruits and vegetables and whole grains, and drink 64 ounces of water daily.

Passionflower

PROPRANOLOL HYDROCHLORIDE

BRAND NAME *Inderal*

TYPE OF DRUG	Beta blocker
DESCRIPTION	Propranolol is used to treat high blood pressure, angina, and abnormal heart rhythms, and to help prevent a second heart attack. It is also sometimes used to treat bleeding from the stomach or esophagus, migraines, and the symptoms of hyperthyroidism (overactive thyroid gland). In some cases propranolol is used to treat anxiety disorders, schizophrenia, and the side effects of antipsychotic drugs. Propranolol is a powerful drug that can interact adversely with a number of prescription drugs, so use it with caution. Be certain to tell your physician about other prescription and nonprescription drugs and dietary supplements you take.
DON'T MIX WITH	**Black pepper** *(Piper nigrum)*. One study in 1991 suggests that piperine, a chemical found in black pepper, could raise the level of propranolol. Until more information is known, avoid eating large amounts of black pepper. **St. John's wort** *(Hypericum perforatum)*. Monoamine oxidase inhibitors (MAOIs) interact adversely with propranolol. Because St. John's wort works in a way similar to these drugs, do not use it if already taking propranolol.
KEEP IN MIND	• Beta blockers block your use of coenzyme Q_{10} (CoQ_{10} or ubiquinone), which is needed for energy production within your cells. Consider taking supplements (100 mg daily). • The antacid cimetidine *(p. 137)* increases the amount of propranolol in your bloodstream. Choose a different type of antacid.

PSEUDOEPHEDRINE

BRAND NAMES *Actifed, Afrin, Benadryl, Contac, Sinarest, Sudafed, others*

TYPE OF DRUG	Decongestant

DESCRIPTION

Pseudoephedrine is a nonprescription decongestant that is sold by itself (Afrin, Sudafed, others) or in combination with antihistamines and other medications (Benadryl, Contac, others) to treat seasonal allergies and symptoms of colds and flu.

DON'T MIX WITH

Witch hazel

Caffeine-containing herbs. The stimulant effect of caffeine can make the side effects of pseudoephedrine, such as nervousness, restlessness, insomnia, and dizziness, worse. Avoid caffeine-containing herbs, including guarana (*Paullinia cupana*), kola nut (*Cola* spp.), and maté (*Ilex paraguariensis*).

Ephedra (*Ephedra* spp., also known as ma huang). Ephedrine, a drug closely related to pseudoephedrine, was originally isolated from ephedra. Taking ephedra with any product containing pseudoephedrine could increase the side effects of the drug, including nervousness, insomnia, dizziness, high blood pressure, and heart arrhythmias.

Tannin-containing herbs. Herbs that are high in tannin, including black walnut (*Juglans nigra*), red raspberry (*Rubus idaeus*), oak (*Quercus* spp.), uva ursi (*Arctostaphylos uva-ursi*), and witch hazel (*Hamamelis virginiana*), can interfere with the absorption of pseudoephedrine, as can the tannins in tea. Do not consume these substances within two hours of taking this drug.

KEEP IN MIND

• The side effects of pseudoephedrine, such as nervousness, restlessness, insomnia, and dizziness, may be worsened by caffeine's stimulant effect. Coffee, tea, and cola drinks naturally contain caffeine; it is also added to many soft drinks and "energy-boosting" products. Avoid these if taking ephedrine.

PSYLLIUM

BRAND NAMES *Fiberall, Konsyl, Metamucil, others*

TYPE OF DRUG	Bulk laxative

DESCRIPTION

Psyllium (*Plantago* spp.) is a plant-based form of soluble fiber used to treat occasional constipation by increasing the bulk and softness of the stool. People with asthma have occasionally had asthma attacks from inhaling psyllium dust or using psyllium products. If you have asthma, discuss psyllium with your physician.

DON'T MIX WITH

Herbal laxatives. Aloe (*Aloe* spp.), buckthorn (*Rhamnus catharticus*), cascara sagrada (*Rhamnus purshianus*), frangula (*Rhamnus frangula*), also known as buckthorn bark, rhubarb (*Rheum* spp.), and senna (*Cassia* spp.) are powerful laxatives that should be used only when psyllium hasn't helped. If combined with psyllium, they can cause diarrhea and cramping.

KEEP IN MIND

• Frequent use of psyllium can reduce your absorption of many drugs, herbs, and dietary supplements by moving them through your digestive system too quickly. If you must take psyllium on a regular basis, separate it from your other medications and supplements by at least three hours.

RANITIDINE	BRAND NAMES *Zantac, Zantac 75*
TYPE OF DRUG	H2 blocker
DESCRIPTION	Ranitidine sharply reduces the body's production of stomach acid. In prescription form (Zantac) it is used to treat ulcers and gastroesophageal reflux disease (GERD) and to help prevent internal bleeding from large doses of nonsteroidal anti-inflammatory drugs such as aspirin *(p. 128)*. In nonprescription form (Zantac 75), it is used for mild heartburn.
DON'T MIX WITH	No known herbal interactions.
DO TAKE WITH	**Deglycyrrhizinated licorice** (DGL, derived from *Glycyrrhiza glabra*). DGL can speed ulcer healing as it stimulates the production of mucus that protects the stomach lining and also has an anti-inflammatory effect. Consider taking supplements (250 mg 2 to 4 times daily).
KEEP IN MIND	• Ranitidine and other H2 blockers reduce your absorption of a number of vitamins and minerals including folic acid (folate), vitamin B_{12} (cobalamin), zinc, and iron. If you use these drugs on a regular basis, consider taking a multivitamin and mineral supplement, along with additional folic acid (400 mcg daily) and vitamin B_{12} (500 mcg daily). Take these supplements at least two hours apart from ranitidine. • Magnesium supplements and calcium-, magnesium-, and magnesium/aluminum-based antacids may block your absorption of ranitidine. Take them at least two hours apart from ranitidine.

ROFECOXIB	BRAND NAME *Vioxx*
TYPE OF DRUG	Cyclooxygenase-2 (COX-2) inhibitor nonsteroidal anti-inflammatory drug (NSAID)
DESCRIPTION	COX-2 inhibitors are used to treat arthritis. They work by blocking the body's production of an enzyme that regulates pain and inflammation. COX-2 inhibitors are slightly less likely than are other NSAIDs to cause stomach irritation; they also don't thin blood like other NSAIDS do. Rofecoxib is also used to treat painful menstruation and acute pain.
DON'T MIX WITH	**Salicylate-containing herbs.** In combination with rofecoxib, these herbs could cause severe stomach irritation. They include meadowsweet *(Filipendula ulmaria)*, white willow bark *(Salix alba)*, and wintergreen *(Gaultheria procumbens)*.
DO TAKE WITH	**Milk thistle** *(Silybum marianum)*. Silymarin, an active compound in the herb milk thistle, may help protect your liver against irritation caused by rofecoxib. Consider taking supplements (150 mg 3 to 4 times daily).
KEEP IN MIND	• Many NSAIDs reduce your absorption of folic acid (folate). Although there is no evidence that rofecoxib does this, consider taking supplements (400 mcg daily).

Milk thistle

SERTRALINE

BRAND NAME *Zoloft*

TYPE OF DRUG	Selective serotonin reuptake inhibitor (SSRI)

DESCRIPTION

Sertraline is used to treat depression and obsessive-compulsive disorder. Like all SSRI drugs, sertraline affects the way your body uses the neurotransmitter serotonin.

DON'T MIX WITH

Sedative herbs. When combined with sertraline, these herbs may cause excessive drowsiness. Avoid sedative herbs such as chamomile (*Matricaria recutita*), catnip (*Nepeta cataria*), kava kava (*Piper methysticum*), passionflower (*Passiflora incarnata*), valerian (*Valeriana officinalis*), and others.

St. John's wort

St. John's wort (*Hypericum perforatum*). Although there have been no reports of dangerous interactions, it is possible that combining this herb with sertraline could raise the body's serotonin levels too high. If you wish to take St. John's wort instead of sertraline, discuss it with your physician.

DO TAKE WITH

Ginkgo (*Ginkgo biloba*). Sexual dysfunction in both men and women is a fairly common side effect of sertraline. Gingko may be helpful for reducing this problem. Consider supplements (60 mg gingko extract standardized to 24 percent ginkgo flavone glycosides 3 times daily).

KEEP IN MIND

• Sertraline can cause drowsiness and dizziness. Alcohol can make these side effects worse. Do not consume alcohol if taking this drug.

• Don't use the dietary supplements 5-HTP, tryptophan, or SAMe if you take sertraline. They may cause your serotonin level to rise too high.

SIMVASTATIN

BRAND NAME *Zocor*

TYPE OF DRUG	Statin cholesterol-lowering agent

DESCRIPTION

Simvastatin is prescribed to lower high cholesterol, slow or prevent hardening of the arteries, and reduce the risk of heart attack and stroke.

DON'T MIX WITH

No known herbal interactions.

DO TAKE WITH

Milk thistle (*Silybum marianum*). Although there are no studies to date, silymarin, an active compound in the herb milk thistle may protect against the liver damage that can occur as a side effect of this type of drug. Consider taking supplements (150 mg 3 to 4 times daily).

KEEP IN MIND

• Lovastatin, a drug similar to simvastatin, interacts adversely with grapefruit juice. There are no studies yet of simvastatin and grapefruit juice, but similar problems are possible. Until more is known, do not take simvastatin with grapefruit juice.
• The dietary supplement, red yeast rice, sold as Cholestin, works in a way similar to the statin drugs. Do not use red yeast rice with simvastatin.
• According to one study, statin drugs can gradually raise vitamin A levels. Until more is known, do not take vitamin A supplements.

• Several studies show that taking statin drugs can lower your level of coenzyme Q_{10} (CoQ_{10} or ubiquinone), a substance needed for energy production in your cells. Consider taking CoQ_{10} supplements (100 mg daily).
• Some research suggests that moderate doses of niacin (500 mg twice daily) along with simvastatin could lower cholesterol significantly more than taking the drug alone. Discuss niacin with your physician before you try it, however, because high doses of niacin interact adversely with some statin drugs.

SULFAMETHOXAZOLE

BRAND NAMES *Bactrim, Gantanol, Septra, others*

TYPE OF DRUG	Sulfonamide antibiotic
DESCRIPTION	Sulfamethoxazole is prescribed by itself (Gantanol) or in combination with another antibiotic drug called trimethoprim (Bactrim, Cotrim, Septra, others). The combination is also known as TMP/SMZ. Both drugs are used to treat infections caused by bacteria or protozoa, especially urinary tract infections (UTIs).
DON'T MIX WITH	**Salicylate-containing herbs.** The herbs meadowsweet *(Filipendula ulmaria)*, white willow bark *(Salix alba)*, and wintergreen *(Gaultheria procumbens)* contain salicylates, compounds similar to aspirin *(p. 128)*. Do not take them in conjunction with sulfamethoxazole or TMP/SMZ; it could make your salicylate level rise too high. **Photo-sensitizing herbs.** Sulfamethoxazole can make your skin very sensitive to sun. Because St. John's wort *(Hypericum perforatum)* and dong quai *(Angelica sinensis)* also have this effect when taken for more than a few days, do not combine the drug with these herbs. Avoid direct sun and wear sunscreen.
KEEP IN MIND	• Both sulfamethoxazole and TMP/SMZ block the body's ability to use or absorb folic acid (folate), vitamin B_6 (pyridoxine), and vitamin B_{12} (cobalamin). If you take these drugs on a long-term basis, consider taking supplements (B-50 formula daily). These drugs also decrease the absorption of calcium and magnesium and may affect the level of vitamin K. Consider taking a daily multivitamin with minerals. Take all vitamin and mineral supplements at least two hours apart from sulfamethoxazole. • The dietary supplement PABA may block the action of sulfamethoxazole. Until more is known, do not take PABA supplements when taking this drug. The PABA in sunscreens is unlikely to have any effect on sulfamethoxazole and is safe to use.

SULFASALAZINE

BRAND NAME *Azulfidine*

TYPE OF DRUG	Sulfonamide antibiotic
DESCRIPTION	Sulfasalazine is prescribed to treat rheumatoid arthritis, ulcerative colitis, and Crohn's disease. Although this drug is a type of antibiotic, it is used because it is also reduces inflammation.
DON'T MIX WITH	**Salicylate-containing herbs.** The herbs meadowsweet *(Filipendula ulmaria)*, white willow bark *(Salix alba)*, and wintergreen *(Gaultheria procumbens)* contain salicylates, compounds similar to aspirin *(p. 128)*. Do not take them in conjunction with sulfasalazine; it could raise your salicylate levels too high. **Photo-sensitizing herbs.** Sulfasalazine can make the skin very sensitive to sun. Because St. John's wort *(Hypericum perforatum)* and dong quai *(Angelica sinensis)* also have this effect when taken for more than a few days, do not combine the drug with these herbs. Avoid direct sun and wear sunscreen.
KEEP IN MIND	• The dietary supplement PABA may block the action of sulfasalazine. Until more is known, do not take PABA supplements when taking this drug. The PABA in sunscreens is unlikely to have any effect on sulfasalazine and is safe to use. • Sulfasalazine blocks your absorption of folic acid (folate). Discuss this problem with your physician and consider taking supplements (800 mcg daily). Take them at least two hours apart from the drug. • Iron can bind with sulfasalazine and stop it being absorbed. Take iron supplements two hours apart from sulfasalazine.

SUMATRIPTAN

BRAND NAME *Imitrex*

TYPE OF DRUG	Triptan-type antimigraine

DESCRIPTION

Sumatriptan is prescribed to help prevent and relieve migraines. It works by affecting serotonin receptors in the brain. Sumatriptan and other triptan drugs should not be used if you have or are at risk for heart disease – heart problems have developed in people using this drug. Triptan drugs can interact adversely with MAOI drugs such as phenelzine *(p. 180)* and with other drugs, including oral contraceptives. Be certain to tell your physician about all prescription and nonprescription drugs and dietary supplements you take.

DON'T MIX WITH

Feverfew

Feverfew *(Tanacetum parthenium).* Recent studies have shown that the herb feverfew can help prevent migraines. There are no studies showing possible interactions between feverfew and sumatriptan, but you should discuss feverfew with your physician before you take it with sumatriptan.

St. John's wort *(Hypericum perforatum).* St. John's wort and sumatriptan may work in similar ways. Combining them could cause your serotonin levels to become too high. Until more information is known, do not take St. John's wort with sumatriptan.

KEEP IN MIND

• The natural sedatives 5-HTP, tryptophan, and SAMe all affect your serotonin levels, as does sumatriptan. Do not combine them with this drug.

TAMOXIFEN

BRAND NAME *Nolvadex*

TYPE OF DRUG	Antiestrogen

DESCRIPTION

Tamoxifen blocks the use of the hormone estrogen. It is used to treat breast cancers that grow more quickly in the presence of estrogen, and to help prevent recurrences. Tamoxifen is also used for some other types of cancer such as pancreatic cancer and endometrial cancer.

DON'T MIX WITH

Estrogenic herbs. The herbs black cohosh *(Cimicifuga racemosa),* dong quai *(Angelica sinensis),* chaste tree *(Vitex agnus-castus),* and red clover *(Trifolium pratense)* all have estrogenlike effects. Do not use them in combination with tamoxifen.

Black cohosh

DO TAKE WITH

Milk thistle *(Silybum marianum).* Silymarin, an active compound in the herb milk thistle, may help protect your liver against irritation caused by tamoxifen. Consider taking supplements (200 mg daily).

KEEP IN MIND

• Studies in laboratory animals suggest that soy isoflavones (estrogenlike substances) may help tamoxifen work better. The research is controversial, however, and the long-term value of taking soy isoflavones is still unknown.

• High doses of melatonin, a natural hormone, may also help tamoxifen work better, especially in patients who are not helped by tamoxifen alone. Discuss both of these supplements with your physician before trying them.

TETRACYCLINE
BRAND NAMES *Ala-Tet, Panmycin, Sumycin, Tetracap, Tetracyn, others*

TYPE OF DRUG
Tetracycline antibiotic

DESCRIPTION
Tetracycline is prescribed for bacterial infections, including tick-borne infections, acne, and as an alternative antibiotic for people allergic to penicillin.

DON'T MIX WITH
Berberine-containing herbs. Goldenseal (*Hydrastis canadensis*), barberry (*Berberis vulgaris*), and Oregon grape (*Berberis acquiflolium*) contain berberine, an antibacterial chemical that may interfere with the body's absorption of tetracycline. Do not use these herbs if you are taking tetracycline.

KEEP IN MIND
• The aluminum, calcium, and magnesium in antacids can interfere with the body's absorption of tetracycline, as can the calcium, iron, magnesium, zinc, and other minerals in supplements and multivitamins with minerals, and the calcium in milk and other dairy products. Take these antacids and supplements at least two hours apart from taking tetracycline, and discuss your intake of calcium-rich foods with your medical practitioner.

• Tetracycline can block your absorption or use of many B vitamins. Consider supplements (B-50 formula once daily).
• Tetracycline kills not only the harmful bacteria that cause illness but also the good bacteria normally found in your intestines; this can cause diarrhea. Consider taking probiotic supplements (at least 1.5 billion live organisms daily, including a mixture of *Lactobacillus acidophilus, Bifidobacterium bifidum,* and *Saccharomyces boulardii*).

THEOPHYLLINE
BRAND NAMES *Bronkodyl, Slo-bid, Theolair, Theo-Dur, Uniphyl, others*

TYPE OF DRUG
Bronchodilator

DESCRIPTION
Theophylline is prescribed to treat asthma and also emphysema, bronchitis, chronic obstructive pulmonary disease (COPD), and some other conditions.

DON'T MIX WITH
Caffeine-containing herbs. Caffeine can increase the action and side effects of theophylline. Avoid caffeine-containing herbs, including guarana (*Paullinia cupana*), kola nut (*Cola* spp.), and maté (*Ilex paraguariensis*), and other products that contain caffeine.
Cayenne (*Capsicum frutescens*). Eating large amounts of cayenne pepper could increase your absorption of theophylline and raise your blood level too high. Quantities consumed as part of a normal diet are unlikely to cause problems.
Ephedra (*Ephedra* spp., also known as ma huang). Taking ephedra with theophylline raises blood pressure and can cause heart arrhythmias and other serious side effects. Similarly, avoid the drugs ephedrine (p. 152) and pseudoephedrine (p. 185), which are found in many nonprescription cold and allergy remedies.
St. John's wort (*Hypericum perforatum*). This may lower blood levels of theophylline. Until more information is known, do not combine these.
Tannin-containing herbs. Herbs that are high in tannin include black walnut (*Juglans nigra*), red raspberry (*Rubus idaeus*), oak (*Quercus* spp.), uva ursi (*Arctostaphylos uva-ursi*), and witch hazel (*Hamamelis virginiana*). Tea can also interfere with the absorption of theophylline. Do not use these herbs when taking theophylline.

Cayenne

KEEP IN MIND
• Studies have shown that theophylline depletes vitamin B6 (pyridoxine) levels. Discuss vitamin B6 with your physician and consider taking supplements (50 mg daily).
• Theophylline may also deplete levels of potassium and magnesium. Discuss supplements with your physician.

THIAZIDE

BRAND NAMES *Aquatensen, Diuril, Diurese, Exna, Metahydrin, others*

TYPE OF DRUG	Potassium-wasting diuretic

DESCRIPTION Thiazide diuretics are used most often to treat high blood pressure. These drugs are often called "potassium-wasting" diuretics because they increase elimination of potassium – and also magnesium, sodium, and zinc – from the body.

DON'T MIX WITH

Digitalis (*Digitalis purpurea*, also known as foxglove). This dangerous herb is very similar to the heart drug digoxin, which is derived from digitalis and can lower your potassium level. In combination with a thiazide diuretic, digitalis could make your potassium level dangerously low.

Herbal diuretics. In combination with a thiazide diuretic, herbal diuretics could make your potassium level drop too low. Avoid herbal diuretics, including bilberry leaf (*Vaccinium myrtillus*), buchu (*Barosma betulina*), burdock (*Arctium lappa*), couch grass (*Agropyron repens*), damiana (*Turnera diffusa*), dandelion (*Taraxacum officinale*), fennel seed (*Foeniculum vulgare*), goldenrod (*Solidago virgaurea*), horsetail (*Equisetum arvense*), kava kava (*Piper methysticum*), kola nut (*Cola* spp.), marshmallow (*Althaea officinalis*), maté (*Ilex paraguariensis*), parsley (*Petroselinum* spp.), sarsaparilla (*Smilax* spp.), saw palmetto (*Serenoa repens*), uva ursi (*Arctostaphylos uva-ursi*), vervain (*Verbena* spp.), and yarrow (*Achillea millefolium*).

Licorice (*Glycyrrhiza glabra*). Large amounts of licorice can reduce potassium levels. In combination with a thiazide diuretic, this could make your potassium level dangerously low. This effect does not occur with deglycyrrhizinated licorice (DGL) or artificial licorice flavoring.

Bilberry

TICLOPIDINE

BRAND NAME *Ticlid*

TYPE OF DRUG	Anticoagulant

DESCRIPTION Ticlopidine is an anticoagulant ("blood-thinning") drug used to prevent blood clots and reduce the risk of strokes. It is also used to treat intermittent claudication (poor circulation in the legs) and some other conditions, such as sickle cell anemia. H2 blockers, such as cimetidine (p. 137), slow the body's elimination of ticlopidine, which raises the amount in the bloodstream and increases the risk of side effects. Ask your physician or pharmacist to help you choose a different type of antacid.

DON'T MIX WITH

Blood-thinning herbs. A number of herbs have known or possible anticoagulant action and could increase the effect of ticlopidine. Avoid dan shen (*Salvia miltiorrhiza*), devil's claw (*Harpagophytum procumbens*), dong quai (*Angelica sinensis*), fenugreek (*Trigonella foenum-graecum*), garlic (*Allium sativum*), ginger (*Zingiber officinale*), ginkgo (*Ginkgo biloba*), ginseng (*Panax ginseng*), horse chestnut (*Aesculus hippocastanum*), red clover (*Trifolium pratense*), and sweet woodruff (*Galium odoratum*). Foods containing garlic and ginger in moderate amounts are unlikely to cause any problems.

Salicylate-containing herbs. The herbs meadowsweet (*Filipendula ulmaria*), white willow bark (*Salix alba*), and wintergreen (*Gaultheria procumbens*) contain salicylates, compounds similar to aspirin, which can thin the blood. There is a slight chance that taking these herbs with ticlopidine could thin your blood too much.

Devil's claw

KEEP IN MIND • Magnesium and calcium reduce your absorption of ticlopidine. Take antacids or supplements containing these minerals two hours apart from the drug.

TIMOLOL

BRAND NAMES *Betimol, Blocadren, Timoptic*

TYPE OF DRUG	Beta blocker
DESCRIPTION	Timolol is used to treat high blood pressure and abnormal heart rhythms; it is also used to treat glaucoma. Timolol is a powerful drug that can interact adversely with a number of prescription drugs, so use it with caution. Be certain to tell your physician about any other prescription and nonprescription drugs and dietary supplements you take.
DON'T MIX WITH	**St. John's wort** *(Hypericum perforatum)*. Monoamine oxidase inhibitors (MAOIs) interact adversely with timolol. Because St. John's wort works in a way that is similar to these drugs, do not use it if taking timolol.
KEEP IN MIND	• Beta blockers block your use of coenzyme Q_{10} (CoQ$_{10}$ or ubiquinone), which is needed for energy production within your cells. Consider taking CoQ$_{10}$ supplements (20–50 mg daily). • The antacid cimetidine *(p. 137)* and related H2-blockers such as famotidine *(p. 155)*, and ranitidine *(p. 186)* may increase the amount of timolol in your bloodstream. Ask your physician or pharmacist to help you choose a different type of antacid. • A small amount of the timolol in eyedrops (Timoptic) enters your bloodstream, but is not enough to cause any of the problems associated with beta blockers.

St. John's wort

TRAMADOL

BRAND NAME *Ultram*

TYPE OF DRUG	Nonnarcotic pain reliever
DESCRIPTION	Tramadol is prescribed to relieve moderate to severe pain.
DON'T MIX WITH	**St. John's wort** *(Hypericum perforatum)*. Both St. John's wort and tramadol reduce the uptake of serotonin, a neurotransmitter, into the body's nerves. Combining the two may cause the serotonin level to become too high, which could lead to a serious condition known as serotonin syndrome.
KEEP IN MIND	• The supplements 5-HTP, tryptophan, and SAMe all effect your uptake of serotonin. Do not combine them with tramadol, as your serotonin level may rise too high. • Tramadol can cause drowsiness and impair mental ability and coordination. Alcohol can make these side effects worse. Do not consume alcohol if taking this drug.

TRAZODONE

BRAND NAME *Desyrel*

TYPE OF DRUG	Antidepressant
DESCRIPTION	Trazodone is prescribed for depression, panic disorder, agoraphobia (fear of open spaces), and some other disorders. It is also used to treat cocaine addiction.
DON'T MIX WITH	**Digitalis** (*Digitalis purpurea*, also known as foxglove). This dangerous herb is very similar to the heart drug digoxin, which, when taken with trazodone, could raise the digoxin in your blood to a dangerous level. Until more is known, do not take digitalis with trazodone. **St. John's wort** (*Hypericum perforatum*). Although there have been no reports of interactions, physicians recommend against combining the antidepressant herb St. John's wort with antidepressant drugs such as trazodone.
KEEP IN MIND	• Trazodone can cause drowsiness and dizziness. Alcohol can make these side effects worse. Do not consume alcohol while taking this drug.

Foxglove

TRIAMTERENE

BRAND NAMES *Dyazide, Dyrenium, Maxzide*

TYPE OF DRUG	Potassium-sparing diuretic
DESCRIPTION	Triamterene is a diuretic prescribed alone (Dyrenium) or in combination with hydrochlorothiazide (Dyazide, Maxzide) to treat high blood pressure, heart failure, and some other conditions. Triamterene is a "potassium-sparing" diuretic because it does not cause your body to eliminate excess potassium, in contrast with some other classes of diuretics that are known as "potassium-wasting."
DON'T MIX WITH	**Herbal diuretics.** Combining triamterene and diuretic herbs increases the risk of side effects such as electrolyte disturbances and dehydration. Avoid herbal diuretics including bilberry leaf (*Vaccinium myrtillus*), buchu (*Barosma betulina*), burdock (*Arctium lappa*), couch grass (*Agropyron repens*), damiana (*Turnera diffusa*), dandelion (*Taraxacum officinale*), fennel seed (*Foeniculum vulgare*), goldenrod (*Solidago virgaurea*), horsetail (*Equisetum arvense*), kava kava (*Piper methysticum*), kola nut (*Cola* spp.), marshmallow (*Althaea officinalis*), maté (*Ilex paraguariensis*), parsley (*Petroselinum* spp.), sarsaparilla (*Smilax* spp.), saw palmetto (*Serenoa repens*), uva ursi (*Arctostaphylos uva-ursi*), vervain (*Verbena* spp. and *V. hastata*), and yarrow (*Achillea millefolium*), as well as any other prescription or nonprescription diuretics.
KEEP IN MIND	• Triamterene can increase the amount of potassium in your body. Do not take potassium supplements or use salt substitutes (which are generally high in potassium) with this drug. Discuss your consumption of potassium-rich foods, such as bananas and orange juice, with your physician. • Triamterene might increase your magnesium level. Avoid magnesium supplements and magnesium-containing antacids.

Parsley

VENLAFAXINE

BRAND NAMES *Effexor, Effexor XR*

TYPE OF DRUG	Antidepressant
DESCRIPTION	Venlafaxine is prescribed to treat depression. This drug probably works by reducing the uptake of serotonin, a neurotransmitter, into the body's nerves, but it is not related to selective serotonin reuptake inhibitor (SSRI) drugs such as fluoxetine *(p. 155).*
DON'T MIX WITH	**St. John's wort** (*Hypericum perforatum*). Because St. John's wort is also thought to work by affecting your serotonin levels, don't combine it with venlafaxine. This may cause the serotonin level in your blood to rise too high, which can result in the serious condition serotonin syndrome.
KEEP IN MIND	• The supplements 5-HTP, tryptophan, and SAMe all affect serotonin levels. Do not combine them with venlafaxine as this may cause your serotonin levels to rise too high. • Venlafaxine can cause drowsiness and impair mental ability and coordination. Alcohol can make these side effects worse. Do not consume alcohol if taking this drug.

VERAPAMIL

BRAND NAMES *Calan, Covera HS, Isoptin, Verelan*

TYPE OF DRUG	Calcium channel blocker
DESCRIPTION	Verapamil is prescribed for high blood pressure, angina, abnormal heart rhythms, and cardiomyopathy. It is also sometimes prescribed to treat nighttime leg cramps, asthma, migraines, and bipolar disorder. Verapamil is a calcium channel blocker, a drug that blocks the movement of calcium into muscles, which allows them to relax, and widens blood vessels.
DON'T MIX WITH	No known herbal interactions.
DO TAKE WITH	**Milk thistle** *(Silybum marianum).* Silymarin, an active compound in the herb milk thistle, may protect against liver damage from verapamil. Consider taking supplements (150 mg 3 to 4 times daily).
KEEP IN MIND	• A substance in grapefruit or grapefruit juice may cause the liver to reduce the rate of elimination of other calcium channel blocker drugs such as felodipine (Plendil) and nifedipine *(p. 173).* This can increase the amount of these drugs in your body to dangerous levels. Although there have been no reports of a similar effect with verapamil, until more is known, do not eat grapefruit or drink grapefruit juice when taking this drug. • Calcium from supplements or antacids may block the effects of verapamil, and vitamin D may reduce the drug's effectiveness. Discuss any supplements or drugs containing calcium or vitamin D with your medical practitioner first. • To avoid constipation from verapamil, eat plenty of fresh fruits and vegetables and whole grains and drink plenty of water (at least 64 ounces a day).

Milk thistle

WARFARIN

TYPE OF DRUG	Anticoagulant

DESCRIPTION

Warfarin is an anticoagulant ("blood-thinning") drug used primarily to prevent and treat blood clots and to reduce the risk of strokes. Warfarin is a dangerous drug that can interact adversely with a very wide range of other drugs, herbs, vitamins, and other dietary supplements. If at all possible, do not use any herbs, dietary supplements, or nonprescription drugs if taking warfarin. However, if you are taking any herbs, supplements or nonprescription drugs, do not discontinue them until you have discussed it with your physician.

DON'T MIX WITH

Ginger

Blood-thinning herbs. A number of herbs may have anticoagulant action and could increase the effect of warfarin. Avoid dan shen *(Salvia miltiorrhiza)*, devil's claw *(Harpagophytum procumbens)*, dong quai *(Angelica sinensis)*, fenugreek *(Trigonella foenum-graecum)*, garlic *(Allium sativum)*, ginger *(Zingiber officinale)*, ginkgo *(Ginkgo biloba)*, ginseng *(Panax ginseng)*, horse chestnut *(Aesculus hippocastanum)*, red clover *(Trifolium pratense)*, and sweet woodruff *(Galium odoratum)*. Foods containing garlic and ginger in moderate amounts are unlikely to cause any problems.

Salicylate-containing herbs. The herbs meadowsweet *(Filipendula ulmaria)*, willow bark *(Salix alba)*, and wintergreen *(Gaultheria procumbens)* contain salicylates, compounds similar to aspirin that may also have a blood-thinning effect. Taking these herbs with warfarin could thin your blood too much.

St. John's wort *(Hypericum perforatum)*. This herb may reduce your absorption of warfarin. Until more is known, do not combine St. John's wort with warfarin.

KEEP IN MIND

• Warfarin works by blocking your use of vitamin K, which is needed to make your blood clot. Do not take vitamin K supplements with warfarin. Discuss your intake of foods rich in vitamin K with your physician.

ZOLPIDEM

TYPE OF DRUG	Sedative/hypnotic

DESCRIPTION

Zolpidem is a sleeping pill prescribed for the short-term treatment of insomnia. Although zolpidem works in ways very similar to benzodiazepine drugs such as diazepam *(p. 146)*, it is not related to these drugs and does not relax muscles.

DON'T MIX WITH

Passionflower

Sedative herbs. When combined with zolpidem, these herbs may cause excessive drowsiness. Avoid using sedative herbs such as chamomile *(Matricaria recutita)*, catnip *(Nepeta cataria)*, kava kava *(Piper methysticum)*, passionflower *(Passiflora incarnata)*, and valerian *(Valeriana officinalis)*.

St. John's wort *(Hypericum perforatum)*. The combination of zolpidem and selective serotonin reuptake inhibitor (SSRI) drugs such as fluoxetine *(p. 155)* has been reported to cause hallucinations in some people. Because St. John's wort is thought to work in a way similar to SSRI drugs, it should not be used when taking zolpidem.

KEEP IN MIND

• Because of the interaction between zolpidem and selective serotonin reuptake inhibitor (SSRI) drugs *(see Don't mix with, above)* experts advise against taking the natural sedatives 5-HTP, tryptophan, and SAMe when taking zolpidem because these supplements affect serotonin levels.

• Zolpidem causes drowsiness. Alcohol makes this effect stronger. Do not consume alcohol if taking this drug.

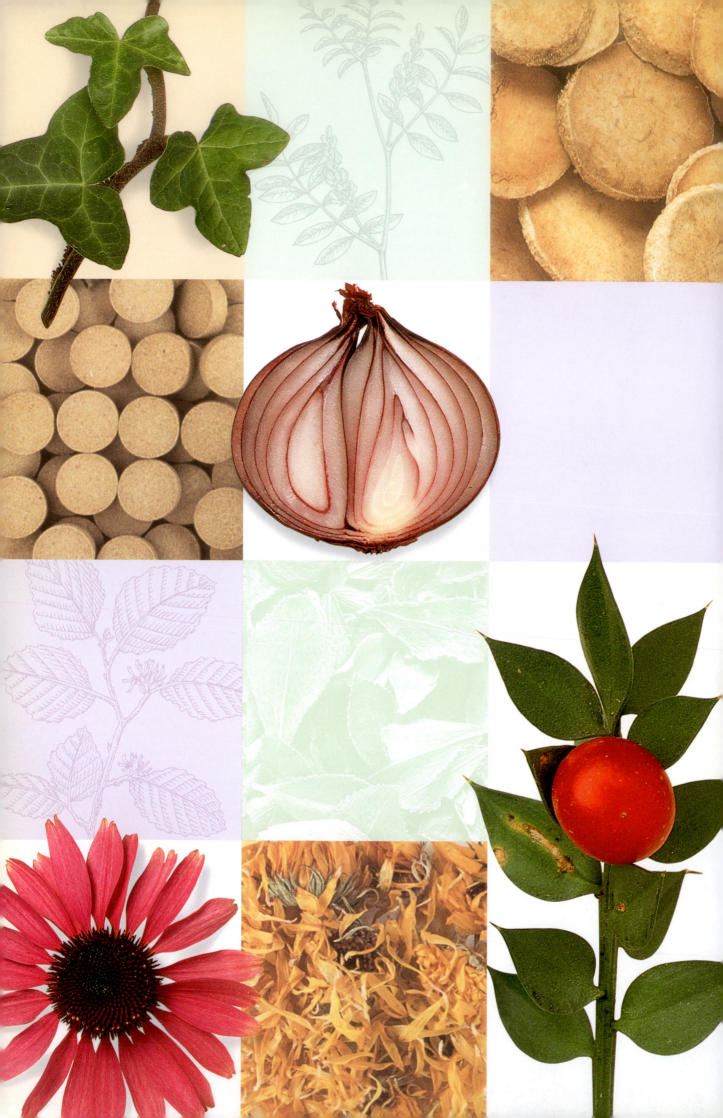

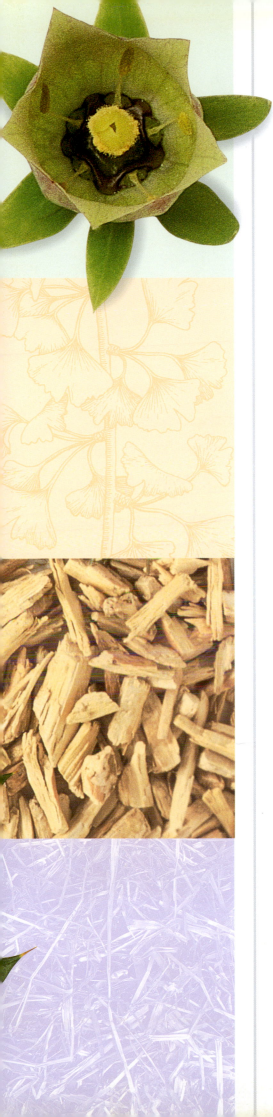

CHAPTER 6

HERBS FOR SPECIAL CASES

CERTAIN GROUPS OF PEOPLE require special consideration when it comes to herbal safety. For children and older adults, many herbs can be used safely in reduced dosages, but other herbs can pose risks for them. Pregnant and nursing women, however, need to be especially cautious about using herbs – even those herbs considered safe in other cases can be dangerous for an unborn baby.

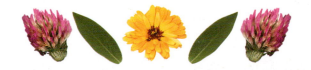

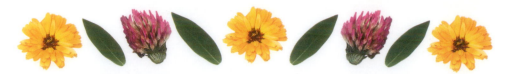

UNDERSTANDING SPECIAL CASES

ERBS ARE GENERALLY known to be gentler remedies than drugs. As a result, some parents may prefer to treat their children with herbs instead of drugs, and older people may value them for their mildness. But some herbs are too powerful for these groups, and pregnant and nursing mothers should be extremely cautious about herbs and their effect on growing babies.

Calendula

❖ HERBS FOR CHILDREN ❖

Many minor childhood illnesses, such as mild sore throats, coughs, and minor skin conditions including scrapes, bruises, and burns can be treated safely with herbs.

When you find a safe herb you would like to give your child, check the entry in Chapter 1 for complete information about the herb, including actions, cautions, and standardization information. To calculate the right dose for your child, multiply the adult dose by the child's weight and divide the result by 150. For example, if the adult dose is 1 teaspoon and your child weighs 35 pounds, the dose would be 0.23 of a teaspoon, or nearly ¼ teaspoon.

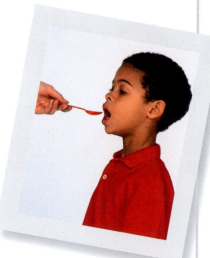

TREATING CHILDREN
Herbs can be used to treat a variety of minor illnesses in children.

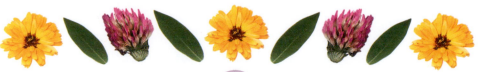

HERB	WHY IT'S USED	COMMENTS & CAUTIONS
MYRRH *Commiphora molmol*	To treat inflammation of the throat, such as tonsillitis.	May cause gastrointestinal irritation.
GUGGUL *Commiphora mukul*	To reduce cholesterol.	May cause diarrhea in children.
CORIANDER SEED *Coriandrum sativum*	To treat digestive problems such as stomach cramps or diarrhea.	May cause gastrointestinal irritation in children.
TURKEY TAIL *Coriolus versicolor*	To stimulate the immune system.	Should be used only under a physician's supervision.
HAWTHORN BERRY, HAWTHORN FLOWER *Crataegus* spp.	To treat heart conditions and high blood pressure.	May cause a dangerous drop in blood pressure and altered heart function.
PUMPKIN SEED *Curcurbita pepo*	A traditional bedwetting and tapeworm remedy.	May cause gastrointestinal irritation.
CARDAMOM SEED *Eletteria cardamomum*	To treat digestive problems and respiratory ailments.	Can interfere with digestion in children.
ELEUTHERO *Eleutherococcus senticosus*	To relieve stress. Also used as a mild stimulant.	May cause overstimulation and altered hormonal balance in children.
HORSETAIL *Equisetum arvense*	To improve bone and nail strength.	May cause gastrointestinal upset. Do not give to children who have kidney disease. Homeopathic preparations are safe as such small quantities are used.
CALIFORNIA POPPY *Eschscholzia californica*	To relieve anxiety and insomnia.	May cause excessive drowsiness in children.
MEADOWSWEET *Filipendula ulmaria*	To reduce fever, relieve pain, and treat cold and flu symptoms.	This herb contains salicylates that have been associated with Reye syndrome, a serious illness.
FENNEL *Foeniculum vulgare*	To treat digestive problems such as heartburn, nausea, and cramps.	Mild fennel tea is safe for children over six. Larger amounts can cause hormonal imbalance.
GENTIAN ROOT *Gentiana lutea*	To treat digestive problems such as loss of appetite and gas.	Can cause severe gastrointestinal irritation.
GINKGO *Ginkgo biloba*	Improves circulation and memory.	Use only under a physician's supervision; may cause headaches and lowered blood pressure in children.
SOY ISOFLAVONES, SOY LECITHIN *Glycine max*	To reduce cholesterol.	May cause hormonal imbalance and diarrhea in children.
LICORICE *Glycyrrhiza glabra*	To treat ulcers, AIDS, upper respiratory infections, and digestive problems.	May cause dangerously high blood pressure in children.
GUMWEED *Grindelia robusta*	To treat coughs from colds and bronchitis.	May cause diarrhea in children.
GYMNEMA *Gymnema sylvestre*	Asian medicinal remedy for mild cases of Type 2 diabetes.	Use only under a physician's supervision.

Blessed thistle

HERB	WHY IT'S USED	COMMENTS & CAUTIONS
WITCH HAZEL *Hamamelis virginiana*	To treat minor injuries such as scrapes, bruises, and insect bites.	May cause skin irritation in children with very sensitive skin.
DEVIL'S CLAW *Harpagophytum procumbens*	To treat digestive problems, arthritis, gout, and back pain.	May cause stomach upset and vomiting in children.
IVY LEAF *Hedera helix*	To relieve coughs resulting from colds, flu, and bronchitis.	May cause skin irritation in children.
HOPS *Humulus lupulus*	To treat anxiety, insomnia, and digestive problems.	Fresh hops may cause excessive drowsiness in children.
ST. JOHN'S WORT *Hypericum perforatum*	To treat depression, anxiety, and insomnia.	Use under a physician's supervision. Homeopathic preparations are safe as such small quantities are used.
MATÉ *Ilex paraguariensis*	Mild stimulant used to relieve fatigue and headaches.	This herb contains caffeine, which may overstimulate children.
WALNUT LEAF *Juglans regia*	Used topically to treat inflammatory conditions such as eczema and sunburn.	May cause skin irritation in children.
LAVENDER *Lavandula* spp.	To treat mild anxiety, muscle soreness, and digestive problems.	May cause skin irritation in children.
MOTHERWORT *Leonurus cardiaca*	To treat heart problems such as irregular or rapid heartbeat.	Can adversely affect heart function in children.
BUGLEWEED *Lycopus virginicus*	To treat hyperthyroidism (overproduction of thyroid hormones).	Can adversely affect thyroid function in children.
ALFALFA *Medicago sativa*	To lower cholesterol and treat mild cases of Type 2 diabetes.	Do not give this herb to children who have diabetes or autoimmune diseases.
MINT OIL *Mentha* spp.	For digestive problems, colds and flu, sore muscles and joints.	May cause choking and skin irritation in children.
BITTER MELON *Momordica charantia*	To treat mild cases of Type 2 diabetes, and to provide immune system support for HIV patients.	Use only under a physician's supervision.
CATNIP *Nepeta cataria*	To relieve anxiety, insomnia, digestive problems, and coughs.	Catnip tincture is safe for treating coughs in children when used under a physician's supervision.
OREGANO OIL *Origanum vulgare*	To treat fungal infections such as ringworm and athlete's foot.	External use only; may cause skin irritation in children. Internal use causes severe gastrointestinal irritation.
GINSENG *Panax ginseng, P. quinquefolium*	To reduce stress and boost energy.	May cause overstimulation in children.
PASSIONFLOWER *Passiflora incarnata*	To relieve anxiety and insomnia.	May cause excessive drowsiness.
GUARANA *Paullinia cupana*	To treat headaches and fatigue.	This herb contains caffeine, which may overstimulate children.

HERB	WHY IT'S USED	COMMENTS & CAUTIONS
PARSLEY *Petroselinum crispum*	To treat urinary tract infections, kidney stones, and minor digestive problems.	This herb is a diuretic and may dehydrate children. Moderate dietary use is safe.
BOLDO LEAF *Peumus boldus*	To treat digestive problems such as cramps and mild nausea.	This herb is a diuretic; it may dehydrate children. Use only ascaridole-free products.
KAVA KAVA *Piper methysticum*	Used primarily to help treat anxiety and insomnia.	May cause excessive drowsiness.
MASTICA *Pistacia lentiscus*	To treat ulcers and maintain gum health.	May cause diarrhea in small children.
PLANTAIN *Plantago* spp.	To treat sore throat, coughs, and minor skin inflammation including sunburn.	Raw leaves may cause skin irritation.
FO-TI *Polygonum multiflorum*	To treat high cholesterol, insomnia, and constipation.	May cause diarrhea in children.
POPLAR BUD *Populus balsamifera*	The cream is used for minor skin injuries; the gargle is used for laryngitis.	This herb contains salicylates that have been associated with Reye syndrome, a serious illness.
BLACKTHORN *Prunus spinosa*	To treat sore throat, respiratory infections, or mouth irritation.	May cause dangerously severe diarrhea in children.
PYGEUM *Pygeum africanum*	To treat male urinary problems.	May cause hormonal imbalance.
BUCKTHORN BARK *Rhamnus frangula*	To treat constipation.	Can cause dangerously severe diarrhea in children.
CASCARA SAGRADA *Rhamnus purshiani*	To treat constipation.	Can cause dangerously severe diarrhea in children.
ROSEMARY LEAF *Rosmarinus officinalis*	To treat digestive problems, joint pain, and sore muscles.	Moderate dietary use is safe; external use of oil may cause skin irritation.
RASPBERRY LEAF *Rubus idaeus*	To treat diarrhea, sore throat, and mouth irritation.	May cause diarrhea in children.
YELLOW DOCK *Rumex crispus*	To treat constipation.	May cause diarrhea in children.
BUTCHER'S BROOM *Ruscus aculeatus*	To treat hemorrhoids and varicose veins.	This herb is a diuretic; it may cause dehydration in children.
WILLOW BARK *Salix alba*	To treat headaches, arthritis, and fever.	This herb contains salicylates that have been associated with Reye syndrome, a serious illness.
SAGE *Salvia officinalis*	To treat digestive problems, sore throat, and mouth irritation.	Moderate dietary consumption is safe. Do not give to children with a fever.
BLOODROOT *Sanguinaria canadensis*	Used in dental products to prevent plaque and gum disease.	Poisonous if taken internally. Because small children may swallow toothpaste or mouthwash, do not use any products containing this herb.

Ivy leaves

HERB	WHY IT'S USED	COMMENTS & CAUTIONS
SCHISANDRA *Schisandra chinensis*	To treat liver problems, especially hepatitis.	May cause skin rash and stomach upset.
SAW PALMETTO *Serenoa repens*	To treat male urinary problems.	May cause hormonal imbalance in children.
SARSAPARILLA *Smilax spp.*	To treat skin conditions, arthritis, and irritable bowel syndrome.	May cause irritation of the skin, kidneys, and gastrointestinal tract.
GOLDENROD *Solidago virgaurea*	To treat bladder infections and kidney stones.	This herb is a diuretic and may cause dehydration.
STEVIA *Stevia rebaudiana*	Used as a calorie-free sugar substitute.	May cause reduced blood pressure in children; use only under a physician's supervision.
CLOVE, CLOVE OIL *Syzygium aromaticum*	To treat digestive problems, bad breath, and gum disease.	Clove oil may cause skin and mouth irritation.
FEVERFEW *Tanacetum parthenium*	To prevent and treat migraines.	May cause gastrointestinal irritation in children.
DANDELION *Taraxacum officinale*	To treat digestive problems such as nausea, bloating, and gas.	This herb is a diuretic and may cause dehydration.
RED CLOVER *Trifolium pratense*	To reduce cholesterol.	May cause liver damage in children.
FENUGREEK *Trigonella foenum-graecum*	To treat blood sugar and cholesterol control in diabetes.	Discuss this herb with your physician before giving it to children with diabetes.
STINGING NETTLE LEAF *Urtica dioica*	To treat kidney stones, pollen allergies, and UTIs.	May cause hormonal imbalance. Safe in homeopathic preparations.
USNEA *Usnea spp.*	To relieve coughs, sore throats, bacterial and yeast infections.	Safe if grown organically to avoid contamination with heavy metals.
VALERIAN *Valeriana officinalis*	To relieve insomnia.	May cause excessive drowsiness in children.
VERVAIN *Verbena officinalis*	To relieve mild pain, particularly from headaches.	May cause excessive drowsiness in children.
CHASTEBERRY *Vitex agnus-castus*	To treat PMS symptoms and irregular menstruation.	May cause hormonal imbalance in children.
ASHWAGANDHA *Withania somnifera*	To improve overall health, energy, and immunity.	May cause hormonal imbalance in children.
YUCCA *Yucca spp.*	To treat arthritis. An ingredient in shampoos and soaps.	May cause an upset stomach in children; can block the absorption of other medications.
CORN SILK *Zea mays*	To treat bladder problems.	This herb is a diuretic and may cause dehydration.
GINGER ROOT *Zingiber officinale*	To treat nausea, motion sickness, arthritis, and migraines.	Moderate dietary use is safe. Medicinal use may cause stomach upset.

UNSAFE HERBS FOR PREGNANT AND NURSING WOMEN

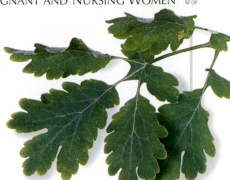

HERB	WHY IT'S USED	COMMENTS & CAUTIONS
YARROW *Achillea millefolium*	To staunch bleeding and to treat colds, flu, and menstrual problems.	Can cause miscarriage.
AGAVE *Agave americana*	No common medicinal uses.	Can cause uterine bleeding and miscarriage.
ALKANNA *Alkanna tinctoria*	To speed wound healing.	Can cause liver damage to the mother and harm to the unborn baby.
GARLIC *Allium sativum*	To relieve cardiovascular and circulatory problems.	Large doses may cause uterine bleeding and miscarriage; dietary moderation is strongly advised.
ALOE VERA *Aloe vera*	To treat skin and digestive problems.	External use of the gel is safe; internal use can cause uterine bleeding and miscarriage.
BLAZING STAR *Alteris farinosa*	To relieve digestive problems such as nausea, gas, or loss of appetite.	This herb is a uterine stimulant that can cause miscarriage.
KHELLA, BISHOP'S WEED *Ammi visnaga*	To treat heart conditions, such as angina, and kidney stones.	This herb is a uterine stimulant that can cause miscarriage.
CELERY *Apium graveolens*	To treat rheumatoid arthritis and gout.	This herb is a uterine stimulant that can cause miscarriage. Moderate dietary consumption is safe.
BURDOCK ROOT *Arctium lappa*	To treat urinary tract infections (UTIs), skin conditions, and rheumatoid arthritis.	This herb is a uterine stimulant that can cause miscarriage.
UVA URSI *Arctostaphylos uva-ursi*	To treat urinary tract infections (UTIs) and bladder conditions.	May cause uterine contractions while pregnant or nursing.
BETEL NUT *Areca catechu*	To treat diarrhea and intestinal parasites.	This herb can cause birth defects.
BIRTHWORT *Aristolochia clematitis*	To support immune function and fight viruses.	This herb is a uterine stimulant that can cause miscarriage.
HORSERADISH *Armoracia rusticana*	To relieve sore throat, colds, flu, and urinary tract infections (UTIs).	Avoid dietary horseradish if you have a high risk of miscarriage, uterine bleeding, or any other bleeding disorder.
ARNICA *Arnica montana*	To relieve minor injuries such as bruises, bumps, and swelling, and sore muscles and joints.	External remedies are generally considered safe if you are not at high risk; consult your physician before using this herb.
PLEURISY ROOT *Ascelpias tuberosa*	To treat coughs and diarrhea.	This herb can cause uterine stimulation and miscarriage.

Horseradish

HERB	WHY IT'S USED	COMMENTS & CAUTIONS
BUCHU *Barosma* spp.	To relieve kidney and bladder conditions and PMS-related bloating.	May cause miscarriage.
OREGON GRAPE *Berberis acquifolium, Mahonia acquifolium*	To relieve the symptoms of psoriasis.	May cause uterine bleeding and miscarriage.
BARBERRY *Berberis vulgaris*	To relieve sore throat, mouth irritation, digestive problems.	This herb can cause uterine bleeding and miscarriage.
BEET LEAF *Beta vulgaris*	To treat digestive problems and support liver and gallbladder.	May increase the chances of uterine bleeding and miscarriage. Dietary moderation is strongly advised.
BORAGE OIL *Borago officinalis*	To treat PMS, skin problems, and rheumatoid arthritis.	May cause liver damage to the mother and harm to the fetus.
CABBAGE, COLEWORT *Brassica oleracea*	To treat ulcers and provide dietary fiber.	Can interfere with mental development in the fetus.
KOUSSO *Brayera anthelmintica*	Used traditionally to treat intestinal parasites.	May cause miscarriage.
BRYONY *Bryonia* spp.	To treat arthritis and asthma.	This herb is highly toxic and is used cautiously by physicians.
CALENDULA *Calendula officinalis*	To relieve skin problems including cuts, rashes, and wounds.	External use is safe. Internal use can cause uterine bleeding and miscarriage.
GREEN TEA *Camellia sinensis*	Used as a stimulant.	Moderate dietary consumption is safe.
SHEPHERD'S PURSE *Capsella bursa-pastoris*	To prevent menstrual irregularities and nosebleeds and treat minor skin abrasions.	May cause uterine bleeding or miscarriage.
CAYENNE *Capsicum frutescens*	To treat loss of appetite, cramps, and gas.	Moderate dietary consumption is safe.
PAPAYA *Carica papaya*	To treat loss of appetite, cramps, and gas.	May cause uterine bleeding or miscarriage.
SAFFLOWER OIL *Carthamus tinctorius*	To lower cholesterol levels.	Large amounts may cause uterine bleeding and miscarriage. Dietary moderation is strongly advised.
SENNA *Cassia* spp.	To relieve constipation.	May cause birth defects if pregnant or breast-feeding.
MADAGASCAR PERIWINKLE *Catharanthus roseus*	Used in some cancer treatments under a physician's supervision.	Can cause miscarriage and birth defects.
GOTU KOLA *Centella asiatica*	To treat varicose veins, poor leg circulation, and hemorrhoids.	May cause miscarriage, particularly in the first trimester.
IPECAC *Cephaelis ipecacuanha*	To induce vomiting.	May stimulate the uterus, increasing the chance of miscarriage.

HERB	WHY IT'S USED	COMMENTS & CAUTIONS
HELONIAS *Chamaelirium luteum*	Traditionally used to induce vomiting.	May cause miscarriage.
ROMAN CHAMOMILE *Chamaemelum nobile*	To relieve nausea, intestinal cramps, anxiety, and insomnia.	Moderate dietary consumption and topical use are safe. Large doses can increase the risk of complications in pregnancy.
CELANDINE *Chelidonium majus*	To relieve digestive problems and irregular menstruation.	May cause liver damage and also cause uterine stimulation.
CHICORY *Cichorium intybus*	To relieve digestive problems and support gallbladder and liver.	Moderate dietary consumption is safe. Large amounts could cause uterine bleeding and miscarriage.
BLACK COHOSH ROOT *Cimicifuga racemosa*	To treat menopausal symptoms, headache, irritability, or insomnia.	May cause miscarriage.
CINCHONA *Cinchona pubescens*	To treat poor appetite, bloating, and gas.	May cause uterine bleeding and miscarriage.
CAMPHOR *Cinnamomum camphora*	To treat sore muscles, chest congestion, and coughing.	May cause uterine bleeding, miscarriage, and birth defects.
CINNAMON *Cinnamomum verum*	To relieve poor appetite, nausea, and gas.	Moderate dietary consumption is safe. Large amounts may cause uterine bleeding and miscarriage.
BITTER APPLE *Citrulus colocynthis*	Traditional remedy for constipation.	This herb is highly poisonous, and may cause uterine bleeding and miscarriage.
CITRUS FRUITS *Citrus* spp.	To provide fiber and vitamin C.	Moderate dietary consumption is safe. Excess intake can result in uterine stimulation.
BITTER ORANGE PEEL *Citrus aurantium*	To relieve heartburn, nausea, poor appetite, bloating, and gas.	Can cause birth defects, uterine bleeding, and miscarriage.
ERGOT *Claviceps purpurea*	Traditional headache remedy.	Can cause uterine bleeding and miscarriage.
COFFEE *Coffea arabica*	Used as a stimulant.	Contains caffeine, which has been linked to miscarriage, low birth weight, premature delivery, and birth defects.
KOLA NUT *Cola acuminata*	Used as a stimulant.	Contains caffeine, which has been linked to miscarriage, low birth weight, premature delivery, and birth defects.
COLEUS *Coleus forskohlii*	To treat asthma, eczema, psoriasis, high blood pressure, and angina.	May cause uterine bleeding or miscarriage.
MYRRH *Commiphora molmol*	To treat sore throat, mouth inflammation, gum disease.	May cause uterine bleeding or miscarriage.
GOLDTHREAD *Coptis trifolia*	To relieve digestive problems including nausea and poor appetite.	May cause miscarriage.

Calendula

HERB	WHY IT'S USED	COMMENTS & CAUTIONS
SAFFRON *Crocus sativus*	To relieve digestive problems such as nausea or poor appetite.	Large doses can cause miscarriage and uterine bleeding. Dietary moderation is strongly advised.
TURMERIC *Curcuma longa*	To relieve arthritis pain and digestive problems.	Large doses can cause miscarriage and uterine bleeding. Dietary moderation is strongly advised.
CITRONELLA, LEMON GRASS *Cymbopogon* spp.	To treat mild stomach upset and poor appetite. Also used as an insect repellent.	Large doses can cause miscarriage and uterine bleeding.
QUEEN ANNE'S LACE *Daucus carota*	Traditional remedy for digestive problems.	May cause uterine bleeding and miscarriage.
MALE FERN, SWEET BRAKE *Dryopteris filix-mas*	To treat intestinal parasites.	May cause vomiting and miscarriage.
ECHINACEA *Echinacea angustifolia, E. pallida, E. purpurea*	To prevent colds and flu.	May trigger autoimmune disorders.
HORSETAIL *Equisetum arvense*	To treat arthritis and urinary tract infections (UTIs). Also strengthens nails and bones.	May interfere with metabolism of B vitamins.
CALIFORNIA POPPY *Eschscholzia californica*	Used to relieve insomnia.	May increase the risk of miscarriage.
FENNEL SEED *Foeniculum vulgare*	To relieve poor appetite, nausea, heartburn, bloating, and gas.	This herb is a uterine stimulant that may cause contractions.
WINTERGREEN *Gaultheria procumbens*	To relieve sore muscles and joint pain, and stimulate digestion.	Large doses can cause uterine bleeding and miscarriage. Dietary moderation is strongly advised.
YELLOW JASMINE *Gelsemium sempervirens*	Traditional remedy for heartburn, headaches, digestive conditions.	This herb is a uterine stimulant that can cause miscarriage.
LICORICE ROOT *Glycyrrhiza glabra*	To treat ulcers, AIDS, colds, flu, coughs, and digestive problems.	Use only under a physician's supervision; can cause high blood pressure and uterine bleeding.
COTTON ROOT *Gossypium herbaceum*	Traditional headache remedy.	May cause uterine bleeding and miscarriage.
LIVERWORT *Hepatica nobilis*	To treat liver disease and gallstones.	This herb can cause severe gastrointestinal irritation and should not be used during pregnancy.
MASTERWORT *Heracleum anatum*	To treat diarrhea, nausea, and poor appetite.	May cause uterine bleeding and uterine contractions.
HIBISCUS *Hibiscus rosa-sinensis*	To relieve constipation and coughs.	May cause miscarriage.
SEA BUCKTHORN *Hippophae rhamnoides*	To treat constipation.	May cause birth defects and miscarriage.
ST. JOHN'S WORT *Hypericum perforatum*	To treat depression, seasonal affective disorder (SAD), anxiety, and insomnia.	May cause uterine bleeding and miscarriage.

HERB	WHY IT'S USED	COMMENTS & CAUTIONS
HYSSOP *Hyssopus officinalis*	To relieve colds, fevers, liver and gallbladder problems.	May cause uterine bleeding and miscarriage.
MATÉ *Ilex paraguariensis*	Used as a stimulant.	Pregnant and nursing women should avoid caffeine (present in maté), which is linked to miscarriage, low birth weight, premature delivery, and birth defects.
ELECAMPANE *Inula helenium*	To relieve coughs due to colds, flu, and bronchitis.	Use only under a physician's supervision; may cause miscarriage.
JALAP *Ipomoea orizabensis*	To relieve constipation.	May cause uterine bleeding.
IRIS, ORRIS ROOT *Iris germanica*	To treat coughs.	May cause uterine bleeding and miscarriage.
COLOMBO *Jateorhiza palmata*	Traditional remedy for digestive disorders.	May cause paralysis and uterine contractions.
BUTTERNUT *Juglans cinerea*	To relieve constipation.	May cause birth defects.
LAVENDER *Lavandula* spp.	To relieve symptoms of anxiety, sore muscles, skin conditions, and treat digestive problems.	Internal use may cause uterine bleeding.
MOTHERWORT *Leonurus cardiaca*	To treat heart problems and hyperthyroidism.	May cause uterine bleeding and miscarriage.
LOVAGE *Levisticum officinale*	Diuretic used to treat kidney and bladder problems.	May cause uterine bleeding and miscarriage.
OSHA *Ligusticum porteri*	To treat cold and flu symptoms and digestive disorders.	May cause uterine bleeding and miscarriage.
FLAXSEED *Linum usitatissimum*	Provides essential fatty acids and fiber; relieves constipation.	Limit dietary intake, especially in the first trimester of pregnancy.
HOREHOUND *Marrubium vulgare*	To treat coughs and digestive problems.	May cause miscarriage.
GERMAN CHAMOMILE *Matricaria recutita*	To relieve nausea, intestinal cramps, anxiety, and insomnia.	Moderate dietary consumption and topical use are safe. Large doses can increase the risk of complications in pregnancy.
LEMON BALM *Melissa officinalis*	To prevent and treat herpes outbreaks; also to relieve digestive problems.	External use is safe; internal use may lead to altered hormone balance and uterine bleeding.
BEE BALM, BERGAMOT, OSWEGO TEA *Monarda didyma*	To treat digestive disorders and symptoms of premenstrual syndrome (PMS).	May cause uterine bleeding and miscarriage.
NUTMEG *Myristica fragrans*	To relieve digestive problems including nausea and gas.	Limit dietary intake; large amounts can lead to miscarriage.
NARD *Nardostachys jatamansi*	Traditionally used to treat digestive problems.	Can cause uterine bleeding and miscarriage.

Lavender

HERB	WHY IT'S USED	COMMENTS & CAUTIONS
WATERCRESS *Nasturtium officinale*	To relieve coughs. It is also used as a mild diuretic.	Dietary moderation is strongly advised; large amounts can cause uterine bleeding and miscarriage.
CATNIP *Nepeta cataria*	To relieve anxiety, insomnia, digestive problems, and menstrual discomfort.	May cause miscarriage.
TOBACCO *Nicotiana tabacum*	Addictive substance used to relieve anxiety.	Smoking during pregnancy causes low birth weight and may cause birth defects and premature delivery.
BASIL *Ocimum basilicum*	Traditional remedy for digestive problems.	May increase risk of birth defects.
MARJORAM *Origanum marjorana*	Traditional remedy for digestive problems.	Limit dietary intake; large amounts can cause uterine bleeding and miscarriage.
WOOD SORREL *Oxalis acetosella*	To treat liver and digestive problems.	May cause uterine bleeding and miscarriage.
PEONY *Paeonia officinalis*	To treat coughs, anal fissures, and arthritis.	May cause uterine bleeding.
GINSENG *Panax spp.*	To reduce stress and boost energy.	May alter hormonal balance; use only under a physician's supervision.
CORN POPPY *Papaver rhoeas*	To relieve pain, anxiety, and insomnia.	May cause miscarriage and infant death.
POPPY *Papaver somniferum*	To relieve pain and severe coughs.	May cause miscarriage and infant death.
GUARANA *Paullinia cupana*	Used as a stimulant and to treat diarrhea and headaches.	Contains caffeine, which has been linked to miscarriage, low birth weight, premature delivery, and birth defects.
PARSLEY *Petroselinum crispum*	To relieve digestive problems; also used as a diuretic for urinary and kidney disorders.	May cause uterine bleeding, uterine contractions, and miscarriage. Dietary moderation is strongly advised.
BITTERWOOD, QUASSIA *Picrasma excelsa*	To relieve digestive problems.	May increase the risk of miscarriage.
JABORANDI *Pilocarpus microphyllus*	Traditional remedy for glaucoma.	This herb is toxic; it may cause birth defects and miscarriage.
KAVA KAVA *Piper methysticum*	To treat anxiety and insomnia.	This herb is toxic; it may cause birth defects and miscarriage.
BISTORT, SNAKEWEED *Polygonum bistorta*	To treat diarrhea.	May cause miscarriage.
APRICOT *Prunus armeniaca*	Used as a source of dietary fiber and vitamin C.	Moderate dietary consumption is safe; the pits contain cyanide and should be avoided.
PEACH *Prunus persica*	Used as a source of dietary fiber and vitamin C.	Moderate dietary consumption is safe; the pits contain cyanide and should be avoided.
CHERRY *Prunus serotina*	Used as a source of dietary fiber and vitamin C.	Moderate dietary consumption is safe; the pits and bark contain cyanide and should be avoided.

Herb	Why it's used	Comments & cautions
Malay Tea *Psoralea corylifolia*	Traditionally used to treat psoriasis.	May increase the risk of miscarriage.
Pasque Flower *Pulsatilla pratensis*	Traditional remedy for headache and insomnia.	May cause miscarriage
Pomegranate *Punica granatum*	Used as a source of dietary fiber and vitamin C.	May cause uterine bleeding.
Buckthorn Fruit *Rhamnus catharticus*	To relieve constipation.	May cause miscarriage.
Buckthorn Bark *Rhamnus frangula*	To relieve constipation.	May trigger contractions.
Cascara Sagrada *Rhamnus purshiana*	To relieve constipation.	May trigger contractions.
Rhubarb *Rheum palmatum*	To relieve constipation.	May cause miscarriage.
Poison Ivy *Rhus toxicodendron*	Traditional remedy for allergies and inflammation.	May cause miscarriage.
Rosemary Leaf *Rosmarinus officinalis*	To relieve digestive problems, joint pain, and sore muscles.	Moderate dietary consumption is safe.
Sage *Salvia officinalis*	To relieve digestive problems, sore throat, and mouth irritation.	Moderate dietary consumption is safe; large doses could cause uterine contractions.
Sandalwood *Santalum album*	To treat kidney and bladder conditions.	May cause miscarriage.
Milk Thistle *Silybum marianum*	To protect the liver and treat liver disease.	May cause uterine bleeding.
Sarsaparilla *Smilax* spp.	To relieve psoriasis, irritable bowel syndrome eczema, and arthritis.	May cause miscarriage.
Strophanthus *Strophanthus hispidus*	Traditional remedy for heart conditions.	May cause dangerous heart rhythm problems and uterine contractions.
Feverfew *Tanacetum parthenium*	To help prevent and treat migraine headaches.	May cause miscarriage.
Dandelion *Taraxacum officinale*	To relieve digestive problems and swelling; provide liver support.	Its safety has not yet been determined.
Cocoa *Theobroma cacao*	Used as a stimulant in beverages and chocolate.	Contains caffeine, which has been linked to miscarriage, low birth weight, premature delivery, and birth defects.
Thyme *Thymus vulgaris*	To relieve coughing and digestive problems.	Dietary moderation is strongly advised; large amounts may cause uterine bleeding and miscarriage.

Poppy

HERB	WHY IT'S USED	COMMENTS & CAUTIONS
FENUGREEK SEED *Trigonella foenum-graecum*	To control blood sugar and cholesterol levels and treat digestive problems.	May cause uterine bleeding and miscarriage.
BIRTHROOT, BETH ROOT *Trillium erectum*	To treat menstrual problems, varicose veins, and hemorrhoids.	May cause uterine bleeding and miscarriage.
STINGING NETTLE LEAF *Urtica dioica*	To relieve urinary tract inflammation, kidney stones, and seasonal pollen allergies.	May cause uterine bleeding, uterine contractions, and miscarriage.
VERVAIN *Verbena officinalis*	To relieve mild pain, particularly from headaches.	May cause miscarriage.
SPEEDWELL *Veronica officinalis*	To relieve coughs, digestive conditions, kidney and liver problems, and arthritis.	May cause miscarriage and birth defects.
CHASTEBERRY *Vitex agnus-castus*	To relieve breast tenderness, irregular menstruation, and menopausal symptoms.	Can cause hormonal changes and uterine bleeding.
ASHWAGANDHA *Withania somnifera*	To improve overall health, energy, and immunity.	May cause miscarriage.
PRICKLY ASH *Zanthoxylum americanum*	To reduce fever and inflammation.	May cause uterine bleeding and miscarriage. Do not use while breast-feeding as it may irritate an infant's digestion.
GINGER *Zingiber officinale*	To treat nausea, motion sickness, arthritis, and migraine.	Dietary moderation is strongly advised; large amounts may cause uterine bleeding and miscarriage. Avoid completely if the risk of miscarriage is high.
JUJUBE *Ziziphus spinosa*	To reduce blood pressure.	May cause uterine bleeding.

Prickly Ash

SAFE HERBS FOR OLDER ADULTS

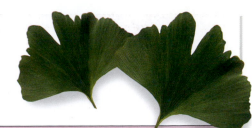

HERB	WHY IT'S USED	COMMENTS & CAUTIONS
YARROW *Achillea millefolium*	To prevent colds and flu and to stop bleeding from nosebleeds and cuts.	May cause sun sensitivity and allergic reactions.
HORSE CHESTNUT *Aesculus hippocastanum*	To relieve varicose veins, leg swelling from poor circulation, hemorrhoids, and bruising.	Discuss with your physician if you have liver or kidney disease.
COUCH GRASS *Agropyron repens*	To treat urinary tract problems including cystitis and enlarged prostate.	Do not diagnose or treat enlarged prostate yourself. Consult a physician.
ONION *Allium cepa*	To prevent atherosclerosis by lowering cholesterol and thinning blood.	Do not eat large amounts of onions in combination with blood-thinning drugs such as warfarin (*p. 195*) without consulting your physician.
GARLIC *Allium sativum*	To relieve cardiovascular disease, infection, and inflammation.	Do not combine with blood-thinning drugs such as warfarin (*p. 195*) without consulting your physician.
MARSHMALLOW LEAF & ROOT *Althaea officinalis*	To treat colds and coughs.	Because the leaves and root are high in sugar, people who have diabetes should use them with caution.
ALOE VERA JUICE & GEL *Aloe vera*	Juice combats infection; gel relieves skin irritations.	Do not confuse juice with aloe vera latex, a dangerous laxative.
BROMELAIN *Ananas comosus*	To treat digestive problems and pain from shingles and arthritis.	Do not use if you have gastritis, ulcers, or esophagitis, or take blood-thinning drugs (*e.g., warfarin, p. 195*). If you have high blood pressure or heart disease, consult your physician first before taking bromelain.
DILL SEED *Anethum graveolens*	To relieve digestive problems.	May cause heartburn or acid reflux in some people.
ANGELICA ROOT *Angelica archangelica*	To relieve digestive problems and menopausal symptoms.	Prolonged used may cause sun sensitivity.
DONG QUAI *Angelica sinensis*	To help relieve menopausal symptoms, especially hot flashes.	If you are using hormone replacement therapy, discuss dong quai with your physician.
BURDOCK ROOT *Arctium lappa, A. minus*	To treat urinary tract infections, skin infections, psoriasis, rheumatoid arthritis.	This herb may act as a diuretic and cause dehydration.
UVA URSI *Arctostaphylos uva-ursi*	To treat urinary tract and bladder infections.	Use for up to five days; do not combine with vitamin C or cranberry juice.
HORSERADISH *Armoracia rusticana*	To relieve upper respiratory infections, sinus congestion, and allergies.	Do not use if you have hypothyroidism, ulcers, or kidney disease. Do not use for more than seven days, and do not consume in high doses.

Garlic

HERB	WHY IT'S USED	COMMENTS & CAUTIONS
ARNICA *Arnica montana*	To relieve bruises, swelling, and soreness.	For homeopathic and external use only; avoid broken skin and mucous membranes.
MUGWORT *Artemisia vulgaris*	To treat minor digestive problems including loss of appetite, cramps, and diarrhea.	Use this herb cautiously and in small doses.
ASPARAGUS ROOT *Asparagus officinalis*	To treat urinary tract infections and prevent kidney stones.	Do not use if you have kidney or heart disease.
SHATAVARI *Asparagus racemosus*	To relieve menopausal symptoms and inflammation.	If you are using hormone replacement therapy, discuss shatavari with your physician.
ASTRAGALUS *Astragalus membranaceus*	To prevent and treat infection.	Do not combine with immunosuppressant drugs used to treat cancer or autoimmune illnesses such as lupus.
OAT BRAN *Avena sativa*	To prevent and treat constipation; regular consumption can also reduce cholesterol.	May reduce your absorption of supplements and drugs; take two hours before or after them.
OAT STRAW *Avena sativa*	To treat skin conditions such as eczema, seborrhea, poison ivy, chicken pox, and sunburn.	Add to bath water to relieve itching and irritation; do not use if you are allergic to grains.
WILD OATS *Avena sativa*	To relieve anxiety and insomnia and to increase libido.	Do not use if you are allergic to grains.
BUCHU *Barosma betulina,* *B. crenulata, B. serratifolia*	To treat kidney and bladder problems.	This herb may cause dehydration; take with plenty of water.
OREGON GRAPE *Berberis acquifolium,* *Mahonia acquifolium*	To relieve the itching and burning of psoriasis.	Do not combine oregon grape with other berberine-containing herbs such as goldenseal (*Hydrastis canadensis, p. 39*).
BARBERRY *Berberis vulgaris*	To treat sore throat, mouth irritation, minor digestive problems including nausea, cramps, constipation.	Use cautiously in small doses. Do not use if you have heart or liver disease or jaundice.
BEET LEAF *Beta vulgaris rubra*	To relieve digestive problems such as poor appetite, bloating, and gas.	Do not use if you have gallstones, gallbladder disease, or biliary duct disease.
BORAGE OIL *Borago officinalis*	To treat diabetic neuropathy, skin problems such as eczema, and rheumatoid arthritis.	Select only pyrrolizidine alkaloid (PA) free products. Do not use if you have liver disease.
BOSWELLIA *Boswellia serrata*	To treat joint problems such as arthritis, tendinitis, and bursitis.	If you are already taking medication for joint problems, discuss boswellia with your physician.
BUPLEURUM *Bupleurum* spp.	To treat liver disease, including hepatitis.	Stop using this herb if it causes a stomach upset or diarrhea.
CALENDULA *Calendula officinalis*	To treat skin problems such as cuts, rashes, and slow-healing wounds.	For external use only; avoid deep wounds and mucous membranes. Discontinue use if any irritation occurs.

HERB	WHY IT'S USED	COMMENTS & CAUTIONS
GREEN TEA *Camellia sinensis*	To protect against cancer and heart disease.	To avoid caffeine, look for decaffeinated green tea leaves or capsules.
SHEPHERD'S PURSE *Capsella bursa-pastoris*	To soothe skin wounds and reduce blood pressure.	Do not use internally without a physician's supervision.
CAPSAICIN CREAM *Capsicum annuum*	To treat pain from shingles, trigeminal neuralgia, diabetic neuropathy, arthritis, and psoriasis.	Use with caution; avoid eyes, broken skin, and mucous membranes. Discontinue if irritation occurs.
CAYENNE PEPPER *Capsicum annuum, C. frutescens*	To treat digestive problems and prevent stomach irritation from nonsteroidal anti-inflammatory drugs.	Do not use if you have ulcers, gastritis, or esophagitis; discontinue use if a digestive upset occurs.
PAPAYA *Carica papaya*	To treat minor digestive problems such as nausea and diarrhea.	Do not use if you have gastritis, acid reflux, or ulcers, or are taking blood-thinning drugs such as warfarin *(p. 195)*.
CARAWAY *Carum carvi*	To treat digestive problems including loss of appetite, heartburn, nausea, and gas.	For occasional use only; overuse can cause kidney and liver damage.
GOTU KOLA *Centella asiatica*	To treat hemorrhoids, varicose veins, and poor leg circulation.	Benefits may take four to six weeks to become apparent.
CAROB *Ceratonia siliqua*	To treat diarrhea, especially traveler's diarrhea.	Take with plenty of liquid. May reduce absorption of other supplements; take two hours before or after them.
ICELAND MOSS *Cetraria islandica*	To treat poor appetite, upset stomach, and upper respiratory tract infections with dry cough.	Buy only from a reputable manufacturer; poor quality products may contain toxic levels of lead.
CHAMOMILE *Chamaemelum nobile* (Roman), *Matricaria recutita* (German)	To relieve digestive problems, stress, and insomnia.	Do not use if you take blood-thinning drugs such as warfarin *(p. 195)*, or if you are allergic to ragweed or plants in the daisy family, such as mugwort *(p. 22)*.
CHICORY *Cichorium intybus*	To relieve gallbladder disease, protect the liver, and treat minor digestive problems.	Long-term use may cause sun sensitivity.
BLACK COHOSH ROOT *Cimicifuga racemosa rhizoma*	To treat menopausal symptoms including hot flashes, headaches, irritability, vaginal dryness, and insomnia.	Do not take for more than six months continuously. If you are using hormone replacement therapy, discuss black cohosh root with your physician.
CHINESE CINNAMON BARK *Cinnamomum aromaticum*	To treat digestive problems including poor appetite, cramps, gas, and diarrhea.	May cause a digestive upset in sensitive individuals or in those with a history of ulcers or gastritis.
CAMPHOR *Cinnamomum camphora*	To relieve sore muscles, chest congestion, and coughing.	For external use only. Use commercial products, which contain less than 11 percent camphor.
CINNAMON *Cinnamomum verum*	To treat digestive problems including poor appetite, nausea, cramps, and gas.	May cause a digestive upset in sensitive individuals or those with a history of ulcers or gastritis.

Cayenne pepper

HERB	WHY IT'S USED	COMMENTS & CAUTIONS
BLESSED THISTLE *Cnicus benedictus*	To treat digestive problems such as loss of appetite or bloating.	Do not use if you are allergic to plants in the daisy family such as cornflower, mugwort, or milk thistle.
COLEUS *Coleus forskohlii*	To treat asthma, eczema, psoriasis, high blood pressure, and angina.	Use this herb only under a physician's supervision.
MYRRH *Commiphora molmol*	To prevent and treat sore throat, minor mouth irritation, and gum disease.	Use as a mouthwash; start with a small dose and gradually increase it.
GUGGUL *Commiphora mukul*	To reduce cholesterol and prevent atherosclerosis.	Benefits may take up to eight weeks to become apparent.
CORIANDER *Coriandrum sativum*	To treat digestive problems including poor appetite, gas, cramps, and diarrhea.	Do not use this herb if you have ulcers, gastritis, or frequent heartburn.
TURKEY TAIL *Coriolus versicolor,* *Trametes versicolor*	To stimulate the immune system during cancer treatment.	Discuss turkey tail with your physician before you try it.
HAWTHORN *Crataegus oxyacantha*	To maintain cardiovascular health, relieve mild angina symptoms, and lower high blood pressure.	Discuss this herb with your physician before taking it, even if you don't take any medication.
TURMERIC ROOT *Curcuma longa*	To treat digestive problems including poor appetite, gas, and rheumatoid arthritis.	Do not use if you have ulcers, gallstones, gallbladder disease, or take a blood-thinning drug such as warfarin (*p. 195*).
PUMPKIN SEED *Curcurbita pepo*	To relieve irritable bladder and symptoms of enlarged prostate.	Do not diagnose or treat enlarged prostate without consulting a physician.
ARTICHOKE LEAF *Cynara scolymus*	To treat digestive problems including loss of appetite, nausea, and gas.	Do not use if you have gallstones, gallbladder disease, or biliary duct disease.
ECHINACEA *Echinacea angustifolia,* *E. purpurea*	To prevent colds and infections.	Do not use if you have an autoimmune disease or if you are allergic to plants in the daisy family such as mugwort (*p. 22*).
CARDAMOM *Elettaria cardamomum*	To treat digestive problems and respiratory infections.	Do not use if you have gallstones, gallbladder disease, or biliary duct disease.
ELEUTHERO *Eleutherococcus senticosus*	To combat the effects of stress and prevent infection.	Do not use if you have high blood pressure or heart problems.
HORSETAIL *Equisetum arvense*	To strengthen nails and bones, and to treat arthritis	This herb may cause dehydration; take with plenty of water. Use only thiaminase-free products.
YERBA SANTA *Eriodictyon californicum*	To treat respiratory infections such as colds and flu.	This pleasant-tasting herb is used as a flavoring agent.
EUCALYPTUS *Eucalyptus globulus*	To relieve chest congestion, sore muscles, and joint pain.	Never use internally; even small amounts are toxic.
MEADOWSWEET *Filipendula ulmaria*	To relieve inflammation, fever, and pain.	Do not use if you are allergic to salicylates or aspirin, or if you take a blood-thinning drug such as warfarin (*p. 195*).

Herb	Why it's used	Comments & cautions
Fennel Seed & Oil *Foeniculum vulgare*	To treat digestive problems such as heartburn, nausea, and gas.	Do not use if you have a history of reproductive cancer.
Reishi *Ganoderma lucidum*	To combat the effects of stress and prevent infection.	Effects may take up to two weeks to become apparent.
Gentian Root *Gentiana lutea*	To treat digestive problems such as loss of appetite or bloating.	Do not use if you have gallstones, gallbladder disease, biliary duct disease, ulcers, or heartburn.
Ginkgo *Ginkgo biloba*	To improve circulation, memory and mental function; treats dizziness and tinnitus.	Do not combine with blood-thinning drugs such as warfarin *(p. 195)*.
Soy Isoflavones *Glycine max*	To relieve menopausal symptoms and reduce cholesterol in women.	If you have thyroid disease or a history of breast or reproductive cancer, consult your physician about soy isoflavones.
Soy Lecithin *Glycine max*	To reduce cholesterol and treat liver disease.	The evidence for the benefits of soy lecithin is not strong.
Licorice Root *Glycyrrhiza glabra*	To treat ulcers, respiratory infections, and digestive upsets.	For ulcers, use only in DGL form. Avoid if you have high blood pressure, kidney disease, or take digoxin.
Maitake *Grifola frondosa*	To combat the effects of stress and prevent infection.	Maitake mushrooms are edible and delicious.
Gumweed *Grindelia* spp.	To relieve coughs related to colds and bronchitis.	Those with ragweed allergies may also be allergic to gumweed.
Gymnema *Gymnema sylvestre*	Used in Asian medicine to treat mild cases of Type 2 diabetes.	If you have diabetes and want to try this herb, discuss it with your physician.
Witch Hazel *Hamamelis virginiana*	To relieve skin abrasions, hemorrhoids, and sore throats.	For external use only; internal use can result in serious digestive upset.
Devil's Claw *Harpagophytum procumbens*	To relieve arthritis, gout, and back pain.	Do not use if you have ulcers or gastritis.
Ivy Leaf *Hedera helix*	To relieve coughs from colds, flu, and bronchitis.	Handling ivy leaves may cause skin rashes.
Hops *Humulus lupulus*	To treat anxiety, insomnia, and digestive problems.	Do not combine with alcohol or other sedative supplements, herbs, or medications.
Goldenseal *Hydrastis canadensis*	To treat sore throat, bladder and fungal infections.	Do not use for more than two weeks unless under your physician's supervision.
St. John's Wort *Hypericum perforatum*	To treat mild to moderate depression, seasonal affective disorder (SAD), anxiety, and insomnia.	Although this herb is generally safe, it must be used with care *(see p. 39, and also drug–herb interactions, e.g., p.127)*.
Walnut Leaf *Juglans regia*	To relieve mild skin abrasions, burns, and eczema.	Begin with small doses and increase gradually as needed.
Larch *Larix decidua*	To boost immunity, and fight and prevent infection.	If you have liver or kidney disease, consult a physician.

Eucalyptus

HERB	WHY IT'S USED	COMMENTS & CAUTIONS
LAVENDER *Lavandula angustifolia*	To relieve anxiety, sore muscles, and skin conditions.	For external use only; internal use can cause severe stomach upset.
MOTHERWORT *Leonurus artemisia,* *L. cardiaca*	To treat heart problems, especially irregular or rapid heartbeat.	Consult your physician for diagnosis and treatment. Do not use if you have a history of breast cancer.
OSHA *Ligusticum porteri*	To treat coughs, sore throat, and minor digestive problems.	Buy only from a reliable source; this herb resembles hemlock, a highly toxic plant.
LIGUSTRUM *Ligustrum lucidum*	To improve immunity and prevent and treat infections.	Do not confuse with other members of the *Ligustrum* family.
FLAXSEED *Linum usitatissimum*	To treat constipation and provide fiber.	Can block your absorption of supplements and medications; take two hours before or after them.
HOREHOUND *Marrubium vulgare*	To relieve coughs and minor digestive problems.	Do not use if you have ulcers or gastritis.
ALFALFA *Medicago sativa*	To relieve menopausal symptoms and reduce cholesterol.	Do not use if you have systemic lupus erythematosus (SLE). Many cases of food poisoning have been traced to fresh alfalfa sprouts; wash them thoroughly.
TEA TREE OIL *Melaleuca alternifolia*	To treat skin abrasions, insect stings, and fungal infections.	For external use only.
LEMON BALM *Melissa officinalis*	To prevent and treat herpes outbreaks, and relieve digestive problems and insomnia.	Do not use lemon balm if you have glaucoma.
PEPPERMINT LEAF *Mentha piperita*	To treat digestive problems including loss of appetite, nausea, cramps, and gas.	Do not use if you have frequent heartburn, liver disease, or biliary duct disease.
BITTER MELON *Momordica charantia*	Used in Asian medicine to treat mild cases of Type 2 diabetes.	If you have diabetes, discuss bitter melon with your physician before you try it.
WATERCRESS *Nasturtium officinale*	Relieves coughs related to colds and flu.	Do not use if you have an ulcer.
CATNIP *Nepeta cataria*	To relieve anxiety and insomnia.	Do not combine with alcohol or other sedative herbs, supplements, or medications.
EVENING PRIMROSE OIL *Oenothera biennis*	To treat diabetic neuropathy and rheumatoid arthritis.	Benefits may take several weeks or longer to become apparent.
OREGANO OIL *Origanum vulgare*	To treat fungal infections including athlete's foot.	Do not use this oil internally unless prescribed by your physician.
GINSENG *Panax ginseng,* *P. quinquefolium*	To prevent infection and improve male sexual function; may help people with diabetes to control their blood sugar.	Do not use for more than two consecutive weeks. Do not combine with caffeine-containing substances such as coffee, tea, maté, or guarana. If you have high blood pressure or diabetes, consult your physician first.
PASSIONFLOWER *Passiflora incarnata*	To relieve anxiety and insomnia.	Do not use in combination with alcohol or other sedative herbs, supplements, medications, or with antidepressant medications.

HERB	WHY IT'S USED	COMMENTS & CAUTIONS
PARSLEY *Petroselinum crispum*	To treat urinary tract infections and kidney stones.	If you have kidney disease or heart disease do not use without consulting your physician first.
KAVA KAVA *Piper methysticum*	To treat anxiety and insomnia.	Do not combine with antihistamines, cold remedies, medications, alcohol, or other sedative herbs.
MASTICA *Pistacia lentiscus*	To treat ulcers.	Do not diagnose an ulcer on your own; consult your physician.
PLANTAIN *Plantago lanceolata, P. major*	To treat sore throat, coughs, and ulcers.	Plantain leaves should never be eaten raw.
PSYLLIUM SEED *Plantago afra, P. ovata*	To treat constipation and irritable bowel syndrome; may reduce cholesterol.	Take with plenty of fluids. May block your absorption of other herbs and supplements; take two hours before or after.
FO-TI *Polygonum multiflorum*	To lower cholesterol, relieve fatigue and constipation, and boost immunity.	Do not take more than 15 grams daily of fo-ti. Large amounts can cause numbness in the arms and legs.
POPLAR BUD *Populus spp.*	To relieve skin conditions including abrasions, burns, and hemorrhoids.	Do not use if you are sensitive to salicylates or are allergic to aspirin.
WILD CHERRY *Prunus serotina*	To relieve coughing related to upper respiratory infections.	Use prepared products only; do not exceed the dosages recommended on the package.
BLACKTHORN *Prunus spinosa*	To relieve mouth irritation, sore throat, and respiratory ailments.	If this herb upsets your digestion, reduce the dose or discontinue use.
MUIRA PUAMA *Ptychopetalum olacoides, P. uncinatum*	To support male sexual function.	Purchase only from a reliable source; this plant is frequently misidentified.
KUDZU *Pueraria lobata*	To treat colds and mild angina.	Before using kudzu for angina, consult your physician.
PYGEUM *Pygeum africanum*	To treat urinary problems, including enlarged prostate.	Do not diagnose or treat enlarged prostate yourself. Consult your physician.
OAK BARK *Quercus alba, Q. petraea, Q. robur*	To relieve diarrhea, mouth and throat irritation, and skin conditions including mild eczema.	May interfere with the absorption of certain medications; if you take any medication, consult your physician.
RADISH *Raphanus sativus*	To improve gallbladder function and relieve coughs.	Stop using this herb if it upsets your digestion.
BUCKTHORN BARK *Rhamnus catharticus, R. frangula*	To relieve constipation.	Do not use if you take cardiac glycoside medication such as digoxin (p. 147).
CASCARA SAGRADA *Rhamnus purshiana*	To treat constipation.	Do not use if you have Crohn's disease, bowel disease, or if appendicitis is suspected.
BLACKCURRANT OIL *Ribes nigrum*	To treat diabetic neuropathy, skin problems including eczema, and rheumatoid arthritis.	Benefits may take several weeks or longer.

Watercress

HERB	WHY IT'S USED	COMMENTS & CAUTIONS
ROSE HIPS *Rosa canina, R. centifolia, R. rugosa*	To treat colds and flu, and constipation. Also used as a source of vitamin C.	Large doses of vitamin C can cause diarrhea.
ROSEMARY LEAF *Rosmarinus officinalis*	To treat digestive problems, joint pain, and sore muscles.	The oil is for external use only.
RASPBERRY LEAF *Rubus idaeus*	To treat diarrhea, sore throat, and mouth irritation.	In very large amounts, may cause nausea or mild diarrhea.
BLACKBERRY LEAF *Rubus fruticosus, R. villosus*	To treat diarrhea, sore throat, mouth irritation, skin abrasions, and hemorrhoids.	In large amounts, may cause mild digestive upset.
YELLOW DOCK *Rumex crispus*	To relieve constipation and improve digestion.	Do not use if you have a history of kidney stones. May cause mild diarrhea.
BUTCHER'S BROOM *Ruscus aculeatus*	To support the circulatory system and relieve hemorrhoids and varicose veins.	This herb is generally well tolerated, but may cause mild nausea in sensitive individuals.
WILLOW BARK *Salix spp.*	To relieve headaches, fever, and arthritis pain.	Do not use if you are allergic to salicylates or aspirin, or if you take blood-thinning drugs such as warfarin (*p. 195*).
SAGE *Salvia officinalis*	To treat digestive problems, colds, sore throat, cold sores, and gum disease.	Do not use if you have a fever.
ELDERBERRY *Sambucus nigra*	To prevent and relieve colds and flu.	Dried elder tree bark is a very powerful laxative that should not be used.
ELDERBERRY FLOWER *Sambucus nigra*	To improve immunity and treat colds, coughs, flu, and fever.	Dried elder tree bark is a very powerful laxative that should not be used.
SCHISANDRA *Schisandra chinensis*	To treat liver problems, especially hepatitis. Also used for immune support.	May cause digestive upset, decreased appetite, or skin rash in sensitive individuals.
SENNA *Senna alexandrina*	To relieve constipation.	This is a powerful laxative that should be used only under a physician's supervision and for no more than seven days in a row.
SAW PALMETTO *Serenoa repens*	To treat enlarged prostate.	Do not diagnose or treat enlarged prostate yourself. Consult your physician.
MILK THISTLE *Silybum marianum*	To treat liver problems including hepatitis, jaundice, cirrhosis; may also relieve psoriasis and gallstones.	Numerous scientific studies demonstrate this herb's effectiveness in treating liver disease.
SARSAPARILLA *Smilax sarsaparilla*	To treat psoriasis, eczema, arthritis, and irritable bowel syndrome.	Do not use this herb if you have gastritis, ulcers, or kidney disease. Do not combine with digoxin (*p. 147*) or pink bismuth (*p. 131*).
GOLDENROD *Solidago spp.*	Used in conjunction with drugs to treat bladder infections and kidney stones.	This herb acts as a diuretic and may cause dehydration.

HERB	WHY IT'S USED	COMMENTS & CAUTIONS
SPILANTHES *Spilanthes oleracea*	To relieve digestive problems.	Usually used in combination with other herbs.
STEVIA *Stevia rebaudiana*	Used as a calorie-free sweetener. May reduce blood pressure and blood glucose.	This herb is a safe sugar substitute, but discuss it with your physician before using it medicinally.
CLOVE *Syzygium aromaticum*	To treat digestive problems, bad breath, gum disease, and mouth pain.	See a dentist regularly if you experience symptoms of gum disease.
CLOVE OIL *Syzygium aromaticum*	To relieve dental pain. Also used as an antiseptic.	See a dentist as soon as possible for toothache.
LAPACHO *Tabebuia avellanedae,* *T. impetiginosa*	To treat mild yeast and bladder infections, colds and flu, and diarrhea.	Buy lapacho only from a reputable manufacturer.
FEVERFEW *Tanacetum parthenium*	To prevent and relieve migraine headaches.	If you take medication for frequent migraines, discuss feverfew with your physician before you try it.
DANDELION *Taraxacum officinale*	To relieve digestive problems and swelling and to provide liver support.	Do not use if you have ulcers, gastritis, gallstones, gallbladder disease, or biliary duct disease.
THYME *Thymus vulgaris*	To relieve coughing and minor digestive problems including heartburn.	Do not use the oil internally, and avoid dental products containing thyme oil.
LINDEN FLOWER *Tilia cordata*	To treat colds, flu, and coughs.	Do not use if you have heart disease.
FENUGREEK SEED *Trigonella foenum-graecum*	May help people who suffer from diabetes reduce blood sugar and cholesterol levels.	If you have diabetes, discuss this herb with your physician.
SLIPPERY ELM *Ulmus fulva*	To soothe sore throat and coughs.	May interfere with absorption of other supplements or drugs; take it two hours before or after them.
CAT'S CLAW *Uncaria tomentosa*	To reduce inflammation, combat viral illnesses, and treat arthritis.	If you have an autoimmune illness such as lupus, discuss cat's claw with your physician.
STINGING NETTLE LEAF *Urtica dioica*	To relieve urinary tract inflammation, kidney stones, and seasonal allergies.	This herb may cause dehydration; take with plenty of water.
STINGING NETTLE ROOT *Urtica dioica*	To treat urinary problems including enlarged prostate.	Do not diagnose or treat enlarged prostate yourself. Consult your physician.
USNEA *Usnea barbata, U. florida,* *U. hirta, U. plicata*	To treat coughs, sore throat, minor mouth and throat irritation.	This herb is sometimes used under a physician's supervision to treat bacterial or yeast infections.
CRANBERRY *Vaccinium macrocarpon*	To prevent and treat urinary tract infections.	Use cranberry capsules or pure, unsweetened cranberry juice.

Dandelion

HERB	WHY IT'S USED	COMMENTS & CAUTIONS
BILBERRY *Vaccinium myrtillus*	To improve night vision and prevent age-related macular degeneration.	The effect of bilberry on night vision is almost immediate but lasts only for about two hours.
BLUEBERRY *Vaccinium* spp.	To treat bladder infections, colds, sore throat, and mild diarrhea.	For diarrhea, used dried berries. If diarrhea continues for more than 24 hours, contact your physician.
VALERIAN *Valeriana officinalis*	To relieve insomnia.	Do not use in combination with alcohol or other sedative herbs, supplements, drugs, or sleep aids.
MULLEIN *Vebascum thapsus*	To relieve coughs, sore throat, and ear infections.	Use mullein oil for an ear infection only if the eardrum is not punctured.
VERVAIN *Verbena officinalis, V. hastata*	To relieve mild pain, headaches, and coughs.	Vervain has a very mild anti-inflammatory effect.
CHASTEBERRY *Vitex agnus-castus*	To treat menopausal symptoms, especially hot flashes.	If using hormone replacement therapy, discuss chasteberry with your physician.
GRAPESEED EXTRACT *Vitis vinifera*	To treat a variety of circulatory problems; may also help some diabetic conditions *(see p. 60)*.	If you take a blood-thinning drug such as warfarin *(p. 195)*, discuss grape seed extract with your physician before you try it.
ASHWAGANDHA *Withania somniferum*	Used in Asian medicine to boost energy and immunity.	Do not use in combination with alcohol or sedative herbs, supplements, or medications.
YUCCA *Yucca* spp.	To relieve pain and inflammation from arthritis.	Can block vitamin absorption; do not use for more than three months. High doses may cause diarrhea.
CORN SILK *Zea mays*	Used as a diuretic to treat bladder problems.	Do not use in combination with diuretic drugs, blood-thinning drugs such as warfarin *(p. 195)*, or with drugs to treat high blood pressure or diabetes.
GINGER ROOT *Zingiber officinale*	To relieve nausea, motion sickness, rheumatoid arthritis, and migraines.	Consult your physician for the proper dose for migraines.

Chasteberry

POTENTIALLY DANGEROUS HERBS FOR OLDER ADULTS

HERB	WHY IT'S USED	COMMENTS & CAUTIONS
AGRIMONY *Agrimonia eupatoria*	To treat sore throat, mouth irritation, diarrhea, mild skin irritation.	Can cause digestive problems. Do not use in a poultice, as skin irritation can occur.
CELANDINE *Chelidonium majus*	To treat digestive problems, especially liver and gallbladder disease.	Do not use if you have liver disease or gallstones, or are taking glaucoma medication.
BITTER ORANGE PEEL *Citrus aurantium*	To treat digestive problems including indigestion, loss of appetite, and nausea.	May make your skin sensitive to light.
KOLA NUT *Cola acuminata or C. nitida*	Used as a stimulant.	Do not take use if you have ulcers or should avoid caffeine.
CALIFORNIA POPPY *Eschscholzia calfornica*	To relieve anxiety.	Dangerous when used in combination with alcohol and other sedatives.
FENNEL OIL *Foeniculum vulgare*	To treat minor digestive problems including heartburn, loss of appetite, and nausea.	Do not use if you have a history of reproductive cancer or have acid reflux.
MATÉ *Ilex paraguariensis*	Caffeine-containing stimulant used to relieve headaches caused by fatigue.	Do not use this herb if you should avoid caffeine because you have high blood pressure, diabetes, heart disease, or other condition.
BUGLEWEED *Lycopus virginicus*	To treat hyperthyroidism (overproduction of thyroid hormones).	Use only under your physician's supervision.
MINT OIL *Mentha arvensis*	To treat minor digestive problems such as nausea or gas.	Do not use if you have acid reflux, gallbladder disease, gallstones, or liver disease.
GUARANA *Paullinia cupana*	Caffeine-containing stimulant used to treat headaches and diarrhea.	Do not use if you should avoid caffeine because of high blood pressure, diabetes, heart disease, or other condition.
BOLDO *Peumus boldus*	To treat minor digestive problems such as loss of appetite, cramps, and nausea.	Do not use if you have gallstones, gallbladder disease, biliary duct disease, kidney disease, or elevated liver enzymes.
BLOODROOT *Sanguinaria canadensis*	To prevent plaque and gum disease.	Never swallow products containing bloodroot. Do not use in any form if your health is poor.
RED CLOVER *Trifolium pratense*	To treat menopausal symptoms, particularly hot flashes, and to lower cholesterol.	Do not use if you are taking hormone replacement therapy (HRT) or blood-thinning drugs such as warfarin (*p. 195*) or daily aspirin.

Red clover

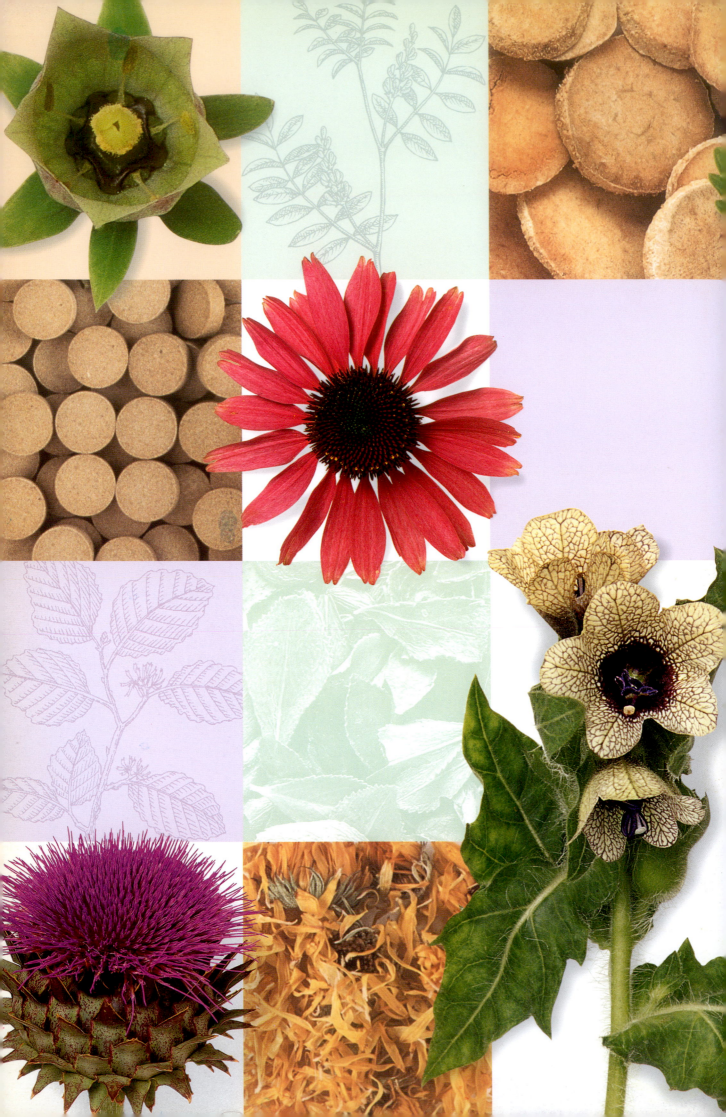

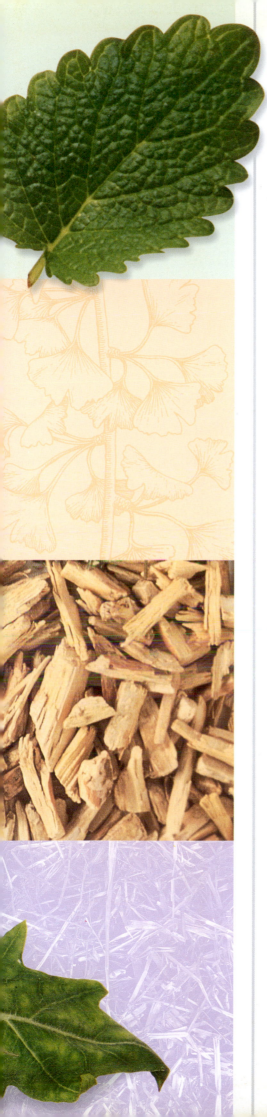

CHAPTER 7

BUYER BEWARE

M OST COMMON HERBS ARE quite safe and effective when they are used properly. But some herbs are so powerful they should be used only under the supervision of your physician. This chapter examines these herbs and also those that are highly toxic, even in small doses. These dangerous herbs are sometimes used as garden ornamentals or gathered in the wild, and should never be ingested.

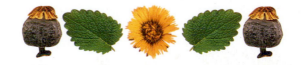

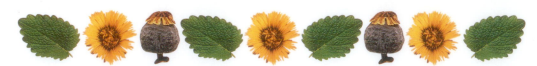

HERBAL SAFETY BASICS

SOME HERBS are so powerful and fast-acting, they should only be used under the supervision of your physician. Others are so dangerous they should never be used at all. When herbal specialists aren't completely certain that an herb is safe, they prefer to err on the side of caution and label it as unsafe.

Some toxic herbs are common backyard plants, such as yew *(Taxus baccata, p. 240)*, clematis *(Clematis recta, p. 235)*, and buttercup *(Ranunculus acris, p. 238)*. If young children play in your backyard, consider removing these plants so the children can't accidentally eat or brush up against them.

YEW
The slow-growing evergreen yew tree, which thrives in northern temperate zones, is so toxic that it is rarely used in herbal medicine.

❖ DANGEROUS HERBS ❖

Dangerous herbs are often used out of ignorance. Outdated reference works may recommend herbs that are now known to be harmful or ineffective. For instance, sassafras *(Sassafras albidum, p. 239)*, a pleasant-

---

WORDS OF CAUTION

OTHER potential sources of dangerous herbs include imported and wild-crafted products (herbs gathered in the wild). Poor quality control or lack of knowledge by the gatherer could lead to mislabeled or misidentified herbs. Always check the label for the scientific, or Latin, name of the herb. If the scientific name is not given, or if it doesn't match the usual common name for that herb, stay away from the product. Always purchase herbs from a reliable manufacturer at a reputable store *(see p. 243 for a list of reliable herbal manufacturers and distributors)*. If you are ever in any doubt about an herb, do not buy the product.

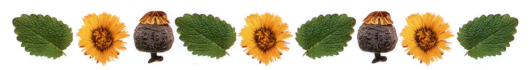

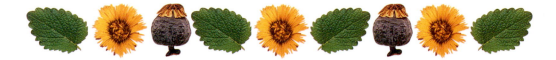

tasting root once used to flavor root beer, was also used to treat conditions such as arthritis. In the 1960s, research showed that sassafras contains the compound safrole, which causes cancer in laboratory animals, and the herb was banned by the FDA for food use.

Some toxic herbs are the source of modern drugs – for example, autumn crocus *(Colchicum autumnale, p. 235)*, the source of the gout medication colchicine *(p. 142)*; foxglove *(Digitalis purpurea, p. 236)*, used to make the heart medication digoxin *(p. 147)*; and belladonna *(Atropa belladonna, p. 234)*, the source of the powerful muscle relaxants scopolamine and atropine *(p. 129)*. These herbs are extremely powerful, fast-acting, and potentially fatal. Physicians occasionally use these herbs, but they should never be used in self-treatment.

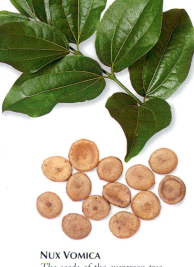

NUX VOMICA
The seeds of the evergreen tree nux vomica contain strychnine, a lethal poison that can cause muscle spasms and death.

HOW TO USE THIS CHAPTER

THIS chapter contains herbs that may cause severe side effects if used unsupervised. Of the herbs listed, some are considered safe only when used in homeopathic preparations or under the supervision of a physician. Commercial homeopathic remedies typically contain a highly diluted form of the herb that is generally considered safe to take.

HERB	REASONS TO AVOID IT	COMMENTS & CAUTIONS
ACONITE *Aconitine napellus*	Aconiti, the active ingredient in this plant, is a deadly poison. Even small amounts of aconiti are highly toxic.	The use of this herb is prohibited by the FDA. The entire plant is known to be toxic. Aconite is also known as wolfsbane and monkshood.
CALAMUS *Acorus calamus*	Calamus root has been used to treat mild digestive problems such as loss of appetite and stomach cramps. Some studies have shown that it causes cancer.	This herb should be used only under the supervision of an experienced physician. Calamus is also known as sweet flag.
AGA *Amanita muscaria*	This mushroom is highly toxic and hallucinogenic.	Aga is sometimes used in homeopathy, but it should never be used in herbal medicine. It is also known as fly agaric.

Common and scientific name of herb

"Reasons to avoid it" lists the potential dangers of harmful herbs

Read "Comments and cautions" to check whether you can consult your physician about using an herb

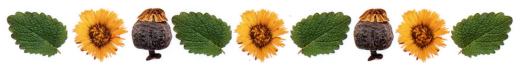

HERBS TO AVOID

HERB	REASONS TO AVOID IT	COMMENTS & CAUTIONS
ACONITE *Aconitum napellus*	Aconitine, the active ingredient in this plant, is a deadly poison. Even small amounts of aconitine are highly toxic.	The use of this herb is prohibited by the FDA. The entire plant is known to be toxic. Aconite is also known as wolfsbane and monkshood.
CALAMUS *Acorus calamus*	Calamus root has been used to treat mild digestive problems such as loss of appetite and stomach cramps. Some studies have shown that it causes cancer.	This herb should be used only under the supervision of an experienced physician. Calamus is also known as sweet flag.
AGA *Amanita muscaria*	This mushroom is highly toxic and hallucinogenic.	Aga is sometimes used in homeopathy, but it should never be used in herbal medicine. It is also known as fly agaric.
VIRGINIAN SNAKEROOT *Aristolochia serpentaria*	This herb contains volatile oils and alkaloids that can cause severe vomiting, abdominal cramps, dizziness, and respiratory failure.	This herb should be used only under the supervision of an experienced physician.
SOUTHERNWOOD *Artemisia abrotanum*	This plant contains a strong-smelling oil called absinthol that is sometimes used to treat intestinal parasites; like its close relative wormwood *(Artemisia absinthium, below)*, southernwood can cause serious side effects, including vomiting and gastrointestinal distress.	This herb should be used only under the supervision of an experienced physician. Although the leaves and flowers are said to be aphrodisiac, there is no evidence of this. The leaves can be used to keep moths out of closets and drawers.
WORMWOOD *Artemisia absinthium*	Wormwood is high in a volatile oil that contains the poisonous substance thujone. Large doses of this herb can cause vomiting, abdominal cramps, dizziness, and damage to the central nervous system.	This herb should be used only under the supervision of an experienced physician. Wormwood is used to flavor absinthe and other alcoholic beverages. These drinks are banned in many countries.
ASARUM *Asarum canadense*	Asarum root contains oils that can cause severe vomiting and uterine bleeding. Although asarum is sometimes recommended for treating bronchitis and asthma, there are no reliable studies to show that it is helpful.	This herb should be used only under the supervision of an experienced physician. Asarum is also known as wild ginger. Dried asarum root resembles dried valerian root.
BELLADONNA *Atropa belladonna*	Belladonna contains powerful substances that have a strong relaxant effect on the muscles.	Although it is an ingredient in several useful drugs, the plant itself is highly poisonous and should never be used.
BLACK MUSTARD *Brassica nigra*	This traditional remedy can cause skin blisters, eye irritation, sneezing, wheezing, and asthma attacks.	Use mustard plasters only under the supervision of a physician; follow directions carefully. In traditional herbal medicine, black mustard seeds are ground, mixed with water to form a paste, and applied to the chest to treat pneumonia, bronchitis, and severe chest congestion.

Wormwood

HERB	REASONS TO AVOID IT	COMMENTS & CAUTIONS
BLUE COHOSH *Caulophyllum thalictroides*	Although blue cohosh is sometimes recommended for relieving menstrual discomfort, this herb contains glycosides, substances that can cause uterine spasms.	This herb should be used only under the supervision of an experienced physician. Blue cohosh is also known as papoose root and squaw root.
WORMSEED OIL *Chenopodium ambrosioides*	Wormseed oil, sometimes used to treat intestinal parasites, contains a dangerous compound called ascaridole. Even in small doses, this substance can cause paralysis and severely damage hearing.	This herb should be used only under the supervision of an experienced physician. Wormseed oil is also known as Mexican tea, American wormseed, and Jesuit's tea.
WATER HEMLOCK *Cicuta maculata*	Water hemlock root is extremely poisonous.	This herb should be used only under the supervision of an experienced physician.
CLEMATIS *Clematis recta*	Juice from this plant causes redness, swelling, and blisters. If taken internally, clematis causes vomiting and stomach pain.	This herb should be used only under the supervision of an experienced physician.
AUTUMN CROCUS *Colchicum autumnale*	Although this herb contains colchicine, a substance used in gout medication, it is a highly toxic plant and can cause severe gastrointestinal irritation and birth defects.	This herb should be used only under the supervision of an experienced physician.
HEMLOCK *Conium maculatum*	Although this herb was occasionally used in traditional herbal medicine to treat arthritis, asthma, and other conditions, hemlock contains coniine, a powerful poison that causes rapid paralysis and death.	Hemlock is extremely dangerous and should never be used. Keep children away from this plant. Hemlock is also known by a variety of names, including water parsley, poison parsley, and poison snakeweed.
LILY-OF-THE-VALLEY *Convallaria majalis*	Although this plant was historically used to treat heart rhythm problems and heart failure, it causes side effects including vomiting and headaches.	This herb should be used only under the supervision of an experienced physician. It should never be combined with other heart medications, including digitalis-type drugs such as digoxin (*p. 147*). Lily-of-the-valley is a popular, fragrant ornamental plant. Keep children away from this plant.
CROTON SEED *Croton tiglium*	In traditional Chinese medicine, croton seeds are used on rare occasions to treat gallbladder disease. The seeds contain a highly toxic oil; even in very small amounts, they can cause severe irritation of the gastrointestinal tract and kidneys, dizziness, vomiting, and death.	This herb should be used only under the supervision of an experienced physician.
GERMAN IPECAC *Cynanchum vincetoxicum*	At one time this herb was used to treat heart failure but it can cause a variety of heart problems.	German ipecac should not be used in herbal medicine.
BROOM *Cytisus scoparius*	Broom contains large amounts of the amino acid tyramine, which can cause a dangerous increase in blood pressure.	This herb should be used only under the supervision of an experienced physician, and never by people with high blood pressure, and those taking MAOI antidepressant drugs such as phenelzine (*p. 180*).

Lily-of-the-valley

HERB	REASONS TO AVOID IT	COMMENTS & CAUTIONS
JIMSONWEED *Datura stramonium*	Jimsonweed is occasionally used to treat asthma and severe coughing. This herb contains powerful muscle-relaxing substances that are used as ingredients in several useful drugs, but overdoses of jimsonweed can cause delirium and hallucinations.	This herb should be used only under the supervision of an experienced physician. Jimsonweed is also known as datura. It is a common roadside weed; the fragrant flowers are poisonous. Keep children away from this plant.
FOXGLOVE *Digitalis lantana, D. purpurea*	This herb is the source of the heart medication digoxin *(p. 147)*; it contains substances that stimulate the contraction of the heart muscle and slow down the heart rate.	This herb should be used only under the supervision of an experienced physician. Foxglove is a popular garden plant; keep it away from children.
WILD YAM ROOT *Dioscorea villosa*	This herb is currently popular for helping relieve premenstrual syndrome (PMS) and menopausal symptoms, but there is little research to support these uses.	Although it is used in some homeopathic remedies, this herb should be used only under the supervision of an experienced physician.
EPHEDRA *Ephedra sinica*	This herb contains ephedrine, a powerful stimulant that is used to treat asthma and certain heart problems, and is an ingredient in many diet aids. It can cause high blood pressure, anxiety and irritability, rapid heartbeat, and heart rhythm problems.	This herb should be used only under the supervision of an experienced physician. A number of deaths have been attributed to the misuse and overuse of this herb. In traditional Chinese medicine, ephedra is known as ma huang.
WAHOO *Euonymus atropurpureus*	This herb is sometimes used as a laxative. However, the bark contains substances that can cause damage to the heart, and the berries contain toxins that can cause death, even in small amounts.	This herb should be used only under the supervision of an experienced physician. It is sometimes planted as an ornamental; keep small children away from it.
EYEBRIGHT *Euphrasia officinalis*	This herb is used as a traditional treatment for eye problems such as conjunctivitis, eyestrain, and bloodshot eyes; there is little evidence it is effective. Since eyedrops and topical products containing eyebright are often made in poorly sterilized environments, they create a chance of eye infection and should not be used.	This herb should be used only under the supervision of an experienced physician.
ASAFOETIDA *Ferula* spp.	Although asafoetida has a mild antiseptic effect and is sometimes used to treat gastritis and other digestive problems, in large doses it can cause serious problems such as diarrhea, headache, convulsions, and uterine bleeding.	This herb should be used only under the supervision of an experienced physician. Asafoetida is an oily resin with a very powerful, unpleasant smell. It is also known as devil's dung.
BLACK HELLEBORE *Helleborus niger*	Black hellebore contains helleborin, a mixture of substances that are extremely irritating to mucous membranes.	This herb should be used only under the supervision of an experienced physician.
HENBANE *Hyoscyamus niger*	Henbane contains powerful substances that have a strong relaxant effect on muscles.	Although these substances are used as ingredients in several useful drugs, the plant itself is highly poisonous and should never be used.

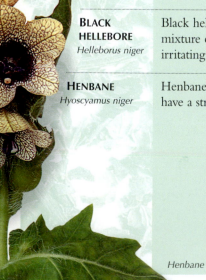

Henbane

HERB	REASONS TO AVOID IT	COMMENTS & CAUTIONS
JUNIPER *Juniperus communis*	Juniper oil is a diuretic that, in large amounts, can cause kidney damage.	This herb should be used only under the supervision of an experienced physician, and never by people with kidney disease.
CHAPARRAL *Larrea divaricata,* *L. tridentata*	Although chaparral is used as a folk remedy for cancer, there is no substantial evidence that it works. Chaparral's active ingredient, nordihydroguaiaretic acid (NGDA), can cause liver and kidney damage.	This herb is highly toxic and should not be used. Chaparral, a native of the deserts of the American southwest, is also known as stinkweed, creosote bush, and greasewood.
LABRADOR TEA *Ledum latifolium*	Labrador tea, made from the leaves of an evergreen shrub, is sometimes used to treat upper respiratory congestion.	Although it is sometimes used in homeopathy, labrador tea should never be used in herbal medicine.
LOBELIA *Lobelia inflata*	Once recommended to treat asthma, lobelia is sometimes recommended as an aid to quitting smoking; there is little evidence that it is helpful for either condition. It also causes side effects, including dry mouth, nausea, vomiting, and diarrhea.	This herb should be used only under the supervision of an experienced physician. Lobeline, the active ingredient in lobelia, is a substance that acts as a mild form of nicotine; it should not be combined with nicotine replacement products designed to help you quit smoking.
MANDRAKE *Mandragora vernalis*	Mandrake root is high in scopolamine, which has a strong relaxant effect on the muscles. High doses can lead to hallucinations, delirium, and even death.	Although mandrake is found in some homeopathic remedies, it should never be used in herbal medication. In ancient times, mandrake root was used for a wide variety of ailments, including asthma, colic, and ulcers.
PENNYROYAL *Mentha pulegium*	Pennyroyal oil is traditionally used to treat digestive problems, but it has been shown to damage the liver and can be fatal in large doses.	This herb should never be used internally. Topical use should only be under the supervision of an experienced physician.
BAYBERRY *Myrica cerifera*	Little is known about the active ingredients in bayberry, but studies have shown it can cause tumors in laboratory animals.	This herb should be used only under the supervision of an experienced physician.
NUTMEG *Myristica fragrans*	Although small amounts of nutmeg are safe, the herb should not be used medicinally.	Moderate dietary consumption of nutmeg is safe.
DAFFODIL *Narcissus pseudonarcissus*	This popular garden bulb is poisonous. Powdered daffodil or daffodil extract has historically been used to treat colds, coughs, and asthma, but overdoses can cause vomiting and diarrhea.	This herb should be used only under the supervision of an experienced physician.
YOHIMBE *Pausinystalia yohimbe*	Yohimbe contains the substance yohimbine (also known as quebrachine), an ingredient in some medications used to treat erectile dysfunction (Yocon and Yohimex). However, the plant can cause side effects, including trembling, rapid heartbeat, and a dangerous rise in blood pressure.	This herb should be used only under the supervision of an experienced physician. Yohimbe is an evergreen tree native to west Africa.

Juniper

HERB	REASONS TO AVOID IT	COMMENTS & CAUTIONS
PETASITES *Petasites hybridus*	Petasites has traditionally been used to relieve coughs, muscle spasms, abdominal cramps, and the pain resulting from kidney stones. However, this plant contains substances that can damage the liver and may increase the risk of cancer.	This herb should be used only under the supervision of an experienced physician.
MISTLETOE *Phoradendron serotinum* (American), *Viscum album* (European)	Mistletoe has traditionally been used to treat a wide variety of ailments, including epilepsy, gout, and asthma. However, both the European and American species of mistletoe contain toxic proteins that can slow the heart rate, raise blood pressure, and cause convulsions and death.	This herb should be used only under the supervision of an experienced physician. Keep children and pets away from this plant.
POKEWEED *Phytolacca americana*	This plant is known to be highly toxic, and extremely irritating to mucous membranes.	This herb should be used only under the supervision of an experienced physician. Pokeweed produces clusters of poisonous purplish berries; keep children away. In Native American herbal medicine, pokeweed was used to treat arthritis and skin diseases.
MAYAPPLE *Podophyllum peltatum*	Mayapple root and resin, historically used in the treatment of warts, are highly irritating to the skin and mucous membranes.	This herb should never be used internally. Topical use should be under the supervision of an experienced physician. Physicians sometimes use a semisynthetic form of this resin to treat certain skin cancers.
SENEGA SNAKEROOT *Polygala senega*	In Native American herbal medicine, senega snakeroot is used to treat coughs. However, overdoses can cause severe nausea, vomiting, diarrhea, and nervous system depression.	This herb should be used only under the supervision of an experienced physician. Senega snakeroot is also known as rattlesnake root and milkwort.
BUTTERCUP *Ranunculus acris*	This plant is poisonous when fresh. Juice from the fresh plant causes redness, swelling, and blisters. If taken internally, buttercup can cause vomiting and stomach pain.	This herb is highly toxic and should not be used. Keep children away from this common yard weed.
RAUWOLFIA *Rauwolfia serpentina*	The modern drug reserpine, used as a sedative and to treat high blood pressure, contains ingredients found in rauwolfia.	This herb should be used only under the supervision of an experienced physician. Rauwolfia root has a long history of use in Ayurveda (traditional Indian medicine), particularly for treating snake bite, fever, and heart failure. Do not use rauwolfia if you are clinically depressed. Rauwolfia should not be taken in combination with alcohol or other sedative herbs, supplements or medications. Drowsiness and depression are common side effects.
CASTOR BEAN *Ricinus communis*	The castor bean plant contains a foul-smelling substance called ricin that acts as a powerful laxative. Ricin is one of the most toxic plant substances known; it can cause severe liver damage.	This herb should be used only under the supervision of an experienced physician. The seeds and seed pods are highly toxic and should never be used. Keep children away from this ornamental plant; eating even a single seed can kill a small child.

HERB	REASONS TO AVOID IT	COMMENTS & CAUTIONS
MADDER *Rubia tinctorum*	Lucidin, a substance in madder, has been reported to help dissolve kidney stones, but it is known to cause cancer.	This herb is highly toxic and should never be used medicinally. It has been used as a natural dye for thousands of years.
CANAIGRE *Rumex hymenosepalus*	This herb has no known therapeutic use; some companies have made unsubstantiated claims that canaigre offers benefits similar to ginseng.	This herb should be used only under the supervision of an experienced physician. This herb is sometimes marketed as red American ginseng or red desert ginseng.
RUE *Ruta graveolens*	Rue leaves and oil are sometimes used to treat menstrual problems and relieve gas and stomach cramps. Large doses can cause vomiting, liver damage, and kidney damage. Contact with the skin can cause irritation or blisters.	This herb should be used only under the supervision of an experienced physician.
SASSAFRAS *Sassafras albidum*	Sassafras contains large amounts of safrole, a substance that has been shown to cause cancer in rats.	This herb should be used only under the supervision of an experienced physician.
SCULLCAP *Scutellaria lateriflora*	Although scullcap is used to relieve muscle spasms, there is little research to support this use. The dangerous herb germander *(Teucrium chamaedrys, p. 240)* is often mistaken for scullcap; for this reason, it must be purchased from a reputable source.	This herb should be used only under the supervision of an experienced physician.
LIFE ROOT *Senecio aureus,* *S. nemorensis*	Life root is used to treat bleeding, menopausal symptoms, diabetes, and high blood pressure, but there is no evidence that it is helpful for any of these conditions.	This herb should never be used internally. Topical use should be under the supervision of an experienced physician.
DUSTY MILLER *Senecio cineraria*	Dusty miller contains substances that can cause liver damage and cancer.	Dusty miller is highly toxic and should never be used in herbal medicine. The plant is an attractive garden ornamental.
RAGWORT *Senecio jacoboea*	This poisonous herb is high in substances that can cause liver damage and cancer.	Although it is sometimes used in lotions to treat rheumatoid arthritis, this herb should never be used internally. Topical use should be under the supervision of an experienced physician.
GROUNDSEL *Senecio vulgaris*	Groundsel has been used to treat intestinal worms and colic, but it contains substances that can cause liver damage and cancer.	This herb is highly toxic and should never be used medicinally.
NUX VOMICA *Strychnos nux vomica*	Nux vomica, traditionally used to treat a wide variety of ailments, is high in strychnine, a toxic substance that can cause liver damage, convulsions, and death.	Nux vomica is used in several homeopathic remedies, but should never be used in herbal medicine.

Ragwort

HERB	REASONS TO AVOID IT	COMMENTS & CAUTIONS
COMFREY *Symphytum officinale*	Comfrey contains substances that can cause liver damage and cancer.	Although it is sometimes used topically to treat bruises and sprains, this herb should never be used internally. Topical use should be under the supervision of an experienced physician.
TANSY *Tanacetum vulgare*	Tansy contains large amounts of a poisonous oil called thujone; this substance can cause skin rashes, vomiting, liver and kidney damage, and death.	This herb is highly toxic and should not be used medicinally.
YEW *Taxus baccata*	Yew leaves are extremely poisonous and can cause cardiac arrest, even in small amounts.	Yew is found in some homeopathic remedies. Its use as an herbal remedy is limited and should only be used under the care of an experienced physician.
GERMANDER *Teucrium chamaedrys*	Germander has been used to treat gallbladder disease, gout, and minor digestive problems, but it can cause serious liver damage.	Germander is found in some homeopathic remedies, but should never be used in herbal medicine. Germander was banned in France in 1992.
THUJA *Thuja occidentalis*	Thuja contains large amounts of a poisonous oil known as thujone. Thujone can cause skin rashes, vomiting, kidney damage, liver damage, and death.	Thuja is used in homeopathic remedies, but the herbal form should be used only under the supervision of an experienced physician. Thuja is also known as arborvitae, hackmatack, and white cedar. It is a popular ornamental evergreen; keep small children away from it.
DAMIANA *Turnera diffusa*	Damiana is said to be an aphrodisiac, but there is little scientific evidence to support this claim.	This herb should be used only under the supervision of an experienced physician.
COLTSFOOT *Tussilago farfara*	Although coltsfoot has been widely used to treat coughs, it contains substances that can cause liver damage and cancer.	This herb should be used only under the supervision of an experienced physician.
WHITE HELLEBORE *Veratrum album*	Although white hellebore root is sometimes recommended for heart problems, it can be extremely toxic and may cause severe side effects, including cardiac and respiratory arrest.	White hellebore is found in some homeopathic remedies, but the herbal form should only be used under the supervision of an experienced physician.
AMERICAN HELLEBORE *Veratrum viride*	This herb is highly toxic and causes severe side effects, even in small doses, including reduced blood pressure and heart rate.	This herb should be used only under the supervision of an experienced physician.

Yew

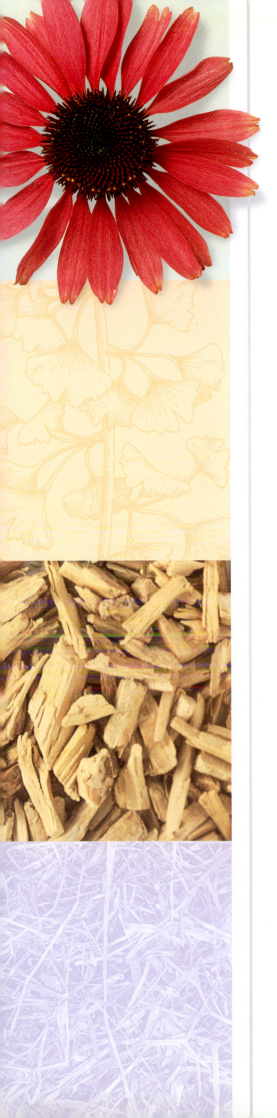

APPENDIX

RELIABLE HERBAL MANUFACTURERS AND SUPPLIERS

It is important to inquire into the company from which you buy herbs and supplements. If you purchase products over the internet, search the company's web site for the following information; if you shop in person, ask the sales clerk:
• Does the company have certificates of analysis (often called C of A's)?
• Is a lot number and expiration date printed on every bottle?
• Does a complete listing of all ingredients appear on every bottle?
Here is a brief list of some reliable companies that offer quality products:

ALLERGY RESEARCH GROUP
800-782-4274
www.nutricology.com

ANABOLIC LABORATORIES
800-445-6849
www.anaboliclabs.com

BEZWECKEN
800-743-2256
www.bezwecken.com

BIONATIVUS
888-NATIVUS
www.bionativus.com

BIOTICS RESEARCH
(Distributor)
www.bioticsresearch.com

CARLSON LABORATORIES
847-255-1600
www.carlsonlabs.com

DAVINCI LABORATORIES
800-325-1776
www.davincilabs.com

ECLECTIC INSTITUTE
800-332-4372
www.eclecticherb.com

ENZYMATIC THERAPIES
877-424-6570
www.getbigger.com

ETHICAL NUTRIENTS
800-668-8743
www.ethicalnutrients.com

FLORA
800-446-2110
www.florahealth.com

GAIA HERBS
800-878-4795
www.gaiaherbs.com

HERB PHARM
800-348-4372
www.herb-pharm.com

HIGHLAND LABORATORIES
508-881-1570
www.highlandlabs.com

JARROW FORMULAS
800-726-0886
www.jarrowformulas.com

KARUNA
800-826-7225
www.karunahealth.com

METABOLIC MAINTENANCE
800-772-7873
www.metabolicmaintenance.com

METAGENICS
800-692-9400
www.metagenics.com

MOUNTAIN TOP HERBS
877-94-HERBS
www.mountaintopherbs.com

NATROL
800-326-1520
www.natrol.com

NATURADE
800-367-2880
www.naturade.com

NATURAL FACTORS
800-322-8704
www.naturalfactors.com

NATURE'S HERBS
800-437-2257
www.naturesherbs.com

NATURE'S PLUS
800-645-9500
www.naturesplus.com

NATURE'S WAY
800-9NATURE
www.naturesway.com

NF FORMULAS
(Distributor)
www.nfformulas.com

OMEGA NUTRITION
800-661-3529
www.omeganutrition.com

OREGON'S WILD HARVEST
800-316-6869
www.oregonswildharvest.com

PHYSIOLOGICS
800-765-6775
www.physiologics.com

PHYTOPHARMICA
(Distributor)
www.phytopharmica.com

PRIORITY ONE
877-863-3922
www.cleansewell.com

QUANTUM
800-448-1448
www.quantumhealth.com

SOLGAR
877-SOLGAR-4
www.solgar.com

THORNE
208-263-1337
www.thorne.com

TRACE MINERALS RESEARCH
877-424-6570
www.getbigger.com

TREE OF LIFE
904-824-2902
www.treeoflife.com/whs.htm

TWIN LABS
631-467-3140
www.twinlabs.com

TYLER
800-931-1709
www.tyler-inc.com

VITANICA
800-572-4712
www.vitanica.com

WEIDER NUTRITION
801-975-5000
www.weidernutrition.com

(The exclusion of a company from this list does not mean they don't offer quality products.)

TOP-SELLING HERBS

HERB	SALES (IN MILLIONS)
1 Multi-Herb Products	1,380
2 Ginkgo biloba	310
3 St. John's wort	290
4 Ginseng	250
5 Garlic	230
6 Echinacea	230
7 Saw palmetto	120
8 Goldenseal	70
9 Aloe	60
10 Cranberry	50
11 Kava kava	50
12 Valerian	50
13 Cat's claw	40
14 Bilberry	40
15 Grape seed extract	40
16 Cascara sagrada	30
17 Cayenne	30
18 Ginger	30
19 Feverfew	30
20 Dong quai	30

Figures current as of 1999. Information courtesy of the Nutrition Business Journal, *a monthly executive journal focusing on nutrition industry and its impact on the food, pharmaceutical, and health care industries.*

INDEX OF SAFE HERBS BY CONDITION

A

ALZHEIMER'S DISEASE
Soy lecithin *Glycine max*
Ashwagandha *Withania somniferum*

ANGINA
Coleus *Coleus forskohlii*
Hawthorn *Crataegus oxyacantha*
Kudzu *Pueraria lobata*

ANXIETY
Wild oats *Avena sativa*
California poppy *Eschscholzia calfornica*
Hops *Humulus lupulus*
St. John's wort *Hypericum perforatum*
Lavender *Lavandula angustifolia*
Motherwort *Leonurus artemisia, L. cardiaca*
Catnip *Nepeta cataria*
Passionflower *Passiflora incarnata*
Kava kava *Piper methysticum*

ARTERIOSCLEROSIS
Guggul *Commiphora mukul*

ARTHRITIS
Boswellia *Boswellia serrata*
Capsaicin *Capsicum annuum*
Guggul *Commiphora mukul*
Horsetail *Equisetum arvense*
Eucalyptus *Eucalyptus globules*
Devil's claw *Harpagophytum procumbens*
Sarsaparilla *Smilax sarsaparilla*
Willow bark *Salix* spp.
Cat's claw *Uncaria tomentosa*
Yucca *Yucca* spp.

ARTHRITIS, RHEUMATOID
Borage oil *Borago officinalis*
Turmeric root *Curcuma longa*
Horsetail *Equisetum arvense*
Evening primrose oil *Oenothera biennis*
Blackcurrant oil *Ribes nigrum*
Ginger root *Zingiber officinale*

ASTHMA
Marshmallow leaf *Althaea officinalis*
Bromelain *Ananas comosus*
Chamomile (Roman) *Chamaemelum nobile*
Coleus *Coleus forskohlii*
Yerba santa *Eriodictyon californicum*
Reishi *Ganoderma lucidum*
Ginkgo *Ginkgo biloba*
Chamomile (German) *Matricaria recutita*
Tylophora *Tylophora asthmatica*

ATHEROSCLEROSIS
Onion *Allium cepa*
Garlic *Allium sativum*

ATHLETE'S FOOT
Tea tree oil *Melaleuca alternifolia*
Oregano oil *Origanum vulgare*

B

BACKACHE
Devil's claw *Harpagophytum procumbens*

BAD BREATH
Dill seed *Anethum graveolens*
Chinese cinnamon bark *Cinnamomum aromaticum*
Cinnamon *Cinnamomum verum*
Parsley *Petroselinum crispum*
Yellow dock *Rumex crispus*
Clove *Syzygium aromaticum*

BEDWETTING
Pumpkin seed *Curcurbita pepo*

BENIGN PROSTATIC HYPERTROPHY (BPH)
Pumpkin seed *Curcurbita pepo*
Pygeum *Pygeum africanum*
Saw palmetto *Serenoa repens*
Stinging nettle root *Urtica dioica*

BIPOLAR DISORDER
Soy lecithin *Glycine max*

BLADDER INFECTIONS
Goldenseal *Hydrastis canadensis*
Goldenrod *Solidago* spp.
Lapacho *Tabebuia avellanedae, T. impetiginosa*
Corn silk *Zea mays*

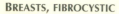

BREASTS, FIBROCYSTIC
Dong quai *Angelica sinensis*

BRONCHITIS
Echinacea *Echinacea angustifolia,*
  E. purpurea
Cardamom *Elettaria cardamomum*
Yerba santa *Eriodictyon californicum*
Eucalyptus *Eucalyptus globules*
Gumweed *Grindelia* spp.
Goldenseal *Hydrastis canadensis*
Elderberry flowers *Sambucus nigra*
Thyme *Thymus vulgaris*

BRUISES
Horse chestnut *Aesculus
  hippocastanum*
Bromelain *Ananas comosus*
Arnica *Arnica chamissonis, A. montana*
Shepherd's purse *Capsella bursa-pastoris*
Witch hazel *Hamamelis virginiana*
Lavender *Lavandula angustifolia*

BURNS
Gotu kola *Centella asiatica*
Witch hazel *Hamamelis virginiana*
Walnut leaf *Juglans regia*
Lavender *Lavandula angustifolia*

BURSITIS AND TENDINITIS
Boswellia *Boswellia serrata*

C

CANCER PREVENTION
Onion *Allium cepa*
Garlic *Allium sativum*
Aloe vera juice *Aloe vera*
Green tea *Camellia sinensis*
Reishi *Ganoderma lucidum*
Lapacho *Tabebuia avellanedae,
  T. impetiginosa*

CANKER SORES
Aloe vera juice *Aloe vera*

CHRONIC FATIGUE SYNDROME
Turkey tail *Coriolus versicolor,
  Trametes versicolor*
Eleuthero *Eleutherococcus senticosus*

CIRCULATORY PROBLEMS
Garlic *Allium sativum*
Gingko *Ginkgo biloba*

COLDS AND FLU
Couch grass *Agropyron repens,
  Elymus repens*
Marshmallow leaf *Althaea officinalis*
Echinacea *Echinacea angustifolia,
  E. purpurea*
Cardamom *Elettaria cardamomum*

Meadowsweet *Filipendula ulmaria*
Licorice root *Glycyrrhiza glabra*
Larch *Larix occidentalis*
Olive leaf *Oleae folium*
Blackthorn *Prunus spinosa*
Rose hips *Rosa canina, R. centifolia,
  R. rugosa*
Elderberry *Sambucus nigra*
Elderberry flowers *Sambucus nigra*
Lapacho *Tabebuia avellanedae,
  T. impetiginosa*
Linden flowers *Tilia cordata*
Blueberry *Vaccinium* spp.

COLITIS, ULCERATIVE
Aloe vera juice *Aloe vera*

CONSTIPATION
Yarrow *Achillea millefolium*
Oat bran *Avena sativa*
Barberry *Berberis vulgaris*
Flaxseed *Linum usitatissimum*
Psyllium seed *Plantago afra, P. ovata*
Fo-ti *Polygonum multiflorum*
Buckthorn bark *Rhamnus catharticus,
  R. frangula*
Cascara sagrada *Rhamnus purshiana*
Rhubarb *Rheum officinale,
  R. palmatum*
Rose hips *Rosa canina, R. centifolia,
  R. rugosa*
Yellow dock *Rumex crispus*
Senna *Senna alexandrina*

COUGHING
Couch grass *Agropyron repens,
  Elymus repens*
Marshmallow root *Althaea officinalis*
Camphor *Cinnamomum camphora*
Cardamom *Elettaria cardamomum*
Yerba santa *Eriodictyon californicum*
Gumweed *Grindelia* spp.
Larch *Larix occidentalis*
Osha *Ligusticum porteri*
Horehound *Marrubium vulgare*
Catnip *Nepeta cataria*
Plantain *Plantago lanceolata, P. major*
Wild cherry *Prunus serotina*
Radish *Raphanus sativus*
Thyme *Thymus vulgaris*
Usnea *Usnea barbata, U. florida,
  U. hirta, U. plicata*
Mullein *Verbascum thapsus*

CROHN'S DISEASE
Aloe vera juice *Aloe vera*
Marshmallow leaf *Althaea officinalis*
Goldenseal *Hydrastis canadensis*

CUTS, SCRAPES, AND ABSCESSES
Yarrow *Achillea millefolium*
Aloe vera gel *Aloe vera*
Shepherd's purse *Capsella*

---

  bursa-pastoris
Chamomile (Roman) *Chamaemelum
  nobile*
Witch hazel *Hamamelis virginiana*
Chamomile (German) *Matricaria
  recutita*
Tea tree oil *Melaleuca alternifolia*
Blackberry leaf *Rubus fruticosus,
  R. villosus*

D

DIABETES, TYPE 2
Salt bush *Atriplex halimus*
Aloe vera juice *Aloe vera*
Gymnema *Gymnema sylvestre*
Alfalfa *Medicago sativa*
Bitter melon *Momordica charantia*
Ginseng *Panax ginseng,
  P. quinquefolium*
Pterocarpus *Pterocarpus marsupium,
  P. santalinus*
Fenugreek seed *Trigonella foenum-
  graecum*

DIARRHEA
Agrimony *Agrimonia eupatoria*
Marshmallow leaf *Althaea officinalis*
Carob *Ceratonia siliqua*
Goldenseal *Hydrastis canadensis*
Guarana *Paullinia cupana*
Oak bark *Quercus alba, Q. petraea,
  Q. robur*
Blackberry leaf *Rubus fruticosus,
  R. villosus*
Raspberry leaf *Rubus idaeus*
Lapacho *Tabebuia avellanedae,
  T. impetiginosa*
Blueberry *Vaccinium* spp.

DIGESTIVE PROBLEMS
Marshmallow leaf *Althaea officinalis*
Bromelain *Ananas comosus*
Dill seed *Anethum graveolens*
Angelica root *Angelica archangelica*
Mugwort *Artemisia vulgaris*
Barberry *Berberis vulgaris*
Beet leaf *Beta vulgaris rubra*
Cayenne pepper *Capsicum annuum,
  C. frutescens*
Papaya *Carica papaya*
Chamomile (Roman) *Chamaemelum
  nobile*
Chicory *Cichorium intybus*
Chinese cinnamon bark
  Cinnamomum aromaticum
Cinnamon *Cinnamomum verum*
Bitter orange peel *Citrus aurantium*
Blessed thistle *Cnicus benedictus*
Turmeric root *Curcuma longa*
Artichoke leaf *Cynara scolymus*
Cardamom *Elettaria cardamomum*

Fennel seed *Foeniculum vulgare*
Gentian root *Gentiana lutea*
Licorice root *Glycyrrhiza glabra*
Devil's claw *Harpagophytum procumbens*
Hops *Humulus lupulus*
Lavender *Lavandula angustifolia*
Osha *Ligusticum porteri*
Horehound *Marrubium vulgare*
Chamomile (German) *Matricaria recutita*
Lemon balm *Melissa officinalis*
Mint oil *Mentha arvensis*
Peppermint leaf *Mentha piperita*
Catnip *Nepeta cataria*
Parsley *Petroselinum crispum*
Boldo *Peumus boldus*
Radish *Raphanus sativus*
Rosemary leaf *Rosmarinus officinalis*
Sage *Salvia officinalis*
Spilanthes *Spilanthes oleracea*
Clove *Syzygium aromaticum*
Dandelion *Taraxacum officinale*
Thyme *Thymus vulgaris*
Fenugreek seed *Trigonella foenum-graecum*

DIVERTICULITIS
Flaxseed *Linum usitatissimum*
Psyllium seed *Plantago afra, P. ovata*

DIZZINESS
Ginkgo *Ginkgo biloba*

E

EARACHE
Echinacea *Echinacea angustifolia, E. purpurea*

EAR INFECTION
Larch *Larix occidentalis*
Olive leaf *Oleae folium*
Mullein *Verbascum thapsus*

EDEMA
Dandelion *Taraxacum officinale*

F

FATIGUE
Eleuthero *Eleutherococcus senticosus*
Ginseng *Panax ginseng, P. quinquefolium*

FERTILITY PROBLEMS
Ashwagandha *Withania somnifera*

FEVER
Neem *Azadirachta indica*
Meadowsweet *Filipendula ulmaria*
Willow bark *Salix* spp.

G

GALL BLADDER PROBLEMS
Chicory *Cichorium intybus*

GALLSTONE
Milk thistle *Silybum marianum*

GASTRITIS
Marshmallow root *Althaea officinalis*
Goldenseal *Hydrastis canadensis*

GINGIVITIS
Chamomile (Roman) *Chamaemelum nobile*
Myrrh *Commiphora molmol*
Echinacea *Echinacea angustifolia, E. purpurea*
Chamomile (German) *Matricaria recutita*
Bloodroot *Sanguinaria canadensis*
Clove *Syzygium aromaticum*

GOUT
Devil's claw *Harpagophytum procumbens*

H

HANGOVER
Guarana *Paullinia cupana*

HAY FEVER
Tylophora *Tylophora asthmatica*
Stinging nettle leaf *Urtica dioica*

HEADACHE
Maté *Ilex paraguariensis*
Guarana *Paullinia cupana*
Willow bark *Salix* spp.
Vervain *Verbena hastata, V. officinalis*

HEADACHE, MIGRAINE
Feverfew *Tanacetum parthenium*
Ginger root *Zingiber officinale*

HEART DISEASE
Garlic *Allium sativum*
Green Tea *Camellia sinensis*
Cayenne pepper *Capsicum annuum, C. frutescens*
Kelp *Fucus versiculosus, Laminaria, Macrocytis, Nereocystis* spp.
Pine bark extract *Pinus maritime*
Grapeseed extract *Vitis vinifera*

HEMORRHOIDS
Horse chestnut *Aesculus hippocastanum*
Gotu kola *Centella asiatica*
Witch hazel *Hamamelis virginiana*
Blackberry leaf *Rubus fruticosus,*

R. villosus
Yellow dock *Rumex crispus*
Butcher's broom *Ruscus aculeatus*

HERPES
Shatavari *Asparagus racemosus*
Lemon balm *Melissa officinalis*
Olive leaf *Oleae folium*
Elderberry flower *Sambucus nigra*
Cat's claw *Uncaria tomentosa*

HIGH BLOOD PRESSURE
Garlic *Allium sativum*
Coleus *Coleus forskohlii*
Hawthorn *Crataegus oxyacantha*
Kelp *Fucus versiculosus, Laminaria, Macrocytis, Nereocystis* spp.
Olive leaf *Oleae folium*
Stevia *Stevia rebaudiana*

HIGH CHOLESTEROL
Garlic *Allium sativum*
Oat bran *Avena sativa*
Guggul *Commiphora mukul*
Artichoke leaf *Cynara scolymus*
Kelp *Fucus versiculosus, Laminaria, Macrocytis, Nereocystis* spp.
Soy isoflavones *Glycine max*
Soy lecithin *Glycine max*
Alfalfa *Medicago sativa*
Olive leaf *Oleae folium*
Psyllium seed *Plantago afra, P. ovata*
Fo-ti *Polygonum multiflorum*
Red clover *Trifolium pratense*
Ashwagandha *Withania somniferum*

HIV INFECTION (AIDS)
Aloe vera juice *Aloe vera*
Bupleurum *Bupleurum* spp.
Codonopsis *Codonopsis* spp.
Reishi *Ganoderma lucidum*
Licorice root *Glycyrrhiza glabra*
Shiitake mushrooms *Lentinus edodes*
Bitter melon *Momordica charantia*
Elderberry flowers *Sambucus nigra*

HYPERTHYROIDISM
Motherwort *Leonurus artemisia, L. cardiaca*

I

IMMUNE SYSTEM
Aloe vera juice *Aloe vera*
Astragalus *Astragalus membranaceus*
Turkey tail *Coriolus versicolor, Trametes versicolor*
Echinacea *Echinacea angustifolia, E. purpurea*
Eleuthero *Eleutherococcus senticosus*
Larch *Larix occidentalis*
Ligustrum *Ligustrum lucidum*

Ginseng *Panax ginseng,
P. quinquefolium*
Elderberry flower *Sambucus nigra*
Ashwagandha *Withania somniferum*

INDIGESTION
Yarrow *Achillea millefolium*
Dill seed *Anethum graveolens*
Angelica root *Angelica archangelica*
Barberry *Berberis vulgaris*
Beet leaf *Beta vulgaris rubra*
Cayenne pepper *Capsicum annuum,
C. frutescens*
Chicory *Cichorium intybus*
Chinese cinnamon bark
Cinnamomum aromaticum
Cinnamon *Cinnamomum verum*
Bitter orange peel *Citrus aurantium*
Blessed thistle *Cnicus benedictus*
Guggul *Commiphora mukul*
Artichoke leaf *Cynara scolymus*
Cardamom *Elettaria cardamomum*
Fennel seed *Foeniculum vulgare*
Fennel seed oil *Foeniculum vulgare*
Gentian root *Gentiana lutea*
Devil's claw *Harpagophytum procumbens*
Catnip *Nepeta cataria*
Boldo *Peumus boldus*
Clove *Syzygium aromaticum*
Dandelion *Taraxacum officinale*

INFECTION, BACTERIAL
Aloe vera juice *Aloe vera*
Usnea *Usnea barbata, U. florida,
U. hirta, U. plicata*

INFECTION, FUNGAL
Burdock root *Arctium lappa, A. minus*
Goldenseal *Hydrastis canadensis*
Tea tree oil *Melaleuca alternifolia*
Oregano oil *Origanum vulgare*

INFECTION, MICROBIAL
Garlic *Allium sativum*

INFECTIONS, VIRAL
Aloe vera juice *Aloe vera*
Osha *Ligusticum porteri*
Elderberry flower *Sambucus nigra*

INFERTILITY, MALE
Ginseng *Panax ginseng,
P. quinquefolium*

INFLAMMATORY BOWEL DISEASE
Peppermint leaf *Mentha piperita*

INSOMNIA
Catnip *Nepeta cataria*
Chamomile (Roman) *Chamaemelum
nobile*
Chamomile (German) *Matricaria
recutita*

Dill seed *Anethum graveolens*
Fo-ti *Polygonum multiflorum*
Hops *Humulus lupulus*
Kava kava *Piper methysticum*
Lemon balm *Melissa officinalis*
Mugwort *Artemisia vulgaris*
St. John's wort *Hypericum perforatum*
Valerian *Valeriana officinalis*

IRRITABLE BOWEL SYNDROME
Oat bran *Avena sativa*
Fennel seed *Foeniculum vulgare*
Flaxseed *Linum usitatissimum*
Mint oil *Mentha arvensis*
Psyllium seed *Plantago afra, P. ovata*
Sarsaparilla *Smilax sarsaparilla*
Slippery elm *Ulmus fulva, U. rubra*

K

KIDNEY PROBLEMS
Asparagus root *Asparagus officinalis*
Buchu *Barosma betulina,
B. crenulata, B. serratifolia*

KIDNEY STONES
Parsley *Petroselinum crispum*
Goldenrod *Solidago* spp.
Stinging nettle leaf *Urtica dioica*

L

LIVER PROBLEMS
Bupleurum *Bupleurum* spp.
Artichoke leaf *Cynara scolymus*
Soy lecithin *Glycine max*
Shiitake mushrooms *Lentinus edodes*
Schisandra *Schisandra chinensis*
Milk thistle *Silybum marianum*

MACULAR DEGENERATION
Pine bark extract *Pinus maritime*
Bilberry *Vaccinium myrtillus*
Grapeseed extract *Vitis vinifera*

M

MENOPAUSAL SYMPTOMS
Dong quai *Angelica sinensis*
Shatavari *Asparagus racemosus*
Black cohosh root *Cimicifugae
racemosae rhizoma*
Soy isoflavones *Glycine max*
Alfalfa *Medicago sativa*
Red clover *Trifolium pratense*
Chasteberry *Vitex agnus-castus*

MENSTRUAL BLEEDING
Shepherd's purse *Capsella
bursa-pastoris*

MENSTRUAL CRAMPS
Dong quai *Angelica sinensis*
Cramp bark *Viburnum opulus*

MOTION SICKNESS
Ginger root *Zingiber officinale*

NAUSEA
Ginger root *Zingiber officinale*

N

NICOTINE WITHDRAWAL
Wild oats *Avena sativa*

NIGHT VISION
Bilberry *Vaccinium myrtillus*

PAIN
Meadowsweet *Filipendula ulmaria*

P

PREMENSTRUAL SYNDROME (PMS)
Dong quai *Angelica sinensis*
Buchu *Barosma betulina,
B. crenulata, B. serratifolia*
Borage oil *Borago officinalis*
Evening primrose oil *Oenothera
biennis*
Blackcurrant oil *Ribes nigrum*
Chasteberry *Vitex agnus-castus*

PSORIASIS
Burdock root *Arctium lappa, A. minus*
Capsaicin *Capsicum annuum*
Milk thistle *Silybum marianum*

R

RESPIRATORY PROBLEMS
Marshmallow leaf *Althaea officinalis*
Horseradish *Armoracia rusticana*
Cardamom *Elettaria cardamomum*
Licorice root *Glycyrrhiza glabra*
Mint oil *Mentha arvensis*
Blackthorn *Prunus spinosa*
Elderberry *Sambucus nigra*
Linden flowers *Tilia cordata*

S

SEASONAL AFFECTIVE DISORDER (SAD)
St. John's wort *Hypericum perforatum*

SEXUAL FUNCTION, MALE
Muira puama *Ptychopetalum
olacoides, P. uncinatum*

SHINGLES
Bromelain *Ananas comosus*
Capsaicin *Capsicum annuum*

SINUSITIS
Bromelain *Ananas comosus*
Horseradish *Armoracia rusticana*

SKIN PROBLEMS
Agrimony *Agrimonia eupatoria*
Aloe vera gel *Aloe vera*
Aloe vera juice *Aloe vera*
Burdock root *Arctium lappa, A. minus*
Oat straw *Avena sativa*
Borage oil *Borago officinalis*
Calendula *Calendula officinalis*
Chamomile (Roman) *Chamaemelum nobile*
Coleus *Coleus forskohlii*
Walnut leaf *Juglans regia*
Lavender *Lavandula angustifolia*
Chamomile (German) *Matricaria recutita*
Evening primrose oil *Oenothera biennis*
Oak bark *Quercus alba, Q. petraea, Q. robur*
Blackcurrant oil *Ribes nigrum*
Sarsaparilla *Smilax sarsaparilla*
Red clover *Trifolium pratense*

SORES, MOUTH
Blackberry leaf *Rubus fruticosus, R. villosus*

SORE JOINTS
Arnica *Arnica chamissonis, A. montana*
Boswellia *Boswellia serrata*
Mint oil *Mentha arvensis*
Rosemary leaf *Rosmarinus officinalis*

SORE MUSCLES
Arnica *Arnica chamissonis, A. montana*
Camphor *Cinnamomum camphora*
Lavender *Lavandula angustifolia*
Mint oil *Mentha arvensis*
Rosemary leaf *Rosmarinus officinalis*

SORE THROAT
Agrimony *Agrimonia eupatoria*
Marshmallow root *Althaea officinalis*
Horseradish *Armoracia rusticana*
Barberry *Berberis vulgaris*
Myrrh *Commiphora molmol*
Witch hazel *Hamamelis virginiana*
Goldenseal *Hydrastis canadensis*
Larch *Larix occidentalis*
Osha *Ligusticum porteri*
Blackthorn *Prunus spinosa*
Oak bark *Quercus alba, Q. petraea, Q. robur*
Blackberry leaf *Rubus fruticosus, R. villosus*

Raspberry leaf *Rubus idaeus*
Sage *Salvia officinalis*
Slippery elm *Ulmus fulva*
Usnea *Usnea barbata, U. florida, U. hirta, U. plicata*
Blueberry *Vaccinium* spp.
Mullein *Verbascum thapsus*

STRESS
Chamomile (Roman) *Chamaemelum nobile*
Eleuthero *Eleutherococcus senticosus*
Reishi *Ganoderma lucidum*
Maitake *Grifola frondosa*
Motherwort *Leonurus artemisia, L. cardiaca*
Chamomile (German) *Matricaria recutita*
Ginseng *Panax ginseng, P. quinquefolium*
Passionflower *Passiflora incarnata*
Ashwagandha *Withania somniferum*

SUNBURN
Witch hazel *Hamamelis virginiana*
Walnut leaf *Juglans regia*
Plantain *Plantago lanceolata, P. major*

SWELLING
Arnica *Arnica chamissonis, A. montana*

T

TAPEWORM
Pumpkin seed *Curcurbita pepo*

TINNITUS
Ginkgo *Ginkgo biloba*

TONSILLITIS
Myrrh *Commiphora molmol*
Elderberry *Sambucus nigra*

TOOTHACHE
Clove oil *Syzygium aromaticum*

TOOTH DECAY
Bloodroot *Sanguinaria canadensis*

TRIGEMINAL NEURALGIA
Capsaicin *Capsicum annuum*

U

ULCERS
Marshmallow leaf *Althaea officinalis*
Marshmallow root *Althaea officinalis*
Licorice root *Glycyrrhiza glabra*
Mastica *Pistacia lentiscus*
Plantain *Plantago lanceolata, P. major*

URINARY TRACT PROBLEMS
Couch grass *Agropyron repens, Elymus repens*
Burdock root *Arctium lappa, A. minus*
Uva ursi *Arctostaphylos uva-ursi*
Horseradish *Armoracia rusticana*
Asparagus root *Asparagus officinalis*
Buchu *Barosma betulina, B. crenulata, B. serratifolia*
Horsetail *Equisetum arvense*
Parsley *Petroselinum crispum*
Goldenrod *Solidago* spp.
Stinging nettle leaf *Urtica dioica*
Cranberry *Vaccinium macrocarpon*
Blueberry *Vaccinium* spp.

V

VARICOSE VEINS
Horse chestnut *Aesculus hippocastanum*
Gotu kola *Centella asiatica*
Pine bark extract *Pinus maritime*
Butcher's broom *Ruscus aculeatus*
Grape seed extract *Vitis vinifera*

Y

YEAST INFECTIONS
Echinacea *Echinacea angustifolia, E. purpurea*
Olive leaf *Oleae folium*
Lapacho *Tabebuia avellanedae, T. impetiginosa*
Usnea *Usnea barbata, U. florida, U. hirta, U. plicata*

ADDITIONAL READING

If you'd like to learn more about herbal medicine, consult these resources.

ALLMEDCARE'S WEB SITE:
www.naturalmed.net.

THE COMPLETE GERMAN COMMISSION E MONOGRAPHS: THERAPEUTIC GUIDE TO HERBAL MEDICINES.
Blumenthal, M., et al.
Austin, Texas: American Botanical Council, 1998.

THE TOXICOLOGY OF BOTANICAL MEDICINE, 3RD EDITION.
Brinker, F.
Sandy, Oregon: Eclectic Medical Publications, 2000.

HERB CONTRAINDICATIONS AND DRUG INTERACTIONS, 2ND EDITION.
Brinker, F.
Sandy, Oregon: Eclectic Medical Publications, 1998.

FORMULAS FOR HEALTHFUL LIVING, 2ND EDITION.
Brinker, F.
Sandy, Oregon: Eclectic Medical Publications, 1998.

THE PEOPLE'S PHARMACY GUIDE TO HOME AND HERBAL REMEDIES.
Graedon, J., and Graedon, T.
New York: St. Martin's Press, 2001.

A–Z GUIDE TO DRUG-HERB-VITAMIN INTERACTIONS.
Lininger, S.W., et al.
Rocklin, California: Prima Publishing, 1999.

THE NATURAL PHARMACY, 2ND EDITION.
Lininger, S.W., et al.
Rocklin, CA: Prima Publishing, 1999.

INTERACTION BETWEEN DRUGS AND NATURAL MEDICINES: WHAT THE PHYSICIAN AND PHARMACIST MUST KNOW ABOUT VITAMINS, MINERALS, FOODS AND HERBS.
Meletis, C.D., and Jacobs, T.
Sandy, Oregon: Eclectic Medical Publications, 1999.

HERBAL MEDICINALS: A CLINICIAN'S GUIDE.
Miller, L.G., and Murray W.J., eds.
New York: Pharmaceutical Products Press, 1998.

THE HEALING POWER OF HERBS, 2ND EDITION.
Murray, Michael T.,
Rocklin, CA: Prima Publishing, 1995.

THE NATURAL PHARMACIST WEB SITE:
www.tnp.com.

PDR FOR HERBAL MEDICINE, 2ND EDITION.
Montvale, New Jersey: Medical Economics Company, 2000.

HONEST HERBAL: A SENSIBLE GUIDE TO THE USE OF HERBS AND RELATED REMEDIES, 4TH EDITION.
Tyler, V.E., and Foster, S. Tyler.
New York: Haworth Press, 1999.

BOTANICAL INFLUENCES ON ILLNESS, 2ND EDITION.
Werbach, M.
Tarzana, California: Third Line Press, 2000.

ABOUT THE NATIONAL COLLEGE OF NATUROPATHIC MEDICINE (NCNM)

Established in 1956, NCNM is the country's premier institution for the certification and licensing of physicians specializing in naturopathy, a distinct system of health care that integrates mainstream and alternative medical skills known to enhance the body's natural ability to heal itself and maintain wellness.

Located in Portland, Oregon, the college offers Doctor of Naturopathic Medicine (N.D.) and Master of Science in Oriental Medicine (M.S.O.M.) degrees, and has an active program of research into the efficacy of therapeutics in the treatment of acute and chronic diseases.

To find out more about NCNM, call 503-499-4343, or visit **www.ncnm.edu.**

INDEX